FOURTH EDITION

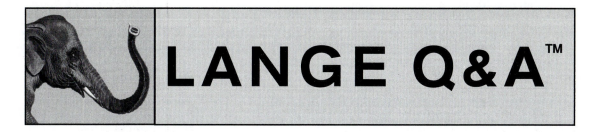

LANGE Q&A™

INTERNAL MEDICINE

Yashesh Patel, MD, MSc, FRCPC
Assistant Professor
University of Toronto
Division of General Internal Medicine
Mount Sinai Hospital
Toronto, Ontario
Canada

Barry J. Goldlist, MD, FRCPC, FACP
Professor and Head
Division of Geriatric Medicine
University of Toronto
Toronto, Ontario
Canada

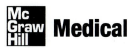
McGraw Hill Medical

New York Chicago San Francisco Lisbon London Madrid Mexico City Milan
New Delhi San Juan Seoul Singapore Sydney Toronto

Lange Q&A™: Internal Medicine, Fourth Edition

1 2 3 4 5 6 7 8 9 0   QPD/QPD   0 9 8 7

ISBN-13: 978-0-07-147364-4
ISBN-10: 0-07-147364-5

This book was set in Palatino by International Typesetting and Composition.
The editors were Marsha S. Loeb and John Williams.
The production supervisor was Sherri Souffrance.
Project management was provided by International Typesetting and Composition.
Quebecor World Dubuque was printer and binder.

This book is printed on acid-free paper.

Library of Congress Cataloging-in-Publication Data

Patel, Yash.
   Lange Q & A. Internal medicine / Yash Patel.—4th ed.
      p. ; cm.
   Rev. ed. of: Appleton & Lange's review of internal medicine / Barry J.
Goldlist. 3rd ed. c2003.
   Includes bibliographical references and index.
   ISBN-13: 978-0-07-147364-4 (pbk. : alk. paper)
   ISBN-10: 0-07-147364-5 (alk. paper)
      1. Internal medicine—Examinations, questions, etc.   I. Goldlist, Barry J.
Appleton & Lange's review of internal medicine.   II. Title.   III. Title: Lange Q and A. Internal medicine.
IV. Title: Q & A. Internal medicine.   V. Title: Internal medicine.
      [DNLM: 1. Internal Medicine—Examination Questions. WB 18.2 P295L   2007]
   RC58.G59   2007
   616.0076—dc22
                                                                             2007003356

Contents

Preface

The practice of internal medicine requires both breadth and depth of knowledge. To acquire mastery of the subject requires extensive reading and clinical experience. The knowledge base is also constantly expanding and changing as medicine enters the era of molecular biology and large randomized clinical trials. This textbook provides a review of the major issues in internal medicine by presenting a wide variety of typical examination questions and referenced answers.

The text is organized by topic to facilitate in-depth review but contains a large comprehensive test that mimics the typical examination format. The content has been organized to reflect the areas tested on Step 2 of the United States Medical Licensing Examination (USMLE Step 2). The format of the questions is modeled after the format used on the USMLE, making it an ideal study guide for individuals preparing for licensing examinations.

The questions and answers reflect the increasing growth of knowledge in the field of internal medicine. As a result, reviewing the answers gives the reader a "mini review" of basic concepts and pathophysiology in internal medicine, allowing the reader to approach clinical problems in an appropriate manner.

Finally, since the last edition was published, the list of references has been expanded and updated to reflect current knowledge in the field of internal medicine.

Yashesh Patel, MD, MSc, FRCPC
Barry J. Goldlist, MD, FRCPC, FACP

Acknowledgments

I would like to thank the countless medical students and residents who teach me and compel me to learn every day. Thanks to the patience of my family and friends for putting up with my absences while I worked on the book. Finally, thanks to Barry Goldlist for giving me the opportunity to work on the latest edition of the book with him.

Yashesh Patel, MD, MSc, FRCPC

CHAPTER 1

Cardiology
Questions

DIRECTIONS (Questions 1 through 61): Each of the numbered items in this section is followed by answers. Select the ONE lettered answer that is BEST in each case.

1. A 62-year-old man with coronary artery disease (CAD) presents with presyncope. His physical examination is normal except for bradycardia (pulse 56 beats/min) and an irregular pulse. The electrocardiogram (ECG) shows Wenckebach's type atrioventricular (AV) block. Which of the following are you most likely to see on the ECG?

    (A) progressive PR shortening
    (B) progressive lengthening of the PR interval
    (C) tachycardia
    (D) dropped beat after PR lengthening
    (E) fixed 2:1 block

2. A 72-year-old woman had a pacemaker inserted 4 years ago for symptomatic bradycardia because of AV nodal disease. She is clinically feeling well and her ECG shows normal sinus rhythm at a rate of 68/min but no pacemaker spikes. Her pacemaker only functions when the ventricular rate falls below a preset interval. Which of the following best describes her pacemaker function?

    (A) asynchronous
    (B) atrial synchronous
    (C) ventricular synchronous
    (D) ventricular inhibited
    (E) atrial sequential

3. A 42-year-old man develops shortness of breath (SOB) and chest pain 7 days after an open cholecystectomy. His blood pressure is 145/86 mm Hg, pulse is 120/min, respirations 24/min, and oxygen saturation of 97%. Pulmonary embolism is clinically suspected. Which of the following is the most common ECG finding of pulmonary embolism?

    (A) a deep S wave in lead I
    (B) depressed ST segments in leads I and II
    (C) prominent Q wave in lead I, and inversion of T wave in lead III
    (D) sinus tachycardia
    (E) clockwise rotation in the precordial leads

4. A 63-year-old woman develops exertional angina and has had two episodes of syncope. Examination shows a systolic ejection murmur with radiation to the carotids and a soft S_2. Which of the following is the most likely diagnosis?

    (A) mitral stenosis
    (B) mitral insufficiency
    (C) aortic stenosis
    (D) aortic insufficiency
    (E) tricuspid stenosis

5. A 42-year-old man with known valvular heart disease develops a fever for 1 week. He appears unwell; findings include a pansystolic murmur at the apex that radiates to the axilla and a soft S1 sound. He has petechiae on his conjunctival sac, linear hemorrhages under a few fingernails, and painful, tender, and erythematous nodules on some of the distal fingertips. Which of the following is the most responsible mechanism for these physical findings?

(A) direct bacterial invasion
(B) immune response
(C) vascular phenomena
(D) valvular damage
(E) preexisting cardiac dysfunction

6. Which of the following antiarrhythmic drugs mediates its effect by interfering with movement of calcium through the *slow channel*?

(A) phenytoin
(B) verapamil
(C) lidocaine
(D) amiodarone
(E) bretylium

7. A 67-year-old man presents with an anterior myocardial infarction (MI) and receives thrombolytic therapy. Three days later, he develops chest pain that is exacerbated by lying down, and his physical findings are normal except for a friction rub. His ECG shows evolving changes from the anterior infarction but new PR-segment depression and 1-mm ST-segment elevation in all the limb leads. Which of the following is the most likely diagnosis?

(A) reinfarction
(B) pulmonary embolus
(C) viral infection
(D) post-MI pericariditis
(E) dissecting aneurysm

8. Which of the following best describes the effect of calcium ions on the myocardium?

(A) positively inotropic
(B) negatively inotropic
(C) positively chronotropic
(D) negatively chronotropic
(E) excitation contraction uncoupling

9. A 22-year-old primagravida woman develops hypertension at 28 weeks. She is asymptomatic and the examination is normal except for 1+ pedal edema. Her complete blood count, liver enzymes, and electrolytes are normal. The urinalysis is positive for proteinuria. Which of the following is true for this type of hypertension?

(A) improves in the third trimester
(B) leads to large-birth-weight babies
(C) should be controlled with medications
(D) spares the placenta
(E) spares maternal kidney function

10. A 61-year-old man has a non-ST-elevation MI and is admitted to the coronary care unit. The following day, he develops bradycardia but no symptoms. His blood pressure is 126/84 mm Hg, pulse 50/min, and on examination, the heart sounds are normal, with no extra sounds or rubs. His ECG has changed. Which of the following ECG findings is the best indication for this patient to receive a pacemaker?

(A) persistent bradycardia
(B) second-degree AV block Mobitz type I
(C) first-degree AV block
(D) new right bundle branch block
(E) left bundle branch block (LBBB) and second-degree AV block Mobitz type II

11. Auscultation of the heart of a 17-year-old boy reveals an increased intensity of the pulmonary component of the second heart sound. He complains of dyspnea on exertion but no other cardiac or pulmonary symptoms. Which of the following explanations is the most likely cause of his dyspnea? (See Fig. 1–1.)

(A) pulmonary stenosis
(B) aortic stenosis
(C) MI
(D) pulmonary hypertension
(E) systemic hypertension

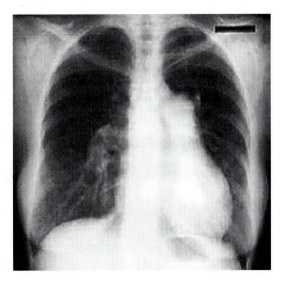

Figure 1–1.

12. A 22-year-old woman complains of palpitations and has a regular heartbeat at a rate of 170/min, with a blood pressure of 110/70 mm Hg. The rate abruptly changes to 75/min after applying carotid sinus pressure. Which of the following is the most likely diagnosis? (See Fig. 1–2.)

(A) sinus tachycardia

(B) paroxysmal atrial fibrillation

(C) paroxysmal atrial flutter

(D) paroxysmal supraventricular tachycardia (PSVT)

(E) paroxysmal ventricular tachycardia

13. A 73-year-old man has angina pectoris on exertion, but an angiogram reveals noncritical stenosis of the coronary arteries. This occurs most frequently with which of the following valvular heart diseases?

(A) mitral stenosis

(B) mitral insufficiency

(C) pulmonary stenosis

(D) aortic stenosis

(E) aortic insufficiency

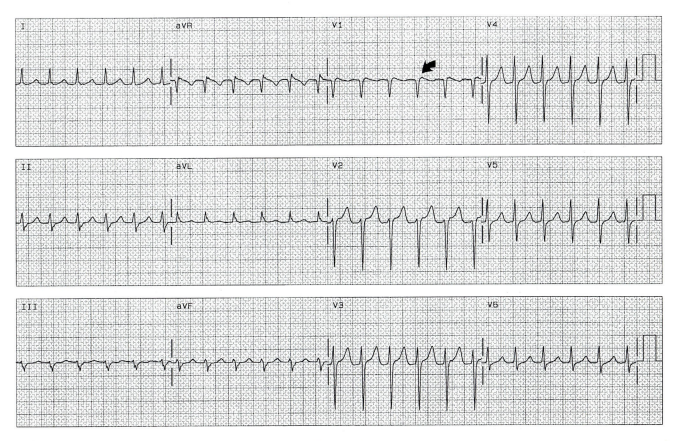

Figure 1–2.
(Reproduced, with permission, from Fuster V, et al., *Hurst's the Heart*, 11th ed. New York: McGraw-Hill, 2004:819.)

14. A patient with new-onset syncope has a blood pressure of 110/95 mm Hg and a harsh systolic ejection murmur at the base, radiating to both carotids. Auscultation of the second heart sound at the base might reveal which of the following findings?

(A) it is accentuated
(B) it is diminished
(C) it is normal in character
(D) it is widely split due to delayed ventricular ejection
(E) it shows fixed splitting

15. A 69-year-old woman complains of easy fatigue and one episode of presyncope. On examination of the jugular venous pressure (JVP), there are irregular large *a* waves. The ECG has fixed PP and RR intervals but varying PR intervals. Which of the following conditions is this most likely caused by? (See Fig. 1–3.)

(A) surgical removal of an atrium
(B) independent beating of atria and ventricles
(C) a reentry phenomenon
(D) a drug effect
(E) a heart rate under 60 beats/min

16. A 57-year-old man has an anterior MI. It is complicated by the development of heart failure. Nitroglycerin would be a useful first medication under which circumstances?

(A) severe pulmonary congestion, blood pressure 80 mm Hg systolic
(B) clear lungs, blood pressure 120 mm Hg systolic
(C) clear lungs, blood pressure 80 mm Hg systolic
(D) clear lungs, blood pressure 160 mm Hg systolic
(E) moderate pulmonary congestion, blood pressure 130 mm Hg systolic

17. A 28-year-old man develops *viridans group streptococci* septicemia. Which of the following cardiac lesions has the highest risk of developing endocarditis?

(A) ventricular septal defect
(B) atrial septal defect, secundum type
(C) mitral valve prolapse with regurgitation
(D) pure mitral stenosis
(E) asymmetric septal hypertrophy

18. A 47-year-old woman has new-onset transient right arm weakness and word finding difficulty symptoms lasting 3 hours. She is also experiencing exertional dyspnea, and had a

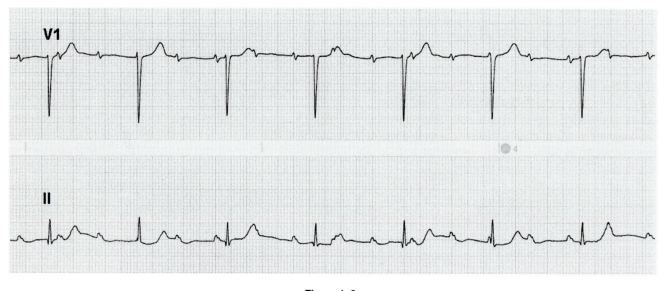

Figure 1–3.
(Reproduced, with permission, from Fuster V, et al., *Hurst's the Heart*, 11th ed. New York: McGraw-Hill, 2004:904.)

syncopal event 1 month ago. Her echocardiogram reveals a cardiac tumor in the left atrium, it is pendunculated and attached to the endocardium. Which of the following is the most likely cause of this lesion?

(A) myxoma
(B) sarcoma
(C) rhabdomyoma
(D) fibroma
(E) lipoma

19. A 72-year-old woman has new-onset atrial flutter with a ventricular rate of 150/min. She is hemodynamically stable with a blood pressure of 155/90 mm Hg, but is experiencing palpitations. Which of the following drugs is the best intravenous choice for controlling the heart rate?

(A) diltiazem
(B) lidocaine
(C) aminophylline
(D) magnesium
(E) atropine

20. Several of the older patients in your practice intend to pursue exercise programs. They have no cardiac symptoms, but some do have vascular risk factors such as diabetes or hypertension. In these patients, which of the following is true about exercise electrocardiography?

(A) it is an invasive procedure
(B) it is contraindicated in patients over 65 years of age
(C) it detects latent disease
(D) it has a morbidity of approximately 5%
(E) it is used in pulmonary embolism

21. A 58-year-old man is undergoing cardiac catheterization for evaluation of chest pain symptoms. He is worried about the risks, and as part of obtaining informed consent, you advise him about the risks and benefits of the procedure. Which of the following aspects of angiography is true?

(A) it is contraindicated in the presence of cyanosis
(B) it is considered noninvasive
(C) it is generally performed with cardiopulmonary bypass
(D) it may cause renal failure
(E) it requires carotid artery puncture

22. A 23-year-old man develops sharp left-sided chest pain, fever, and a friction rub heard at the lower left sternal border, unaffected by respiration. The pain is also aggevated by lying down and relieved by sitting up. He is otherwise well with no other symptoms and the remaining physical examination is normal. Which of the following is the most likely cause for his symptoms?

(A) rheumatic fever
(B) tuberculosis (TB)
(C) herpes simplex virus
(D) MI
(E) coxsackievirus

23. A 72-year-old woman with angina undergoes cardiac catheterization. The pulmonary capillary "wedge" pressure is an approximation of the pressure in which of the following structures?

(A) pulmonary artery (PA)
(B) pulmonary vein
(C) left atrium
(D) right atrium
(E) vena cava

24. A 58-year-old man with hypertension is brought to the emergency room after sudden-onset chest pain that radiates to his back and arms. He is in moderate distress with a blood pressure of 160/90 mm Hg in the left arm and 120/70 mm Hg in the right arm. Cardiac examination reveals a soft second heart sound and a murmur of aortic insufficiency. His ECG shows sinus tachycardia but no acute ischemic changes, and the chest x-ray (CXR) is shown in Fig. 1–4. Which of the following is the most appropriate next step in confirming the diagnosis?

(A) coronary angiography
(B) transthoracic echocardiography
(C) computerized tomography (CT) chest
(D) exercise stress test
(E) cardiac troponin level

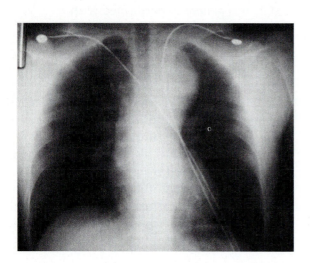

Figure 1–4.

25. A 17-year-old girl develops exertional dyspnea, but has no cough, sputum, or wheezing symptoms. On examination, she has a fixed splitting of her second heart sound and a 3/6 systolic ejection murmur heard best over the left sternal border. An echocardiogram confirms the condition. Which of the following is the best physiologic explanation for her condition?

    (A) pulmonary blood flow is greater than systemic blood flow
    (B) pulmonary blood flow is less than systemic blood flow
    (C) pulmonary blood flow is equal to systemic blood flow
    (D) the left ventricle is enlarged
    (E) the systemic blood pressure is elevated

26. A 19-year-old man develops typical angina pectoris. There is no family history of premature CAD. Which of the following is the most likely diagnosis?

    (A) mitral stenosis
    (B) coronary artery aneurysm
    (C) coarctation
    (D) atrial septal defect
    (E) Werner's syndrome

27. A 32-year-old asymptomatic woman has a rapidly rising, forceful pulse that collapses quickly. Which of the following is the most likely diagnosis?

    (A) mitral stenosis
    (B) mitral regurgitation
    (C) aortic stenosis
    (D) aortic regurgitation
    (E) coarctation of the aorta

28. A 63-year-old woman on digitalis for chronic atrial fibrillation experiences fatigue, nausea, and anorexia. Her pulse is regular at 50 beats/min, and the heart sounds, chest, and abdominal examinations are normal. On the ECG, no P waves are visible and the QRS complexes are narrow and regular. Which of the following is the most appropriate management step? (See Fig. 1–5.)

    (A) an increase in digitalis dose
    (B) complete cessation of digitalis
    (C) withdrawal of digitalis for one dose
    (D) addition of a beta-blocker
    (E) addition of a calcium channel blocker

29. A 47-year-old man is found to have edema, ascites, and hepatosplenomegaly. The examination of his neck veins reveals elevated venous pressure with a deep *y* descent. Heart size on x-ray is normal. Which of the following etiologies is not a possible explanation for this syndrome?

    (A) rheumatic fever
    (B) TB
    (C) unknown cause
    (D) previous acute pericarditis
    (E) neoplastic involvement of the pericardium

30. A 65-year-old man develops palpitations and dizziness. His blood pressure is 80/50 mm Hg and his pulse is regular at 150/min. His ECG shows a "saw-toothed" pattern of P waves. Which of the following procedures is most appropriate in converting him back to sinus rhythm? (See Fig. 1–6.)

    (A) carotid sinus pressure
    (B) gagging procedures
    (C) Valsalva maneuver
    (D) eyeball compression
    (E) electrical cardioversion

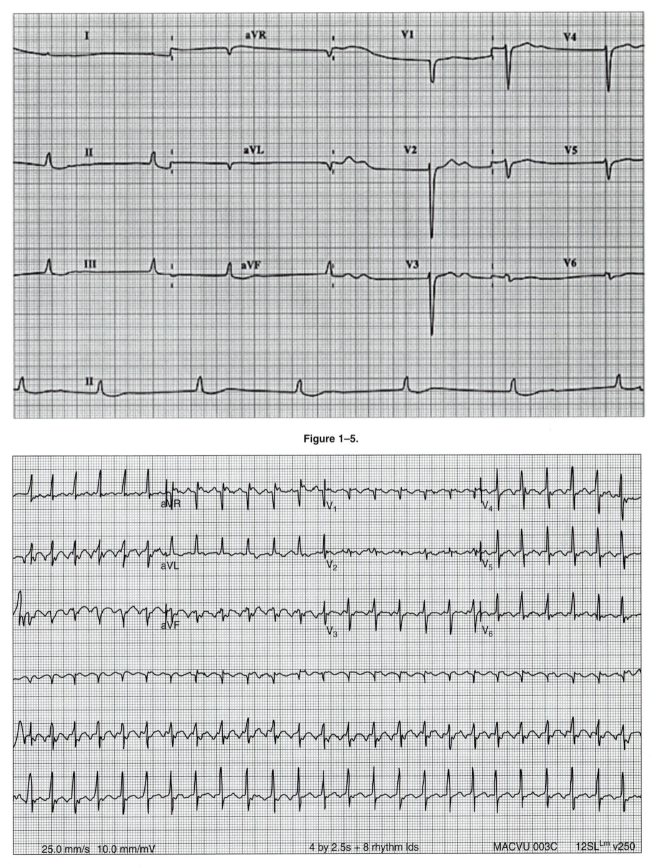

Figure 1–5.

Figure 1–6.
(Reproduced, with permission, from Fuster V, et al., *Hurst's the Heart*, 11th ed. New York: McGraw-Hill, 2004:843.)

31. A 63-year-old woman presents with symptoms of palpitations and atrial flutter on the ECG. Which of the following is the most likely mechanism of this arrhythmia?

(A) atrial asystole
(B) atrial bigeminy
(C) right atrial macro-reentry
(D) AV nodal reentry
(E) accessory pathway

32. A 62-year-old man has progressive symptoms of dyspnea, and more recently noticed difficulty lying supine. Examination shows an elevated JVP at 8 cm, with a third heart sound, pedal edema, and bibasilar crackles on auscultation. Which one of the following may be implicated in fluid retention for this condition?

(A) decreased renin
(B) increased aldosterone
(C) increased estrogen
(D) increased growth hormone
(E) decreased vasopressin

33. Three months after an anterior MI, a 73-year-old man has a follow-up ECG. He is clinically feeling well with no further angina symptoms. His ECG shows Q waves in the anterior leads with persistant ST-segment elevation. The current ECG is most compatible with which of the following diagnosis? (See Fig. 1–7.)

(A) ventricular aneurysm
(B) hibernating myocardium
(C) acute infarction
(D) silent infarction
(E) early repolarization

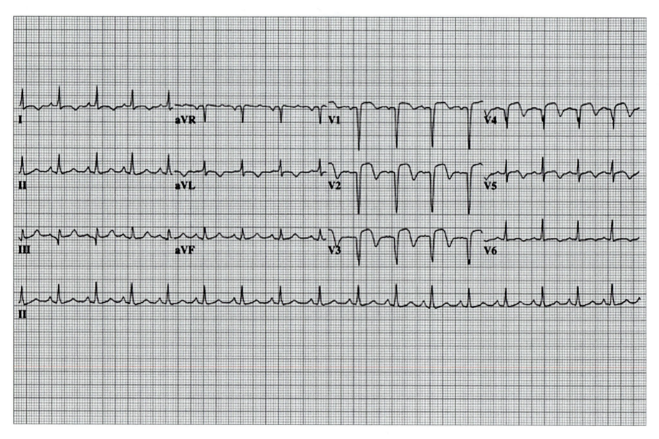

Figure 1–7.

34. A 79-year-old man presents with syncope. On physical examination, he has a slow upstroke in his carotid pulse and a diamond-shaped systolic murmur at the base. His chest is clear. Which of the following findings is his CXR most likely to reveal?

    (A) right ventricular dilatation
    (B) stenosis of the proximal ascending aorta
    (C) left atrial hypertrophy
    (D) normal overall cardiac size
    (E) displaced apex

35. A 49-year-old man has his serum lipids measured. Which pattern suggests the lowest risk for CAD?

    (A) total cholesterol 215 mg/dL, high-density lipoprotein (HDL) cholesterol 28 mg/dL
    (B) total cholesterol 215 mg/dL, HDL cholesterol 43 mg/dL
    (C) total cholesterol 180 mg/dL, HDL cholesterol 29 mg/dL
    (D) total cholesterol 202 mg/dL, HDL cholesterol 45 mg/dL
    (E) total cholesterol 225 mg/dL, HDL cholesterol 40 mg/dL

36. A 16-year-old boy is found to have hypertension on routine evaluation. On examination, the blood pressure in his arms is higher than in his legs by more than 10 mm Hg. Which of the following is the most likely diagnosis?

    (A) aortic insufficiency
    (B) coarctation of the aorta
    (C) normal variant
    (D) ventricular aneurysm
    (E) severe juvenile diabetes

37. A 79-year-old man with a 40-year history of hypertension and cardiomegaly on CXR is likely to show which of the following on his ECG?

    (A) clockwise rotation of the electrical axis
    (B) rSR' pattern in V1
    (C) right axis deviation
    (D) high-voltage QRS complexes in V5 and V6
    (E) prolonged PR interval in the limb leads

38. A 59-year-old woman presents for the first time with untreated congestive heart failure (CHF). Urinalysis and urine biochemistrty is most likely to show which of the following?

    (A) decreased urinary sodium content
    (B) low urine specific gravity
    (C) increased urinary chloride content
    (D) red blood cell (RBC) casts
    (E) proteinuria

39. A 60-year-old woman presents with symptoms of weight loss, anxiety, and palpitations. On examination, she has a thyroid goiter. Which of the following is the most likely cardiac finding?

    (A) prolonged circulation time
    (B) decreased cardiac output
    (C) paroxysmal atrial fibrillation
    (D) pericardial effusion
    (E) aortic insufficiency

40. A 70-year-old woman is found to have an irregular pulse rate on a routine visit. She is experiencing no new symptoms at rest or on exertion. On the ECG, there are no P waves and an irregular RR interval at a rate of 70/min. On her previous ECG from 4 years ago she was in sinus rhythm. Which of the following is the most appropriate next step in management? (See Fig. 1–8.)

    (A) cardioversion
    (B) antiarrhythmic therapy
    (C) beta-blocker
    (D) anticoagulation
    (E) aspirin

41. A 47-year-old woman develops accelerated hypertension (blood pressure 210/105 mm Hg) but no clinical symptoms except frequent headaches. Which of the following findings are most likely on examination of the fundii? (See Fig. 1–9.)

    (A) retinitis obliterans
    (B) cotton wool spots
    (C) retinal detachment
    (D) optic atrophy
    (E) foveal blindness

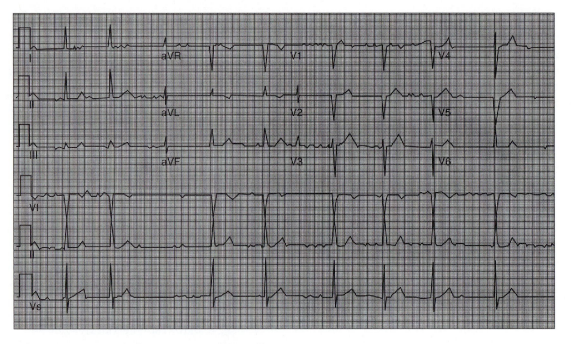

Figure 1–8.

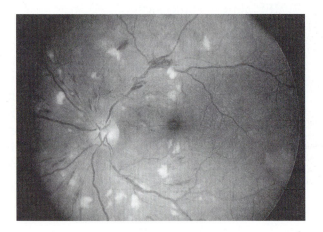

Figure 1–9.
(Reproduced, with permission, from Kasper DL, et al., *Harrison's Principles of Internal Medicine*, 16th ed. New York: McGraw-Hill, 2005:168.)

42. A 32-year-old man presents for routine evaluation. He has no symptoms but has noticed some new "nodules" on his legs. Physical examination reveals lumps on his Achillis tendon, yellow lesions around his eyes, and pigmentation of his iris. Which of the following is the most likely diagnosis? (See Figs. 1–10 a and b.)

   (A) familial hyperlipidemia
   (B) diabetes
   (C) myxedema
   (D) chronic renal disease
   (E) an inherited defect of glycogen utilization

43. A 22-year-old woman develops idiopathic pericarditis, with a resultant pericardial effusion. Which of the following features determines the patient's clinical course and prognosis?

   (A) specific gravity of the fluid
   (B) presence or absence of blood in the fluid
   (C) presence or nature of any underlying disease
   (D) cellular count of the fluid
   (E) viscosity of the fluid

44. A 65-year-old man complains of postural hypotension with dizziness. His blood pressure is 110/80 mm Hg supine and 85/70 mm Hg standing (after 2 minutes), the pulse rate remains the same at 80/min. Which of the following is the most likely diagnosis?

   (A) thyrotoxicosis
   (B) diuretic therapy
   (C) venous varicosities
   (D) possibility of diabetes mellitus (DM)
   (E) essential hypotension

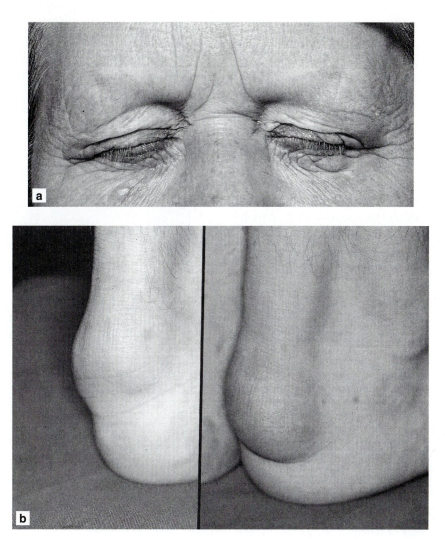

Figure 1–10.
(Reproduced, with permission, from Wolff K and Johnson RA, *Fitzpatrick's Color Atlas & Synopsis of Clinical Dermatology*, 5th ed. New York: McGraw-Hill, 2005:447 & 449.)

45. The echocardiogram of a 22-year-old woman reveals mitral valve prolapse. Which of the following is the most common physical finding in this condition?

(A) diastolic rumble

(B) absent first heart sound

(C) diastolic click

(D) aortic regurgitation

(E) late systolic murmur

46. A 36-year-old man is seen because of palpitations. He admits to precordial discomfort, weakness, and anxiety. His pulse is 150/min, and his blood pressure is 124/70 mm Hg. Heart sounds are normal. Carotid sinus pressure gradually changes the rate to 75/min, but when released, the pulse rate returns to 150/min. Which of the following is the most likely diagnosis?

(A) atrial flutter with 2:1 block

(B) paroxysmal atrial tachycardia with 2:1 block

(C) sinus arrhythmia

(D) atrial fibrillation

(E) nodal tachycardia

47. A 25-year-old man complains of left precordial chest pain that radiates to the left shoulder but not down the left arm. The pain is accentuated by inspiration and relieved by sitting up. The pain is accompanied by fever and chills. His blood pressure is 105/75 mm Hg, pulse 110/min and regular, and temperature 37.5°C. Aside from the tachycardia, there are no abnormal physical findings in the heart or lungs. The ECG shows ST-segment elevation in all leads except aVR and VI. On the third hospital day, the patient's blood pressure falls, JVP rises, and he goes into CHF. Which of the following is the most likely diagnosis?

(A) a second pulmonary embolus

(B) extension of a myocardial infarct

(C) cardiac tamponade

(D) secondary bacterial infection

(E) rupture of a chordae tendineae

48. A 80-year-old man with Type II diabetes and hypertension presents with increasing dyspnea. He appears short of breath, blood pressure is 170/95 mm Hg, pulse 100/min and regular. The JVP is at 7 cm; there is a loud second heart sound and a systolic ejection murmur at the right sternal border, which does not radiate. The lungs have bibasilar crakles up to the scapula. The CXR has bilateral infiltrates and vascular redistribution. His echocardiogram reports aortic sclerosis, concentric left ventricular hypertrophy (LVH), and normal ejection fraction. Which of the following is the most likely mechanism for this condition? (See Fig. 1–11.)

(A) valvular heart disease

(B) diastolic dysfunction

(C) systolic dysfunction

(D) hibernating myocardium

(E) hypertrophic obstructive cardiomyopathy (HOCM)

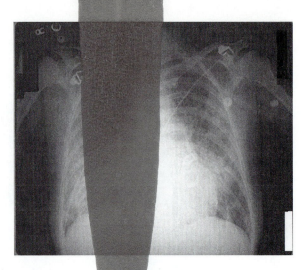

Figure 1–11.

49. A 68-year-woman with hypertension and dyslipidemia presents with 30 minutes of retrosternal chest pain radiating to her neck. She is diaphoretic and in moderate distress. The ECG shows ST-segment elevation in the inferior leads. Which of the following mechanisms is the most likely cause of her condition? (See Fig. 1–12.)

(A) coronary plaque rupture

(B) aortic inflammation

(C) pericardial inflammation

(D) vasculitis

(E) myocarditis

50. A 62-year-old man with a prosthetic aortic valve develops fevers and malaise. His valve was replaced 5 years ago because of aortic stenosis from a bicuspid valve. He has a systolic ejection murmur but no other abnormalities on examination. Blood cultures are most likely to grow which of the following?

(A) fungi

(B) bartonella

(C) diptheroids

(D) *Staphylococcus epidermidis*

(E) *Streptococcus bovis*

RIGHT CORONARY ARTERY

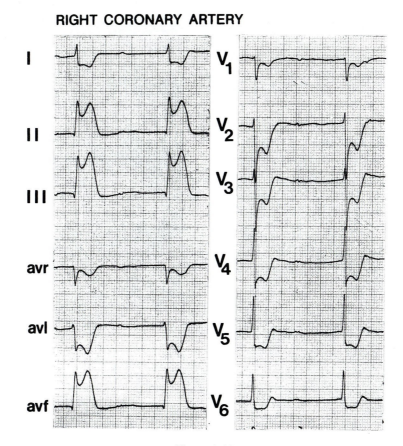

Figure 1–12.
(Reproduced, with permission, from Fuster V, et al., *Hurst's the Heart*, 11th ed.
New York: McGraw-Hill, 2004:1356.)

51. A 58-year-old man with no prior cardiac history presents with retrosternal chest pain starting at rest and lasting 30 minutes. The pain radiates to the left arm and is associated with diaphoresis and dyspnea. His blood pressure is 150/90 mm Hg, pulse 100/min, the heart sounds are normal, and the lungs are clear to auscultation. Which of the following is the next most appropriate investigation?

(A) CT scan—chest
(B) CXR
(C) cardiac troponin
(D) ECG
(E) myocardial perfusion imaging

52. The laboratory results shown in Table 1–1 are obtained from the investigation of a 37-year-old African-American woman who has a blood pressure at rest of 140/100 mm Hg. Which of the following is the most likely diagnosis?

(A) Cushing's syndrome
(B) primary aldosteronism
(C) essential hypertension
(D) pyelonephritis
(E) bilateral renal artery stenosis

TABLE 1–1. LABORATORY INVESTIGATIONS

Urinalysis	
pH	5.2
Albumin	Negative to trace
Serum Na	140 mEq/L
K	3.5 mEq/L
Cl	100 mEq/L
CO_2	25 mEq/L
Creatinine	1.0 mg/100 mL
Fasting sugar	90 mg/100 mL
Calcium	9.0 mg/100 mL
Uric acid	5.0 mg/100 mL

53. Figure 1–13 is the x-ray and MR of an 8-year-old boy who had easy fatigability and a soft, continuous murmur in the upper back. ECG revealed minimal LVH. What is your diagnosis?

   (A) aortic stenosis
   (B) patent ductus arteriosus
   (C) coarctation of the aorta
   (D) pulmonary valvular stenosis
   (E) peripheral pulmonary stenosis

54. Figure 1–14 is an x-ray of an asymptomatic 64-year-old male executive coming in for his regular annual medical checkup. He had an anterior Q wave MI 4 years ago. What is your diagnosis?

   (A) calcific pericarditis
   (B) left ventricular aneurysm
   (C) hydatid cyst
   (D) pleuropericarditis
   (E) normal

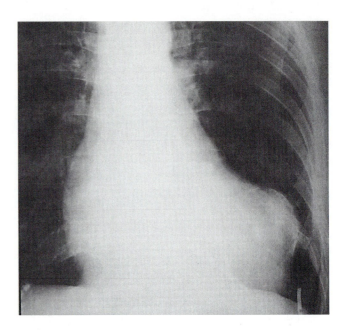

Figure 1–14.

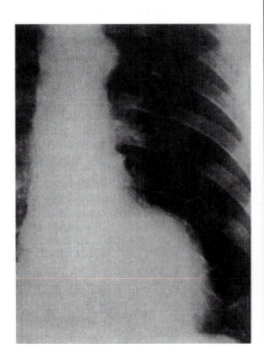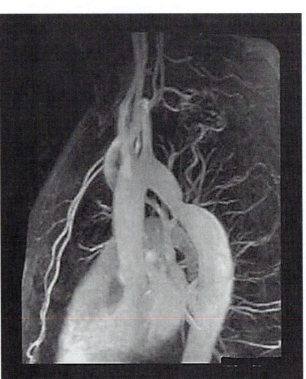

Figure 1–13.

55. A 70-year-old man has dyspnea, orthopnea, and paroxysmal nocturnal dyspnea. He has generalized cardiomegaly and pulmonary and systemic venous hypertension. The ECG is shown in Fig. 1–15. What is the cardiac rhythm?

(A) ectopic atrial tachycardia

(B) atrial flutter with 2:1 AV conduction

(C) sinus tachycardia

(D) supraventricular tachycardia

(E) atrial fibrillation with rapid ventricular response

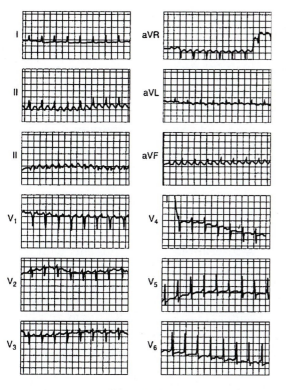

Figure 1–15.

56. A 77-year-old woman comes to the emergency department because of feeling "light-headed and dizzy." Except for the irregular pulse, her physical examination is normal. What is the rhythm in the lead tracing shown in Fig. 1–16?

(A) first-degree heart block

(B) second-degree heart block

(C) third-degree heart block

(D) premature ventricular beats

(E) premature atrial beats

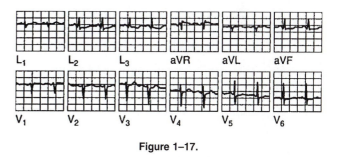

Figure 1–16.

57. A 42-year-old woman has anterior chest pain of a somewhat atypical nature for many years. The patient's pain has been present and relatively stable for a number of years, and the ECG shown in Fig. 1–17 is a stable one. What is the diagnosis?

(A) inferior wall infarction

(B) anterior wall infarction

(C) ventricular aneurysm

(D) nonspecific changes

(E) pericarditis

Figure 1–17.

58. The ECG shown in Fig. 1–18 was obtained during the initial stages of an acute MI. The patient had just received thrombolytic therapy. What is the rhythm?

(A) atrial fibrillation

(B) atrial flutter

(C) second-degree heart block

(D) Wenckebach phenomenon

(E) nonsustained ventricular tachycardia

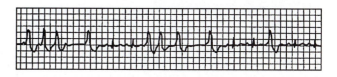

Figure 1–18.

59. A 78-year-old man with advanced renal disease has the ECG shown in Fig. 1–19 (lead II). What is the diagnosis?

(A) hyperkalemia

(B) hypercalcemia

(C) hypernatremia

(D) pericarditis

(E) ventricular aneurysm

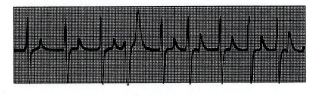

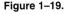

Figure 1–19.

60. A 58-year-old man whom you have followed dies suddenly, spurring you into doing some research on sudden death. Which of the following is the most likely cause for this individual?

(A) extensive coronary atherosclerosis

(B) electrolyte disturbance

(C) pulmonary embolism

(D) acute stroke

(E) CHF

61. You have a large number of patients in your practice with hypertension. If the diagnosis in an individual is essential hypertension, which of the following statements is correct?

(A) over 95% of patients are salt-sensitive

(B) it comprises about 90% of hypertensives in general population

(C) renin levels are invariably high

(D) women have a poorer prognosis

(E) alcohol reduces risk

DIRECTIONS (Questions 62 through 121): Each set of matching questions in this section consists of a list of lettered options followed by several numbered items. For each numbered item, select the appropriate lettered option(s). Each lettered option may be selected once, more than once, or not at all. EACH ITEM WILL STATE THE NUMBER OF OPTIONS TO SELECT. CHOOSE EXACTLY THIS NUMBER.

Questions 62 through 64

(A) shortened PR interval

(B) lengthened PR interval

(C) lengthened QU interval

(D) shortening of the QT interval

(E) shortening of the QU interval

(F) broad-based (>0.20 second) peaked T wave

(G) narrow-based (<0.20 second) peaked T wave

(H) widened QRS

(I) flattened P waves

For each of the following patients, select the characteristic ECG findings.

62. A 80-year-old man presents with nausea, vomiting, and decreased urine output. He has a history of hypertension and chronic renal failure (Stage 3, GFR [glomerular filtration rate] 50 mL/min). He is taking spironolactone and nifedipine for treatment of hypertension. (SELECT FOUR)

63. A 52-year-old woman presents with polyuria, polydypsia, constipation, and fatigue. She has no significant past medical history, and she is not on any medications. She was recently diagnosed with hyperparathyroidism. (SELECT ONE)

64. A 64-year-old man with heart failure is recently started on 80 mg/day of furosemide. He now feels weak and tired, but notes that his heart failure symptoms have improved. There is no change in his urine output and he gets a good diuretic response every time he takes his furosemide. (SELECT ONE)

Questions 65 through 68

(A) low right atrial pressure

(B) normal right atrial pressure

(C) high right atrial pressure

(D) normal or elevated gradient between PA diastolic pressure and wedge pressure

(E) low PA wedge pressure

(F) normal or high PA wedge pressure

(G) low cardiac output

(H) normal or high cardiac output

(I) low systemic vascular resistance

(J) normal or high systemic vascular resistance

(K) normal or high PA diastolic pressure

For the following patients, select the hemodynamic parameters that are most likely to apply.

65. A 52-year-old man with alcoholic cirrhosis develops a variceal bleed with hypotension. His blood pressure is 85/60 mm Hg, pulse 120/min, and heart sounds are normal. The JVP is not visible, the lungs are clear, and his extremities are pale, cool, and clammy. Central hemodynamic monitoring would reveal (SELECT FOUR)

66. A 73-year-old man has an inferior infarct with ST elevation documented on right-sided precordial leads. He is hypotensive (blood pressure 90/70 mm Hg) and tachycardic. The JVP is 10 cm, the heart sounds are normal, lungs are clear, and his extremitites are cool. Central hemodynamic monitoring would reveal (SELECT SIX)

67. A 20-year-old man is being treated for acute lymphoblastic leukemia. While neutropenic, he becomes severely hypotensive with a temperature of 38.5°C. His blood pressure is 80/60 mm Hg, pulse 120/min, and heart sounds are normal. The JVP is below the sternal angle, lungs are clear, and his extremities are warm and flushed. Central hemodynamic monitoring would reveal (SELECT SIX)

68. A 78-year-old woman has an acute anterior wall MI with hypotension and pulmonary congestion. Her blood pressure is 90/70 mm Hg, pulse 110/min, JVP at 8 cm, and the heart sounds are normal. The lungs have bibasilar crackles, and her extremities are cool and diaphoretic. Hemodynamic monitoring would reveal (SELECT FIVE)

Questions 69 and 70

(A) high-pitched holosystolic murmur

(B) early and midsystolic murmur

(C) rapid decompensation with pulmonary edema

(D) diminished S1

(E) may be tolerated without loss of cardiac reserve for years

(F) diminished forward stroke volume

Select the typical auscultation findings for the following patients.

69. An asymptomatic 19-year-old student with a murmur is found to have mitral regurgitation on echocardiogram. The physical findings might include (SELECT THREE)

70. A 60-year-old man with an acute myocardial infarct develops a new murmur. Echocardiogram reveals acute MR. The findings might include (SELECT THREE)

Questions 71 through 75

(A) prolonged PR interval

(B) broad-notched P wave in lead II

(C) short QT interval

(D) short PR interval

(E) LVH

For each of the following patients, select the characteristic ECG finding.

71. A 25-year-old woman develops exertional dyspnea and fatigue. Her past history is significant for rheumatic fever as a child. Auscultation of the heart reveals a loud first heart sound and a low-pitched middiastolic sound. (SELECT ONE)

72. A 70-year-old man with a prior anterior MI comes for his routine evaluation. He feels well and has no symptoms. He is taking metoprolol 100 mg bid, aspirin 81 mg od, enalapril 10 mg bid, and simvastatin 40 mg od for secondary prevention. (SELECT ONE)

73. A 20-year-old woman develops palpitations and dizziness. Her blood pressure is 100/70 mm Hg, pulse 140/min, and heart sounds are normal. She has had symptoms of palpitations for many years. (SELECT ONE)

74. A 64-year-old woman with metastatic breast cancer presents with fatigue and malaise. She recently started noticing polyuria and poly-dypsia. On examination, her JVP is below the sternal angle, heart sounds are normal, and she has tenderness over her thoracic spine. (SELECT ONE)

75. A 78-year-old man develops recent-onset chest pain and dyspnea on exertion. His blood pressure is 150/90 mm Hg, pulse 90/min, and a systolic ejection murmur at the right sternal border that radiates to the carotids. His carotid pulse is also diminished. (SELECT ONE)

Questions 76 through 79

(A) true of metoprolol but not captopril
(B) true of captopril but not metoprolol
(C) true of both captopril and metoprolol
(D) true of neither captopril nor metoprolol

For each of the following statements, select whether it is applicable to metoprolol and/or captopril.

76. Useful in heart failure (SELECT ONE)

77. The effects on the heart result in a prominent negative inotropic effect (SELECT ONE)

78. The treatment of chronic atrial fibrillation (SELECT ONE)

79. Mechanism of action is calcium blockade (SELECT ONE)

Questions 80 through 84

(A) hydralazine
(B) enalapril
(C) spironolactone
(D) metoprolol
(E) nifedipine
(F) digoxin
(G) furosemide
(H) metolazone
(I) amlodipine
(J) nitrates

For each of the following statements, select whether it is applicable to any or all of the above medications.

80. Direct action on vascular smooth muscle (SELECT FOUR)

81. Inhibition of angiotensin converting enzyme I (ACE I) (SELECT ONE)

82. Myocardial stimulant (SELECT ONE)

83. Used for primary pulmonary hypertension (SELECT ONE)

84. May decrease mortality by direct myocardial protective action against catecholamines (SELECT ONE)

Questions 85 through 89

(A) pulsus tardus
(B) pulsus paradoxus
(C) hyperkinetic pulse
(D) bisferiens pulse
(E) dicrotic pulse
(F) pulsus alternans
(G) delayed femoral pulse
(H) pulsus bigeminus

For each of the following patients, select the characteristic arterial pulse finding.

85. A 75-year-old woman with hypertension develops fatigue and dyspnea on exertion. Her blood pressure is 160/60 mm Hg and pulse 80/min. The second heart sound is diminished and there is an early diastolic murmur that radiates from the right sternal border to the apex. Your clinical diagnosis is aortic regurgitation. (SELECT ONE)

86. A 64-year-old man with two previous MIs develops SOB at rest and has difficulty lying down. His blood pressure is 95/70 mm Hg, pulse 100/min, and JVP is 8 cm. The cardiac apex is dilated and displaced laterally, heart sounds are normal, but there is a soft third

heart sound. Your clinical diagnosis is ischemic cardiomyopathy. (SELECT ONE)

87. A 18-year-old man notices occasional light-headedness when standing up quickly. He also has difficulty playing sports because of easy fatigue and SOB. Examination shows normal heart sounds, but a loud systolic ejection murmur at the right sternal border. The murmur decreases with elevating the legs and increases in the standing position. Your clinical diagnosis is hypertrophic cardiomyopathy (HOCM). (SELECT ONE)

88. A 76-year-old woman presents with new-onset syncope. She has also noticed early fatigue on exertion for the past year. On examination, there is a systolic ejection murmur at the right sternal border that radiates to the carotids. Your clinical diagnosis is aortic stenosis. (SELECT ONE)

89. A 62-year-old man with a 40-pack/year history of smoking presents with increased sputum production and marked SOB. On examination, he is using accessory muscles of respiration, and breath sounds are diminished with expiratory wheezes. Your clinical diagnosis is chronic obstructive pulmonary disease (COPD) exacerbation. (SELECT ONE)

Questions 90 through 94

   (A) Cannon *a* wave
   (B) prominent *x* descent
   (C) Kussmaul's sign
   (D) slow *y* descent
   (E) prominent *v* waves
   (F) positive abdominojugular reflux

For each of the following cardiac abnormalities, select the characteristic JVP finding.

90. Tricuspid regurgitation (SELECT ONE)

91. Right atrial myxoma (SELECT ONE)

92. Right ventricular infarction (SELECT ONE)

93. Right-sided heart failure (SELECT ONE)

94. Complete heart block (SELECT ONE)

Questions 95 through 99

   (A) aortic stenosis
   (B) HOCM
   (C) mitral regurgitation (chronic)
   (D) tricuspid regurgitation
   (E) mitral valve prolapse
   (F) pulmonary stenosis

For each patient with a systolic murmur, select the most likely diagnosis.

95. A 25-year-old woman is found to have a midsystolic murmur on routine evaluation. The murmur does not radiate but it does increase with standing. She otherwise feels well and the rest of the examination is normal. (SELECT ONE)

96. A 75-year-old man is bought to the hospital because of a syncopal episode. There was no incontinence or post-event confusion. On examination, his blood pressure is 140/80 mm Hg, pulse 72/min with no postural changes. His second heart sound is diminished and there is a systolic ejection murmur that radiates to the carotids. With the Valsalva maneuver, the murmur decreases in length and intensity. (SELECT ONE)

97. A 22-year-old woman with no past medical history is found to have a systolic ejection murmur on routine physical examination. She has no symptoms and feels well. The murmur is heard along the right and left sternal borders and it decreases with handgrip exercises. (SELECT ONE)

98. A 45-year-old woman has developed increasing SOB on exertion and fatigue. She has a loud systolic ejection murmur heard best at the left sternal border, and the murmur increases with standing. A double apical impulse is also felt. (SELECT ONE)

99. A 65-year-old man with a previous history of an anterior MI comes for follow-up. On examination, he has a systolic murmur heard best at the apex and radiating to the axilla. Transient external compression of both arms with blood pressure cuffs 20 mm Hg over peak systolic pressure increases the murmur. (SELECT ONE)

Questions 100 through 105

    (A) cardiac tamponade
    (B) constrictive pericarditis
    (C) restrictive cardiomyopathy
    (D) right ventricle myocardial infarction (RVMI)

For each patient with SOB and pheripheral edema, select the most likely diagnosis.

100. A 56-year-old man presents with SOB, fatigue, and edema. He has also noticed weight gain, abdominal discomfort, and distension. He has a prior history of lung cancer treated with radiotherapy to the chest. There is no history of liver or cardiac disease in the past. On examination, he has an elvated JVP, prominent y descent of neck veins, and positive Kussmaul's sign. The heart sounds are normal. The CXR shows a normal cardiac silhouette and the ECG has low voltages. (SELECT ONE)

101. A 28-year-old woman recently developed symptoms of chest pain that changed with positioning. It was worse when lying down and relieved when sitting up. The pain is better now but she notices increasing dyspnea and edema. On examination, the blood pressure is 85/60 mm Hg with a positive pulsus paradoxus, low volume pulse at 110/min, and the heart sounds are distant. The JVP is at 7 cm with a negative Kussmaul's sign. There are low voltages on the ECG, and a large cardiac silhouette on the CXR. (SELECT ONE)

102. A 69-year-old woman complains of some atypical chest pain 2 days prior to presentation. On examination, the JVP is at 8 cm, positive Kussmaul's sign, and normal heart sounds. The lungs are clear. The ECG is abnormal, and the CXR shows a normal cardiac silhouette. (SELECT ONE)

103. A 55-year-old woman with metastatic lung cancer presents with dyspnea and pedal edema. On examination, the JVP is at 10 cm, with a negative Kussmaul's sign. The heart sounds are diminished and the lungs have bibasilar crackles. The ECG shows QRS complexes of variable height. (SELECT ONE)

104. A 64-year-old presents with dyspnea and edema. He had previous coronary bypass surgery 5 years ago, which was uncomplicated. Since then he has had no further chest pain. On examination, his JVP is at 8 cm, with prominent Kussmaul's sign. The heart sounds are easily heard but there is an early diastolic filling sound (pericardial knock). (SELECT ONE)

105. A 55-year-old woman is recently diagnosed with amyloidosis. She is now noticing increasing SOB, fatigue, and edema. On examination, the JVP is at 10 cm with a negative Kussmaul's sign but prominent x and y descent. The blood pressure is 90/70 mm Hg, no pulsus paradoxus, pulse 100/min with low volume, and normal heart sounds. (SELECT ONE)

Questions 106 through 110

    (A) focal myocardial necrosis
    (B) proximal aortitis
    (C) endothelial plaques
    (D) systolic scratchy sound
    (E) restrictive cardiomyopathy

For each patient with systemic disease, select the typical cardiovascular involvement.

106. A 45-year-old man develops new symptoms of sudden-onset flushing involving his head and neck lasting a few minutes. He also notices watery diarrhea and abdominal pain when the flushing occurs. Serotonin and its metabolites are elevated in his urine and serum. (SELECT ONE)

107. A 25-year-old man has noticed increasing lower-back and gluteal pain. It is dull and associated with morning stiffness lasting 1 hour, and then it improves after activity. On examination, there are no active inflammatory joints but he has limited forward and lateral flexion of the lumbar spine, as well as decreased chest expansion. X-rays of his pelvis and lumbar spine show changes of sacroiliitis. (SELECT ONE)

108. A 31-year-old woman has new-onset headaches and blood pressure elevation. She also notices that the symptoms come episodically and consist of palpitations, headache, anxiety, and marked blood pressure elevation. She undergoes a workup for secondary causes of hypertension, and is found to have elevated free catecholamines in her urine. (SELECT ONE)

109. A 22-year-old university student notices unintentional weight loss and palpitations for 1 month. She also complains of sweating and feeling hot all the time. On examination, her pulse is regular at 110/min, blood pressure 96/60 mm Hg; she has a diffuse enlargement of the thyroid gland. Her thyroid-stimulating hormone (TSH) is low and free T3 and T4 are elevated. (SELECT ONE)

110. A 60-year-old man presents with SOB, increasing abdominal distention, and lower leg edema. He has no prior history of cardiac, renal, or liver disease. On examination, the JVP is at 8 cm with a negative Kussmaul's sign but prominent x and y descent. The blood pressure is 95/75 mm Hg, no pulsus paradoxus, pulse 100/min with low volume, and normal heart sounds. There is shifting dullness of the abdomen and pedal edema. His blood glucose and hemoglobin A1C are elevated. (SELECT ONE)

Questions 111 through 116

(A) fibric acid derivatives (clofibrate, gemfibrozil)

(B) nicotinic acid

(C) bile acid-binding resins (cholestyramine, colestipol)

(D) hepatic hydroxymethylglutaryl-coenzyme A (HMG-CoA) reductase inhibitors (lovastatin, simvastatin, pravastatin)

(E) lifestyle modification

(F) estrogens (Premarin, estradiol)

For each patient with dyslipidemia, select the most appropriate treatment.

111. A 63-year-old woman with Type II diabetes is seen for follow-up after a fasting lipid profile. She has no other medical conditions and feels well. Her diabetes is well-controlled and the last hemoglobin A1C value was 6.5%. Her total cholesterol (T-chol) is 240 mg/dL, HDL 50 mg/dL, low-density lipoprotein (LDL) 160 mg/dL, and triglycerides 150 mg/dL. (SELECT TWO)

112. A 42-year-old woman, who is an executive at a large company, is seen for her annual evaluation. She is concerned about her risk for future cardiac events since a collegue was just diagnosed with angina. She has no other medical illness and is a lifetime nonsmoker. Her fasting lipid profile is T-chol 240 mg/dL, HDL 55 mg/dL, LDL 160 mg/dL, and triglycerides 140 mg/dL. (SELECT ONE)

113. A 57-year-old man comes to see you for follow-up 4 weeks after being discharged from hospital for unstable angina. His coronary angiogram showed moderate nonstenotic disease in two vessels. The cardiologist asks you to follow up on his fasting lipid profile since it was not checked in the hospital. His T-chol is 240 mg/dL, LDL 120 mg/dL, HDL 50 mg/dL, and triglycerides 130 mg/dL. (SELECT TWO)

114. A 58-year-old woman is admitted to hospital with left-sided hemiparesis. She is diagnosed with an ischemic right cortical stroke, and started on aminosalicylic acid (ASA) for secondary prevention. Her carotid ultrasound reveals no arterial stenosis. She has no other significant past medical history but she does smoke half pack a day. Her fasting lipid profile is T-chol 240 mg/dL, HDL 50 mg/dL, LDL 160 mg/dL, and triglycerides 130 mg/dL. (SELECT TWO)

115. A 56-year-old man is diagnosed with the *metabolic syndrome*, which consists of hypertension, insulin resistance, dyslipidemia, and abdominal obesity. He has no prior history of cardiac or vascular disease and is otherwise well. His fasting T-chol is 270 mg/dL, HDL 50 mg/dL, LDL 150 mg/dL, and triglycerides 150 mg/dL. (SELECT TWO)

116. A 60-year-old woman is concerned about her risk for cardiovascular disease since she is postmenopausal now. She has no symptoms of cardiac or vascular disease and her only cardiac risk factor is hypertension for the past 5 years, which is well-controlled. Her fasting T-chol is 240 mg/dL, HDL 55 mg/dL, LDL 160 mg/dL, and triglycerides 140 mg/dL. (SELECT ONE)

Questions 117 through 121

  (A) thiazides
  (B) spironolactone
  (C) clonidine
  (D) prazosin
  (E) beta-blockers
  (F) hydralazine
  (G) ACE inhibitors
  (H) calcium channel blockers

For each patient with high blood pressure, select the most appropriate medication.

117. A 54-year-old man with diabetes has a persistently elevated blood pressure averaging 150/90 mm Hg. He has complications of pheripheral neuropathy and a urinalysis is positive for microalbuminuria. (SELECT ONE)

118. A 60-year-old woman with no past medical history has an elevated blood pressure of 165/80 mm Hg on routine evaluation. Repeated measurements over the next month confirm the elevated pressure. Physical examination, routine blood count, and biochemistry are all normal. (SELECT ONE)

119. A 26-year-old woman develops new-onset hypertension. She has no other medical problems and is not taking any medications. She undergoes an evaluation for secondary hypertension and is found to have unilateral renal artery stenosis. (SELECT ONE)

120. A 70-year-old man has isolated systolic hypertension. On examination, his blood pressure is 170/80 mm Hg, heart and lungs are normal. He has no other medical conditions. (SELECT ONE)

121. A 57-year-old man has a blood pressure of 155/90 mm Hg on routine evaluation. He had coronary artery bypass grafting 4 years earlier, after which he has had no further chest pain. The rest of the examination is normal, and the elevated blood pressure is confirmed on two repeat visits. (SELECT ONE)

Answers and Explanations

1. **(D)** Wenckebach, or type I second-degree AV block, is characterized on ECG by progressive lengthening of the PR interval until there is a nonconducted P wave. The magnitude of PR lengthening declines with each beat, so the RR intervals characteristically shorten prior to the dropped beat. It is almost always caused by abnormal conduction across the AV node, and the QRS complex is usually of normal duration. *(Fuster, p. 901)*

2. **(D)** The ventricular inhibited (VVI) pacemaker functions when the heart rate falls below a preset interval. If a QRS is detected, the pacemaker is inhibited. If a QRS is not sensed, the pacing stimulus is not inhibited and the ventricle is stimulated. *(Fuster, p. 909)*

3. **(D)** Sinus tachycardia is the most common ECG finding in pulmonary embolism. The specific ECG signs of pulmonary embolism such as the S1, Q3, T3 are rarely seen except in cases of massive pulmonary embolism. In submassive pulmonary emboli, the ECG may show nonspecific ST changes and sinus tachycardia.

    On occasion, pulmonary embolism can precipitate atrial flutter or fibrillation. One of the most useful roles of the ECG is to rule out MI when a massive embolism is present. *(Fuster, pp. 1596–1597)*

4. **(C)** Aortic stenosis is most likely to be associated with angina pectoris, syncope, and exertional dyspnea. Exertional syncope is caused by either systemic vasodilation in the presence of fixed or inadequate cardiac output, an arrhythmia, or both. Syncope at rest is most frequently a result of a transient ventricular tachyarrhythmia. *(Fuster, pp. 1645–1647)*

5. **(C)** Common findings in infective endocarditis include petechiae, Roth's spots, Osler's nodes, Janeway lesions, splinter hemorrhages, stroke, and infarction of viscera, or extremities.

    Many of the complications are thought to be embolic but may include vasculitis. Autopsy studies reveal that many systemic emboli go unrecognized. Brain, lung, coronary arteries, spleen, extremities, gut, and eyes are common locations for emboli. *(Fuster, pp. 2010–2011)*

6. **(B)** The slow channel for calcium assumes considerable importance in the region of the sinus node and AV node. For verapamil, this results in both antiarrhythmic and negative inotropic effects. Different classes of calcium channel blockers have differential effects on these slow channels, explaining the different clinical properties of the various calcium channel blocking drugs. *(Fuster, pp. 950)*

7. **(D)** Pericarditis secondary to transmural infarction is very common and most cases appear within 4 days. The most common manifestation of pericarditis is a friction rub along the left sternal border. It is evanescent, lasting only a few days. The pain is usually perceived by the patient to be different than that of the infarct. It is worsened by inspiration, swallowing, coughing, or lying down. It frequently is associated with a low-grade fever. *(Fuster, p. 1980, 1995–1996)*

8. **(A)** Positively inotropic is the best description of the effect of calcium ions on the myocardium.

Calcium plays a role in excitation–contraction coupling, and in possible drug effects and heart failure. *(Fuster, p. 129)*

9. **(C)** In the past, there was concern that rigorous drug treatment would harm the fetus.

Studies now show benefit in controlling pressure with drugs, but ACE inhibitors are contraindicated because they might cause renal abnormalities in the fetus. Women who develop hypertension during pregnancy have a higher risk of developing hypertension in later life. *(Fuster, p. 2217)*

10. **(E)** There is a possible indication (but not an obligation) to insert a temporary pacemaker if a new LBBB occurs. If LBBB and a Mobitz type II AV block occur, there is general agreement on the usefulness of pacing. Temporary pacemaker is not required for first-degree block.

For second-degree block of the Wenckebach type (usually with an inferior infarction), pacing is only required if symptoms of bradycardia and hypotension cannot be controlled medically. The necessity for temporary pacing during an acute myocardial infarction (AMI) does not necessarily indicate that permanent pacing will be required. *(Fuster, pp. 1323–1324)*

11. **(D)** Pulmonary hypertension is associated with an increased intensity of the second heart sound, which coincides with the end of the T wave on ECG. It is the pulmonic component of the second heart sound that is increased. Pulmonary stenosis can cause dyspnea on exertion but auscultation will reveal a systolic murmur and decreased second heart sound (pulmonic component).

As well, there may be prominent *a* waves in the jugular venous pulse, a right ventricular heave, an ejection click, and a right ventricular fourth heart sound. When signs and symptoms are apparent, the pulmonary hypertension is usually moderate to severe. *(Fuster, pp. 1586–1587)*

12. **(D)** The patient most likely has PSVT, since the tachycardia terminates after carotid sinus massage (CSM). CSM increases vagal tone (parasympathetic) which decreases AV nodal conduction and terminates AV node re-entry arrhythmias. Sinus tachycardia differs from PSVT tachycardia in that it does not start or stop abruptly. In PSVT, the QRS is usually narrow without clearly discernible P waves. A wide QRS in PSVT can result from a preexisting bundle branch block, or a functional bundle branch block secondary to the tachycardia. This can make the distinction from a ventricular arrhythmia quite difficult. *(Fuster, pp. 845–847)*

13. **(D)** In the absence of critical CAD, angina pectoris occurs most frequently with aortic stenosis. AMI is usually due to associated atherosclerotic coronary occlusion. *(Fuster, p. 1645)*

14. **(B)** In aortic stenosis, the first sound is usually normal; the second sound is characteristically diminished because of the increased ventricular pressure and the stenotic valve is less mobile. There can be a single S2 either because A2 and P2 are superimposed or A2 is absent or very soft. Severe aortic stenosis may be accompanied by paradoxical splitting of S2. *(Fuster, p. 1646)*

15. **(B)** AV dissociation is the independent beating of atria and ventricles and is recognized on the ECG by fixed PP and RR intervals but variable PR intervals.

AV block is one cause of AV dissociation. *(Fuster, pp. 904–905)*

16. **(E)** Nitroglycerine is usually used in the setting of severe pulmonary congestion with adequate blood pressure. With significant hypotension, inotropic agents are generally administered prior to nitroglycerine. *(Fuster, pp. 1316–1317)*

17. **(A)** A ventricular septal defect is considered a relatively high-risk lesion for infective endocarditis.

Mitral valve prolapse with regurgitation, asymmetric septal hypertrophy, and pure mitral stenosis are considered an intermediate risk. Atrial septal defects of the secundum type are considered low risk. *(Fuster, p. 2003)*

18. **(A)** The myxoma is a solitary globular or polypoid tumor varying in size from that of a cherry to a peach. About 75% are found in the left atrium, and most of the remainder in the right atrium. The clinical presentation is with one or more of the classical triad of constitution symptoms (fatigue, fever, anemia), embolic events, or obstruction of the valve orifice. *(Fuster, pp. 2081–2082)*

19. **(A)** Diltiazem and verapamil may be of help in both acute paroxysms of atrial flutter and chronic management. The other choices have no effect on the AV node to slow down flutter, and atropine accelerates AV conduction. At times, catheter ablation of the flutter pathway is required in chronic atrial flutter. Surgical ablation is reserved for cases where other surgical interventions are required. *(Fuster, p. 844)*

20. **(C)** Exercise electrocardiography represents an increasingly popular noninvasive method for early detection of latent ischemic heart disease. As with other diagnostic tests, the exercise ECG is of most clinical value when the pretest probability of disease is moderate (i.e., 30–70%). In men over 40 and women over 50 who plan to start vigorous exercise, use of exercise ECG is possibly, but not definitely, supported by the evidence (class IIb). *(Fuster, pp. 477–478)*

21. **(D)** Contrast media used in cardiac catheterization may result in renal impairment. The group at highest risk includes diabetics with renal disease and those with preexisting renal failure. Good hydration is essential. Other manifestations of contrast media include nausea and vomiting (common), and anaphylactoid reactions characterized by low-grade fever, hives, itching, angioedema, bronchospasm, and even shock. Side effects are reduced with the use of new low osmolality contrast media. *(Fuster, p. 489)*

22. **(E)** Pericarditis in clinical practice is commonly idiopathic and frequently assumed to be of possible viral origin. Coxsackieviruses are a common cause, but herpesviruses are not. Although TB, rheumatic fever, and MI can cause pericarditis, they are unlikely in this case. *(Fuster, p. 1979)*

23. **(C)** Left-heart catheterization is a more accurate measurement, but involves a slightly increased risk. End-expiratory PA diastolic pressure is very close (2–4 mm) to wedge pressure as well. A discordance between wedge pressure and PA diastolic pressure suggests the presence of pulmonary hypertension. *(Fuster, p. 512)*

24. **(C)** Aortic dissection is a medical emergency requiring prompt attention. Other cardiac and pulmonary causes of chest pain can be quickly ruled out with ECG and CXR. CT scan of the chest is sensitive (93–100%) in ruling out dissection. Transesophageal echocardiography is equally as sensitive but not a transthoracic echo. *(Fuster, pp. 2312–2313)*

25. **(A)** This is characteristic of an atrial septal defect. Pulmonary blood flow is greater because of increased blood flow from the right atrium, which receives blood from the vena cava and left atrium. *(Fuster, pp. 1797–1798)*

26. **(B)** Angina or infarction in young patients should prompt the physician to consider congenital coronary artery anomaly or congenital coronary artery aneurysm. Acquired coronary artery aneurysm can be caused by atherosclerosis, trauma, angioplasty, atherectomy, vasculitis, mycotic emboli, Kawasaki syndrome, or arterial dissection. *(Fuster, p. 1178)*

27. **(D)** This pulse is seen in aortic regurgitation.
    The pressure in diastole is usually 50 mm Hg or lower. This is known as a water hammer or Corrigan's pulse. A bisferiens pulse (in the bisferiens wave form there are two pressure peaks) may be present as well. Systolic blood pressure is elevated. *(Fuster, p. 1654)*

28. **(B)** Digoxin toxicity may cause any dysrhythmia. Classically, dysrhythmias that are associated with increased automaticity and decreased AV conduction occur (i.e., paroxysmal atrial tachycardia with 2:1 block, accelerated junctional rhythm, or bidirectional ventricular tachycardia [torsade de pointes]). Sinus bradycardia

and other bradyarrhythmias are very common. Slow atrial fibrillation with very little variation in the ventricular rate (regularization of the R-R interval) may occur. This arrhythmia is likely slow atrial fibrillation. Symptoms of digitalis toxicity include anorexia, nausea, fatigue, dizziness, and visual disturbances. The presence of hypokalemia increases the likelihood of digitalis toxicity. *(Fuster, p. 795)*

29. **(A)** Commonly, no cause is found for constrictive pericarditis. Some patients do give a history of previous acute pericarditis. TB is now an uncommon cause. Cancer can cause constriction but is uncommon. Rheumatic fever does not cause pericarditis. *(Fuster, pp. 1989–1991)*

30. **(E)** The maneuvers listed increase the block and are useful for diagnosis, but not for converting the atrial flutter to a sinus rhythm. Electrical cardioversion is the method of choice in patients who are hemodynamically unstable. Often very low amounts of energy during cardioversion will convert atrial flutter. *(Fuster, p. 844)*

31. **(C)** Atrial flutter is characterized by regular atrial activation with an atrial rate of >240 beats/min. The ventricular response depends on the conduction of the AV node, usually there is 2:1 or 3:1 conduction. It is now known that the predominant mechanism for atrial flutter is right atrial macroreentry with circular activation. Atrial flutter typically originates from the right atrium and most often involves a large circuit that travels around the area of the tricuspid valve. This type of atrial flutter is referred to as typical atrial flutter. Less commonly, atrial flutter can result from circuits in other areas of the right or left atrium. *(Fuster, pp. 841–842)*

32. **(B)** Retention of fluid is complex and not due to any one factor, however, hormones may contribute. Growth hormone does not have fluid-retaining properties. The exact mechanisms that initiate renal conservation of salt and water are not precisely understood, but may include arterial volume receptors sensing a decrease in the *effective* arterial blood volume. Aldosterone, renin, and vasopressin are generally increased in heart failure. *(Fuster, p. 713)*

33. **(A)** ST elevation persisting 2 weeks after an infarct, an abnormal pericardial impulse, and a bulge on the left ventricular border on x-ray are characteristic of an aneurysm. Ventricular aneurysms are most often a result of a large anterior infarct. The poor prognosis associated with these aneurysms is due to the associated left ventricular dysfunction, rather than to the aneurysm itself. *(Fuster, pp. 1321–1322)*

34. **(D)** In aortic stenosis, there is normal overall cardiac size, but dilatation of the proximal ascending aorta and blunt rounding of the lower left cardiac contour. Calcification of the valve is often difficult to determine on plain films. Although left atrial enlargement can occur, its presence on the CXR should raise other diagnostic possibilities, such as mitral valve disease. *(Fuster, p. 1647)*

35. **(D)** This combination, although the total cholesterol is borderline, has high HDL cholesterol, which is protective. Nevertheless, a level this high would likely require treatment. *(Fuster, pp. 1099–1100)*

36. **(B)** Besides coarctation of the aorta, aortic occlusive disease, dissection of the aorta, and abdominal aneurysm may lead to differential blood pressure in arms and legs. Coarctation is the third most common form of congenital cardiac disease. One-third of the patients will be hypertensive. The femoral pulses are weak, delayed, and even absent. *(Fuster, p. 1809)*

37. **(D)** He likely has LVH.

    Signs include left axis deviation, high-voltage QRS complexes in V5 and V6, deep S in V1 and V2, and prolonged QRS in the left precordial leads. Age, orientation of the heart in the chest, and noncardiac factors make the ECG an imperfect tool for diagnosing or excluding LVH. The ECG is more accurate and better for following progression or regression of LVH. *(Fuster, pp. 311–312)*

38. **(A)** High urinary specific gravity, nocturia, and daytime oliguria occur in addition to low urinary sodium content in untreated CHF. These changes are the result of the activation of the

renin-angiotensin-aldosterone system. *(Fuster, pp. 713–714)*

39. **(C)** Thyroid disease may affect the heart muscle directly or there may be excessive sympathetic stimulation. Common symptoms of thyrotoxic heart disease include palpitations, exertional dyspnea, and worsening angina. Atrial fibrillation is particularly common in older individuals. *(Fuster, p. 827)*

40. **(D)** Since the duration of atrial fibrillation is not known, it is presumed to be chronic. There is an increased risk of cardioembolic events if restoration of sinus rhythm is attempted before anticoagulating the patient for 3–4 weeks. Aspirin is only modestly effective in reducing cardioembolic events and not the first choice. Beta-blockers are not indicated since the rate is controlled. *(Fuster, pp. 833–834)*

41. **(B)** Cotton wool spots, hemorrhage, and papilledema are common. Fibrinoid necrosis occurs on the arterioles of many organs. Earlier manifestations of arteriosclerosis include thickening of the vessel wall. This is manifested by obscuring of the venous column at arterial crossings. *(Fuster, p. 1541, 1543)*

42. **(A)** Early atherosclerosis with tendon xanthomas, xanthelasma, and arcus senilis are characteristics of familial hypercholesterolemia. The disorder is inherited in an autosomal dominant manner. *(Fuster, pp. 236–237)*

43. **(C)** Acute pericarditis is most often idiopathic and is typically self-limited (usually within 2–6 weeks). While small effusions are common, tamponade is unusual, as are heart failure and constriction. Other diseases causing pericarditis should be searched for, and may influence the prognosis. *(Fuster, p. 1982)*

44. **(D)** Orthostatic hypotension (systolic dropping by 20 mm or more) is particularly common in the elderly and in diabetics because of autonomic neuropathy. Management includes avoidance of precipitating factors, simple adaptive maneuvers, volume expansion, and pharmacologic agents. *(Fuster, pp. 1036–1037)*

45. **(E)** In mitral valve prolapse, the first heart sound is usually preserved followed by a systolic click and late systolic murmur. The click is actually the most common finding. General physical examination may reveal scoliosis, pectus excavatum, straightened thoracic spine, or narrow anteroposterior diameter of chest. *(Fuster, p. 1698)*

46. **(A)** The symptoms and signs are like any sudden paroxysmal tachycardia, but the ventricular rate is the clue, after carotid pressure, to the diagnosis of atrial flutter with 2:1 block. *(Fuster, pp. 841–842)*

47. **(C)** Management of acute viral or idiopathic pericarditis includes analgesia (usually aspirin every 3–4 hours initially) and rest if the pain is severe. Occasionally, nonsteroidal anti-inflammatory drugs (NSAIDs) are required (e.g., ibuprofen or indomethacin). Careful observation for increasing effusion and tamponade are essential. The classic findings of cardiac tamponade include arterial hypotension and pulsus paradoxus. *(Fuster, p. 1985)*

48. **(B)** Diastolic dysfunction is an important cause of heart failure in the elderly. It is commonly associated with a history of hypertension and diabetes. Normal ejection fraction and aortic sclerosis rule out either systolic or valvular heart disease as causes. In HOCM there is nonconcentric hypertrophy. *(Fuster, pp. 710, 2276–2277)*

49. **(A)** Acute rupture of an atherosclerotic plaque is now recognized as the most common cause of ST-elevation MI. Pericarditis has diffuse ST elevation in multiple leads and aortic stenosis does cause angina but not ST elevation. *(Fuster, p. 1226)*

50. **(D)** *S. epidermidis* is still the most frequent early and late cause of endocarditis in patients with prosthetic heart valves. The other organisms are seen less frequently in late prosthetic valve endocarditis. *(Fuster, pp. 2004–2005)*

51. **(D)** This man has acute coronary syndrome (ACS) until proven otherwise. The ECG is the

most useful initial investigation since it identifies individuals with ST-segment elevation who may be candidates for either thrombolysis or primary angioplasty (PCI). The troponins are important in diagnosing myocardial necrosis. The other investigations may be important in looking for alternate causes of chest pain once ST-elevation MI has been ruled out. *(Fuster, pp. 1252, 1256)*

52. **(C)** Essential hypertension is the most likely diagnosis. A secondary cause for hypertension is found in only 10% of patients, with 90% labeled as essential. Current recommendations for initial workup of a hypertensive patient include serum chemistry (glucose, potassium, creatinine), urinalysis, and ECG. *(Fuster, p. 1545)*

53. **(C)** Coarctation of the aorta is the diagnosis.

    There is a *reverse 3* deformity of the esophagus, the belly of which represents the dilated aorta after the coarctation. The border of the descending aorta shows a medial indentation called the *3* or *tuck* sign, the belly of the 3 representing the poststenotic dilation and the upper portion by the dilated subclavian artery and small transverse aortic arch. *(Fuster, p. 1809)*

54. **(B)** Note the abnormal humped contour of the left ventricular border, with a curvilinear calcification following the abnormal cardiac contour. The presence of calcification in the ventricular wall and the abnormal left ventricular contour alerts one to the consideration of a ventricular aneurysm. *(Fuster, pp. 1321–1322)*

55. **(B)** The cardiac rhythm is atrial flutter with 2:1 AV conduction. QRS complexes occur with perfect regularity at a rate of about 150/min. Their normal contour and duration indicate that ventricular activation occurs normally via the AV junction-His-Purkinje system. *(Fuster, pp. 841–842)*

56. **(B)** The PR interval of the first two complexes is normal at 0.20 seconds. The QRS duration is 0.16 seconds. The third P wave is nonconducted. This cycle recurs in the remainder of the strip. This is second-degree heart block of the Mobitz type II variety. Note the wide QRS.

When this type of heart block develops, either de novo or in the course of an AMI, a cardiac pacemaker is usually recommended, as the incidence of complete heart block is high in this situation. *(Fuster, pp. 901–903)*

57. **(D)** The ST is depressed in leads II, III, aVF, and V4–V6. These nonspecific abnormalities do not indicate significant coronary heart disease, especially in an apprehensive young patient. Further evaluations should be guided by clinical circumstances. *(Fuster, pp. 304–305)*

58. **(E)** The underlying rhythm is a regular sinus rhythm with a rate of 85 beats/min. The sinus rhythm is interrupted frequently by bursts of irregular ventricular, premature beats. The sinus rhythm is uninterrupted as can be determined by plotting the PP intervals, which are regular.

    The rhythm may be termed a *chaotic ventricular arrhythmia* or *ventricular tachycardia*. Its gross irregularity is unusual. Antiarrhythmic therapy is usually not indicated for nonsustained VT in the setting of thrombolytic treatment. *(Fuster, pp. 876–877)*

59. **(A)** No atrial activity is detected. The ventricular rate is slightly irregular. Beat number 4 is a ventricular premature contraction. The T waves are tall and markedly peaked. This type of T wave is characteristic of hyperkalemia, as is absence of visible atrial activity.

    The potassium level was 8.2 mmol/L. *(Fuster, p. 313)*

60. **(A)** Sudden death, defined as death within 1 hour of onset of symptoms, is usually caused by cardiac disease in middle-aged and elderly patients, but in younger age groups noncardiac causes predominate. There is a bimodal distribution in the population, with the first peak before 6 months of age (sudden infant death syndrome). The most common coronary artery finding is extensive chronic coronary atherosclerosis, although acute syndromes do occur. *(Fuster, p. 1057)*

61. **(B)** Over 90% of hypertensives in the general population have essential hypertension. Only

about 60% of hypertensives are very sensitive to salt. About 20% of hypertensives have low-renin essential hypertension. This is more common in Blacks. Male sex, Black race, youth, smoking, DM, excess alcohol ingestion, hypercholesterolemia, more severe hypertension, and evidence of end-organ damage are among the factors that suggest a poor prognosis. *(Kasper, pp. 1463–1464)*

62. **(B, G, H, I)** In renal impairment, potassium-sparing diuretics can cause life-threatening hyperkalemia. The characteristic findings of hyperkalemia are a narrow-based, peaked T wave in conjunction with a widened QRS complex. Other causes of widened QRS complexes do not coexist with a narrow-peak T wave. Also, the PR interval prolongs and the P wave flattens with hyperkalemia. *(Fuster, p. 313)*

63. **(D)** With severe hypercalcemia, the QT interval is markedly shortened. There is a correlation between the length of QT interval and the degree of hypercalcemia. *(Fuster, p. 314)*

64. **(C)** Hypokalemia results in prolongation of the QU interval. The delayed repolarization in hypokalemia is best expressed at QU rather than QT prolongation since it can be difficult to separate the T wave from the U wave. In severe cases, the ST segments become depressed. Quinidine, even in therapeutic doses, can cause similar ECG findings. This is felt to be a risk factor for ventricular arrhythmias, including Torsades des pointes. *(Fuster, p. 314)*

65. **(A, E, G, J)** Hypovolemic shock is characterized by a low cardiac output with normal or high systemic vascular resistance. The low right atrial filling pressure and low PA wedge pressure reflect the inadequate venous return. *(Kasper, p. 1615)*

66. **(C, D, F, G, J, K)** This man has a right ventricular MI. Primary right ventricular failure is characterized by a disproportionately high right atrial pressure with normal or high wedge pressure. The PA diastolic pressure is normal or elevated and the gradient between PA diastolic pressure and wedge pressure is usually

increased. Systemic vascular resistance is usually normal. *(Kasper, p. 1615)*

67. **(A, D, E, H, I, K)** In septic shock, right atrial wedge pressures, and systemic vascular resistance are low. PA diastolic pressure is usually normal or high, therefore, resulting in an increased gradient between PA diastolic and wedge pressures. Cardiac output can be normal or high in early sepsis. *(Kasper, p. 1615)*

68. **(C, F, G, J, K)** Cardiogenic shock is characterized by high right atrial pressure (although it can be normal at times), high PA wedge pressure, high PA diastolic pressure, high systemic vascular resistance, and low cardiac output. *(Kasper, p. 1615)*

69. **(A, D, E)** In chronic, compensated mitral regurgitation, there is a holosystolic murmur, which starts with S1 and extends to or past the aortic component of S2. The S1 is diminished, and there is increased splitting of S2.

This condition is often tolerated for years before symptoms develop. *(Fuster, p. 1686)*

70. **(B, C, F)** CAD is the most common cause of acute mitral regurgitation in the United States. The murmur is often midsystolic early on, and a thrill may be present. The apex is usually hyperdynamic but actual forward stroke volume is usually diminished. The presentation is usually dominated by acute pulmonary edema and occurs most often 2–7 days post-MI. *(Fuster, pp. 1680–1682)*

71. **(B)** ECG changes in mitral stenosis are due to enlargement and hypertrophy of the left atrium and asynchronous atrial activation.

The notched P wave is most prominent in lead II. In lead V1, the P wave has a negative terminal deflection. *(Fuster, p. 1673)*

72. **(A)** A prolonged PR interval is a common finding in asymptomatic elderly patients that have age-related degeneration of the AV node. Drugs such as beta-blockers (metoprolol) may exacerbate the condition or even cause PR prolongation in excessive doses. *(Fuster, p. 901)*

73. **(D)** In Wolff-Parkinson-White syndrome, the PR interval is short, the QRS is widened, and there is slurring of the upstroke of the R wave. The shortened PR interval reflects faster than normal conduction through an accessory pathway. The ventricular complex represents a fusion beat. The blurred upstroke of the QRS (delta wave) represents ventricular activation via the accessory pathway. The normal end portion of the QRS represents activation via the normal route through the AV node. *(Fuster, p. 865)*

74. **(C)** Hypercalcemia may prolong the QRS and shorten the ST and QT intervals. Serious arrhythmias rarely occur with hypercalcemia. *(Fuster, p. 314)*

75. **(E)** The ECG in severe aortic stenosis shows LVH, but is not perfectly sensitive and is not specific. Bundle branch blocks and ST-T changes can occur, but some patients have a normal ECG. *(Fuster, p. 1647)*

76. **(C)** Beta-blockers and ACE inhibitors are both indicated in the treatment of heart failure patients with systolic dysfunction. *(Fuster, p. 729)*

77. **(A)** Beta-blockers have a negative inotropic effect on the heart. Despite this they improve survival in patients with left ventricular dysfunction and heart failure *(Fuster, p. 733)*

78. **(A)** In chronic atrial flutter, control of ventricular rate is the goal of therapy. Beta-blockers, $Ca^{2}+$ calcium channel blockers, and digoxin are drugs commonly used. *(Fuster, pp. 836–837)*

79. **(D)** Neither ACE inhibitors or beta-blockers mediate their effects by calcium channel blockade. *(Brunton, pp. 272, 800)*

80. **(A, E, I, J)** Hydralazine has a greater dilator effect on arterioles than on veins, the opposite is true for nitrates. Combined therapy with hydralazine and nitrates has been shown to reduce mortality in patients with heart failure, but not reduce hospitalization for heart failure. Reflex tachycardia with hydralazine is common in patients with hypertension, but less so in heart failure. Tachycardia may precipitate angina. Calcium channel blockers are not generally used in CHF, because of their negative inotropic effect. However, amlodipine can be used for concurrent treatment of angina or hypertension. *(Fuster, pp. 730–738)*

81. **(B)** Enalapril may exert its effect by inhibiting formation of angiotensin II. This lowers systemic vascular resistance. In addition, ACE inhibitors have a natriuretic effect by inhibition of aldosterone secretion. They have been shown to improve mortality and decrease hospitalization in patients with CHF. *(Fuster, pp. 730–738)*

82. **(F)** Digoxin is a direct inotropic agent, but is usually reserved for patients who are symptomatic after treatment with ACE inhibitors and diuretics. It can be used for rate control in atrial fibrillation, although beta-blockers might be preferred. *(Fuster, p. 741)*

83. **(E)** Long-acting nifedipine has been a useful adjunct to the treatment of primary pulmonary hypertension, but great care must be used as even low doses of vasodilators can cause untoward reactions in patients with pulmonary hypertension. Lung transplants have provided a major therapeutic modality for managing severe pulmonary hypertension.
ACE inhibitors and hydralazine have been tried, but are not effective. *(Fuster, p. 1788)*

84. **(D)** There are numerous potential mechanisms that might explain the beneficial effects of beta-blockers in left ventricular dysfunction, and post-MI. The benefit is additive to that provided by ACE inhibitors. *(Fuster, p. 733)*

85. **(C)** A hyperkinetic pulse occurs in the setting of an elevated stroke volume (anemia, fever, anxiety) or an abnormally rapid runoff from the arterial system (aortic regurgitation, patent ductus arteriosus, arteriovenous fistula). *(Fuster, p. 244)*

86. **(E)** A dicrotic pulse has a peak in systole and another in diastole. It occurs in patients with very low stroke volume, especially dilated cardiomyopathy. *(Fuster, p. 244)*

87. (D) The bisferiens pulse, two systolic peaks, occurs in HOCM and aortic regurgitation. In aortic regurgitation, the bisferiens pulse can occur both in the presence or absence of aortic stenosis. *(Fuster, p. 224)*

88. (A) The pulsus tardus of aortic stenosis is the result of mechanical obstruction to left ventricular ejection and often has an accompanying thrill. The characteristic feel of the pulse is caused by a delayed systolic peak. *(Fuster, p. 244)*

89. (B) Pulsus paradoxus, a drop of >10 mm Hg in systolic blood pressure during inspiration, is caused by pericardial tamponade, airway obstruction, or superior vena cava obstruction. At times, the peripheral pulse may disappear completely during inspiration. *(Fuster, p. 245)*

90. (E) Tricuspid regurgitation increases the size of the *v* wave. When tricuspid regurgitation becomes severe, the combination of a prominent *v* wave and obliteration of the *x* descent results in a single, large, positive systolic wave. *(Fuster, p. 248)*

91. (D) Right atrial myxoma, or tricuspid stenosis, will slow the y descent by obstructing right ventricular filling. The y descent of the JVP is produced mainly by the tricuspid valve opening and the subsequent rapid inflow of blood into the right ventricle. *(Fuster, p. 248)*

92. (C) Right ventricular infarction and constrictive pericarditis frequently result in an increase in JVP during inspiration (Kussmaul's sign). Severe right-sided failure can also be a cause. *(Fuster, p. 247)*

93. (F) Right-sided heart failure is the most common cause of a positive abdominojugular reflux (normal JVP at rest, increases during 10 seconds of firm midabdominal compression, and only drops when pressure is released). *(Fuster, p. 247)*

94. (A) Large *a* waves occur with increased resistance to filling (tricuspid stenosis, pulmonary hypertension) or when the right atrium contracts against a tricuspid valve closed by right ventricular systole (*Cannon a* waves) in complete heart block or other arrhythmias. *(Fuster, p. 248)*

95. (E) With standing, most murmurs diminish. The two exceptions are HOCM, which becomes louder, and mitral valve prolapse, which becomes longer and louder. *(Kasper, pp. 1308–1310)*

96. (A) With the Valsalva maneuver, most murmurs will decrease. The exceptions are the murmurs of HOCM and mitral valve prolapse, which increase.

After release of the Valsalva maneuver, right-sided murmurs tend to return to baseline more rapidly. *(Kasper, pp. 1308–1310)*

97. (B) The murmur of HOCM often decreases with submaximal isometric exercise (handgrip). Murmurs across normal or obstructed valves will be increased.

Handgrip can also accentuate an S3 or S4. *(Kasper, pp. 1308–1310)*

98. (B) HOCM often has a bisferiens pulse. It can also be found in pure aortic regurgitation or combined aortic regurgitation and aortic stenosis. *(Kasper, pp. 1308–1310)*

99. (C) This maneuver will increase the murmurs of mitral regurgitation, ventricular septal defect, and aortic regurgitation. Other murmurs are not affected. *(Kasper, pp. 1308–1310)*

100. (B) Constrictive pericarditis is characterized by a prominent y descent of the neck veins and low voltage on ECG. The presence of a positive Kussmaul's sign helps differentiate the syndrome from cor pulmonale and restrictive cardiomyopathies. *(Fuster, p. 1990)*

101. (A) Cardiac tamponade can occur with as little as 200 mL of fluid if the accumulation is rapid. Physical examination reveals a pulsus paradoxus (>10 mm Hg inspiratory decline in systolic arterial pressure), a prominent x descent of the jugular veins, but no Kussmaul's sign. The ECG may show low voltage. *(Fuster, p. 1985)*

102. **(D)** RVMI is characterized by high neck veins, ECG abnormalities, and often a right-sided S3. The low cardiac output associated with RVMI can often be treated by volume expansion. Although a third of patients with inferoposterior infarctions have some degree of right ventricular necrosis, extensive RVMI is uncommon. *(Fuster, p. 1281)*

103. **(A)** Electrical alternans (a beat-to-beat alternation in one or more component of the ECG signal) can occur in pericardial effusion and numerous other conditions. Total electrical alternans (P-QRS-T) and sinus tachycardia is relatively specific for pericardial effusion (often with tamponade). *(Fuster, p. 1985)*

104. **(B)** A pericardial knock is characteristic of constrictive pericarditis. It is in fact an early S3, occurring 0.06–0.12 seconds after aortic closure. S1 and S2 are frequently distant. *(Fuster, p. 1990)*

105. **(C)** The combination of absent pulsus and absent Kussmaul's sign with prominent x descent favors a restrictive cardiomyopathy.

    Unlike constrictive pericarditis, restrictive cardiomyopathies frequently present with an enlarged heart, orthopnea, LVH, and bundle branch blocks. *(Fuster, pp. 1937–1938)*

106. **(C)** The cardiac lesions of gastrointestinal carcinoids are almost exclusively in the right side of the heart and occur only when there are hepatic metastases. Fibrous plaques are found on the endothelium of the cardiac chambers, valves, and great vessels. These plaques can distort cardiac valves; tricuspid regurgitation and pulmonic stenosis are the most common valvular problems. *(Kasper, pp. 1423–1424)*

107. **(B)** The proximal aortitis of seronegative arthritis (ankylosing spondylitis, Reiter syndrome, psoriatic arthritis, or associated with inflammatory bowel disease) can result in aortic regurgitation and AV block. *(Kasper, p. 1424)*

108. **(A)** Focal myocardial necrosis and inflammatory cell infiltration caused by high circulating levels of catecholamines are seen in about 50% of patients who die with pheochromocytoma.

Hypertension can further impair left ventricular function. *(Kasper, p. 1424)*

109. **(D)** The Means-Lerman scratch, a systolic scratchy sound heard at the left second intercostal space during expiration, is thought to result from the rubbing of the hyperdynamic pericardium against the pleura. Palpitations, atrial fibrillation, hypertension, angina, and heart failure are more common cardiac manifestations of hyperthyroidism. *(Kasper, p. 1423)*

110. **(E)** DM can result in a restrictive cardiomyopathy in the absence of large-vessel CAD. Histology reveals increased collagen, glycoprotein, triglycerides, and cholesterol in the myocardial interstitium. Abnormalities may be present in small intramural arteries. *(Kasper, p. 1422)*

111. **(D, E)** Patients with diabetes have the same rates of coronary heart disease events as patients with established CAD. Therefore diabetes is now considered a coronary heart disease, equivalent when assessing risk even if the patient has not had any previous cardiac symptoms. The current guidelines support risk reduction efforts (both lifestyle and drug therapy) in patients with diabetes similar to those recommended for patients with CAD (secondary prevention). The goal for LDL is <100 mg/dL in patients with diabetes and secondary goals include considering fibrates for those with high triglycerides and nicotinic acid for low HDL cholesterol. Lifestyle modification is recommended for everyone irrespective of risk. *(Kasper, pp. 1430–1433)*

112. **(E)** When assessing patients for cardiovascular risk, it is always important to consider recommendations in light of their risk level. For primary prevention (no known symptomatic CAD), there are risk calculators available to estimate an individual's future risk (see *http://www.nhlbi.nih.gov/guidelines/cholesterol/* for a risk calculator based on the Framingham database). The treatment recommendations and goals should match the patient's risk level. In this individual, she has no risk factors for CAD and her 10-year risk for cardiovascular events is low. The goals for LDL in her are

<160 mg/dL, and drug therapy should be only considered if her LDL >190 mg/dL. For her, the best advice is lifestyle modification such as dietary modification, exercise, and weight loss if indicated since these changes will lower triglycerides, raise HDL, and lower LDL. Repeat screening is recommended every 5 years. *(Kasper, pp. 1430–1433)*

113. **(D, E)** For patients with established CAD, their future risk for further cardiovascular events is high (10-year risk >20%). In such individuals, the goals of LDL level are adjusted lower to match the increased risk. For secondary prevention, the LDL level target is <100 mg/dL. For all individuals at increased risk-lifestyle modification is stressed as a key component therapy. In this patient given, the recent diagnosis of CAD and the elevated LDL level treatment with a "statin" is also indicated. *(Kasper, pp. 1430–1433)*

114. **(D, E)** Recent evidence has suggested that lipid modification for patients with ischemic stroke (that is not cardioembolic in origin) by lowering LDL level with statins is beneficial in reducing future stroke risk. This evidence comes from the analysis of cardiovascular statin trials that have a lower rate of ischemic strokes in patients taking the medication as compared to the placebo group. In addition, lifestyle modification is important for this individual especially smoking cessation. *(Kasper, pp. 1430–1433)*

115. **(D, E)** The metabolic syndrome is frequently identified among individuals given the increasing rates of obesity and diabetes in Western society. This individual has multiple atherogenic risk factors (obesity, hypertension, increased LDL) and his 10-year risk for cardiac events is approximated at 10–20% by the risk calculator. At this risk level, the LDL goal is <130 mg/dL and treatment threshold for starting drug therapy is >130 mg/dL. As well lifestyle modification is an important component of the overall treatment. *(Kasper, pp. 1430–1433)*

116. **(E)** Many observational studies have verified the increased risk of CAD in women after menopause, and this formed the basis for recommending estrogen therapy to lower cardiovascular risk in postmenopausal women. Recently two large randomized clinical trials have shown no benefit with estrogen replacement in postmenopausal women as a means of reducing cardiovascular risk. With this evidence, estrogen replacement is not recommended for cardiac risk modification, and is only indicated to treat the symptoms of menopause. For postmenopausal women at increased risk of cardiac disease, statins are considered first-line therapy in modifying risk since there are randomized trial data from multiple trials supporting their effectiveness in women. Since this patient has only one risk factor her future 10-year risk is low (<10%) and lifestyle modification is the best advice. She will require follow-up lipid risk assessment in 5 years. *(Kasper, pp. 1430–1433)*

117. **(G)** ACE inhibitors have no adverse effects on glucose or lipid metabolism and minimize the development of diabetic nephropathy by reducing renal vascular resistance and renal perfusion pressure. The goal for blood pressure control in diabetics is set at 130/80 mm Hg which is lower than in nondiabetics. This lower pressure is important in preventing progression of renal disease and other end-organ damage. *(Kasper, p. 1479)*

118. **(A)** Thiazides have been a cornerstone in most trials of antihypertensive therapy. Their adverse metabolic consequences include renal potassium loss leading to hypokalemia, hyperuricemia from uric acid retention, carbohydrate intolerance, and hyperlipidemia. The current U.S. Joint National Committee (JNC-7) guidelines suggest starting with thiazide diuretics because of their proven efficacy in lowering mortality and morbidity in large clinical trials. Other agents are considered if there are comorbidities such as diabetes or CAD. *(Kasper, pp. 1472, 1478)*

119. **(G)** Although contraindicated in bilateral stenosis, ACE inhibitors are the drug of choice in unilateral renal artery stenosis.

When ACE inhibitors are used in patients with impaired renal function, renal function should be monitored twice a week for the first 3 weeks. *(Kasper, p. 1479)*

120. **(A)** Thiazides seem to work particularly well in Blacks and the elderly. Younger individuals and Whites respond well to beta-blockers, ACE inhibitors, and calcium channel antagonists. Isolated systolic hypertension is a common occurance in the elderly. It is due to arteriosclerosis of the large arteries. Treatment of isolated systolic hypertension with low-dose thiazides results in lower stroke rates and death. The goal for treatment is a blood pressure of 140/90 mm Hg. *(Kasper, pp. 1471, 1480)*

121. **(E)** Beta-blockers are the most appropriate choice for the treatment of hypertension in patients with CAD. They lower mortality in patients with CAD as well as hypertension. ACE inhibitors can also be used, especially if there is left ventricular dysfunction, or the patient has multiple cardiovascular risk factors such as diabetes or dyslipidemia. *(Kasper, p. 1479)*

CHAPTER 2

Skin
Questions

DIRECTIONS (Questions 1 through 5): Each set of matching questions in this section consists of a list of lettered options followed by several numbered items. For each numbered item, select the appropriate lettered option(s). Each lettered option may be selected once, more than once, or not at all. **EACH ITEM WILL STATE THE NUMBER OF OPTIONS TO SELECT. CHOOSE EXACTLY THIS NUMBER.**

Questions 1 and 2

    (A) psoriasis
    (B) eczema
    (C) hypersensitivity reactions
    (D) lichen planus
    (E) toxic erythemas
    (F) lichen planus
    (G) Kaposi sarcoma
    (H) melanotic nodules
    (I) maculopapular rash
    (J) serum-filled bullae

For each patient with a skin lesion, select the most likely diagnosis.

1. A 19-year-old man develops new lesions at the sites of skin trauma. The lesions appear as sharply marginated erythematous papules with silvery-white scales. (SELECT ONE)

2. A 32-year-old man with human immunodeficiency virus (HIV) infection develops skin tumors and patches on the legs with some on the face. They are palpable, firm, and appear violaceous with some nodules appearing purple brownish. (SELECT ONE)

Questions 3 through 5

    (A) rarely involves border of scalp
    (B) discoloration of upper eyelids
    (C) skin atrophy
    (D) never a permanent effect on skin
    (E) potentially aggravated by contact with the skin
    (F) drop-shaped lesions
    (G) exacerbated by exposure to light
    (H) worse on weekends
    (I) high likelihood of malingering
    (J) associated with squamous cell cancer
    (K) extensive large plaques
    (L) pitting of the nails
    (M) lesions at various stages (progression of lesions)

For each patient, select the associated skin and clinical findings.

3. A diagnosis of psoriasis, never previously treated, is made on a 22-year-old man. Findings may include (SELECT THREE)

4. A 63-year-old woman develops skin lesions, and difficulty getting out of a chair. A clinical diagnosis of dermatomyositis is made. Finding may include (SELECT THREE)

5. A 43-year-old woman develops a rash on her arms and hands after starting a new job in a factory. The lesions have well-demarcated erythema and edema with superimposed closely spaced vesicles and papules. Findings might include (SELECT ONE)

DIRECTIONS (Questions 6 through 21): Each of the numbered items in this section is followed by answers. Select the ONE lettered answer that is BEST in each case.

6. A 19-year-old woman with asthma has a chronic rash with distribution on her hands, neck, and elbow creases. It is very itchy, and the skin appears thickened with increased skin markings. There are some areas of fissures in the skin at the elbow creases and hands. Which of the following is the most appropriate advice? (See Fig. 2–1.)

    (A) psychoanalysis
    (B) warm clothing
    (C) dry environment
    (D) environmental manipulation
    (E) vigorous exercise

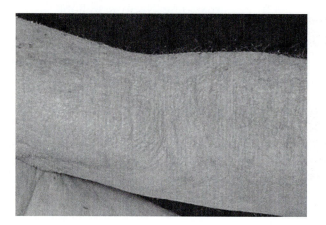

Figure 2–1.

7. A 74-year-old man develops a new single 1.5 cm lesion on his face. It is firm and nodular with a dome shape and central keratotic plug. Excisional biopsy confirms keratoacanthoma. Which of the following best characterizes this lesion?

    (A) rapid growth
    (B) distinct pathology
    (C) usual occurrence on the trunk
    (D) a malignant potential
    (E) a dark brown color

8. A 85-year-old woman has large blistering lesions on the abdomen and thighs that come and go without therapy. Nikolsky's sign is negative. Which of the following is the most likely diagnosis? (See Fig. 2–2.)

    (A) pemphigus vulgaris (PV)
    (B) dermatitis herpetiformis (DH)
    (C) bullous pemphigoid
    (D) herpes gestationis
    (E) erythema multiforme

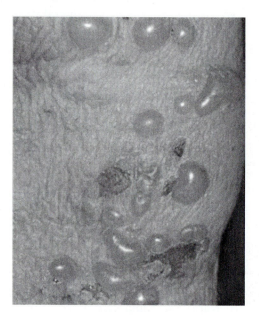

Figure 2–2.

9. A 69-year-old woman develops dark, velvety pigmentation in her axillae. She has noticed 10 lb weight loss over the past 3 months with heartburn and early satiety. She notices no other symptoms. Which of the following conditions should she be studied for? (See Fig. 2–3.)

    (A) a visceral carcinoma
    (B) lymphoma
    (C) diabetes mellitus
    (D) sarcoidosis
    (E) an allergy

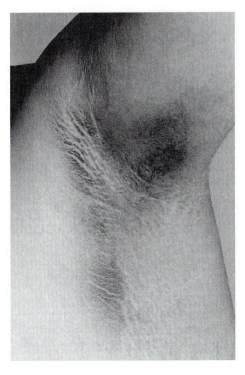

Figure 2–3.
(Reproduced, with permission, from Wolff K and Johnson RA, *Fitzpatrick's Color Atlas & Synopsis of Clinical Dermatology*, 5th ed. New York: McGraw-Hill, 2005:87.)

10. A 22-year-old woman develops an acute contact dermatitis to a household-cleaning agent. Which of the following treatments is most appropriate during the bullous, oozing stage?

   (A) wet dressings
   (B) systemic corticosteroids
   (C) topical anesthetics
   (D) systemic antibiotics
   (E) antihistamines

11. Which of the following is a characteristic of ringworm of the scalp as compared with other dermatophytoses?

   (A) more frequent occurrence in childhood
   (B) high degree of contagiousness
   (C) ability to invade the dermis
   (D) sensitivity to penicillin
   (E) ability to spread to other organs

12. A 27-year-old man develops warts on his hand. Which of the following is a correct statement concerning these skin lesions?

   (A) are viral in etiology
   (B) may be premalignant lesions
   (C) are found mainly in patients with lymphoma
   (D) are contagious in children only
   (E) may be treated with griseofulvin

13. A 27-year-old man develops a painless 1 cm sore on his penis. It appears ulcerated with a raised margin and minimal serous exudates. Which of the following is the most appropriate next step in the diagnosis? (See Fig. 2–4.)

   (A) biopsy
   (B) Gram stain
   (C) serology
   (D) ultrasound
   (E) skin test

14. A 64-year-old woman notices bullous-type lesions over her thighs and axilla. They are itchy, but not painful, and she has no other symptoms. On examination, there are large tense, serous-filled bullae on the affected areas. A biopsy confirms the diagnosis of bullous pemphigoid. Which of the following histologic features is typical of this condition?

   (A) nonspecific changes
   (B) immunoglobulin A (IgA) deposits
   (C) lesions within the epidermis (acantholysis)
   (D) basement membrane lesions
   (E) immunoglobulin M (IgM) deposits.

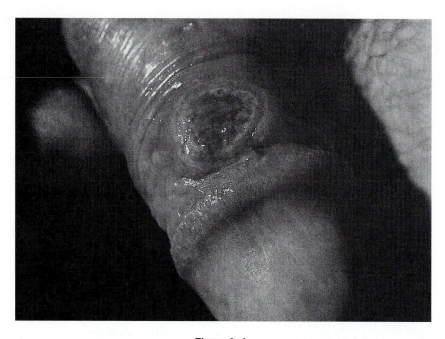

Figure 2–4.
(Reproduced, with permission, from Wolff K and Johnson RA, *Fitzpatrick's Color Atlas & Synopsis of Clinical Dermatology*, 5th ed. New York: McGraw-Hill, 2005:915.)

15. A 27-year-old woman has a 1-year history of loosely formed bowel movements associated with some blood and abdominal pain. She develops multiple painful erythematous nodules on her lower legs. Which of the following is the most likely diagnosis? (See Fig. 2–5.)

(A) erythema multiforme
(B) erythema migrans
(C) erythema nodosum
(D) cutaneous lymphoma
(E) necrobiosis lipoidica

16. Which of the following best describes mycosis fungoides?

(A) fungal infection of the epidermis
(B) benign skin lesion
(C) cutaneous lymphoma
(D) dermatitis
(E) form of eczema

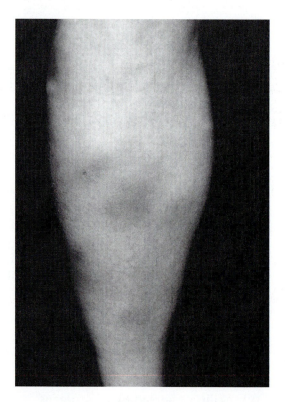

Figure 2–5.
(Reproduced, with permission, from Wolff K and Johnson RA, *Fitzpatrick's Color Atlas & Synopsis of Clinical Dermatology*, 5th ed. New York: McGraw-Hill, 2005:149.)

17. A 58-year-old man complains of an enlarged, pitted nose, and a facial rash that "flushes" in response to drinking hot liquids or alcohol. The rash is on both cheeks, and it is red and flushed in appearance, with some telangiectatica and small papules. Which of the following is the most likely diagnosis? (See Fig. 2–6.)

(A) acne vulgaris
(B) pemphigus
(C) rosacea
(D) psoriasis
(E) seborrheic dermatitis

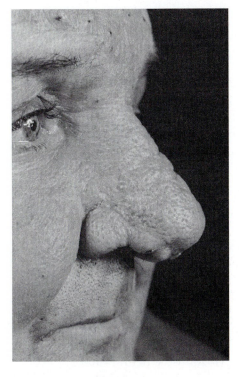

Figure 2–6.
(Reproduced, with permission, from Wolff K and Johnson RA, *Fitzpatrick's Color Atlas & Synopsis of Clinical Dermatology*, 5th ed. New York: McGraw-Hill, 2005:11.)

18. A 81-year-old man presents with pallor, glossitis, cheilitis, and vitiligo. Which of the following is the most likely diagnosis?

(A) sickle cell anemia
(B) cold agglutinin syndrome
(C) methemoglobinemia
(D) pernicious anemia
(E) polycythemia

19. A 70-year-old man develops multiple pruritic skin lesions and bullae mostly in the axillae and around the medial aspects of his groin and thighs. There are some lesions on his forearms and on his lower legs (first appeared in this location), and moderately painful oral lesions. Nikolsky's sign is negative. There is no eye involvement. Which of the following is the most likely diagnosis?

(A) dermatitis herpetiformis (DH)
(B) pemphigus vulgaris (PV)
(C) bullous pemphigoid
(D) cicatricial pemphigoid
(E) epidermolysis bullosa (EB)

20. A man presents with bullous lesions on his face, armpit, and chest. He initially had them only in his mouth. They appear round and oval with serous fluid and some are "flabby." When pressure is applied to the lesion the fluid spreads laterally. A clinical diagnosis of pemphigus vulgaris (PV) is made. Which of the following is the usual age of onset for this condition? (See Fig. 2–7.)

(A) under 10 years of age
(B) 10–20 years of age
(C) 20–40 years of age
(D) 40–60 years of age
(E) 60–80 years of age

21. Which of the following is the most likely drug to cause pemphigus vulgaris (PV)?

(A) captopril
(B) D-penicillamine
(C) sulfonamides
(D) hydralazine
(E) quinidine

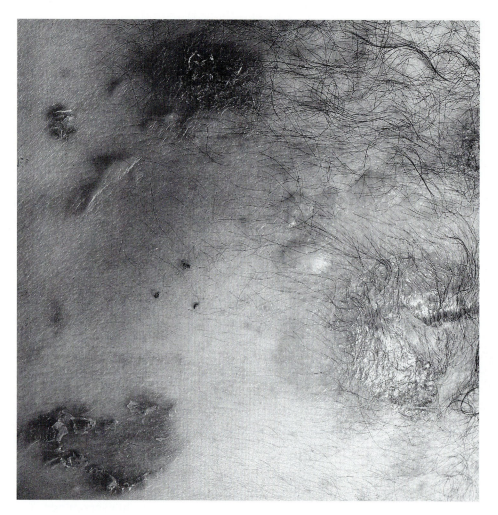

Figure 2–7.
(Reproduced, with permission, from Wolff K and Johnson RA, *Fitzpatrick's Color Atlas & Synopsis of Clinical Dermatology*, 5th ed. New York: McGraw-Hill, 2005:104.)

DIRECTIONS (Questions 22 through 28): Each set of matching questions in this section consists of a list of lettered options followed by several numbered items. For each numbered item, select the appropriate lettered option(s). Each lettered option may be selected once, more than once, or not at all. **EACH ITEM WILL STATE THE NUMBER OF OPTIONS TO SELECT. CHOOSE EXACTLY THIS NUMBER.**

Questions 22 and 23

    (A) other areas of skin pigmentation

    (B) associated with adenocarcinoma

    (C) autosomal dominant inheritance

    (D) insulin resistance

    (E) viral etiology

    (F) adenocarcinoma

    (G) neural tumors most frequently appear during old age

    (H) multiple neural tumors

For each patient with a skin lesion, select the most common associated features.

22. A young child is found to have axillary freckling. The lesions appear light brown with sharp margination and are of variable size from small tiny "freckle"-like macules to larger patches. Other characteristics of this disorder include (SELECT THREE)

23. A 68-year-old woman develops grayish-brown, thickened skin in the axillae. Examination shows increased pigmentation, with accentuated skin lines and the skin appears "dirty."

This skin is thickened and has a velvety texture on palpation. Other findings associated with this disorder may include (SELECT THREE)

Questions 24 through 28

(A) basal cell cancer

(B) basal cell nevus syndrome (BCNS)

(C) melanoma

(D) actinic keratosis

(E) keratoacanthoma

(F) seborrheic keratosis

(G) lipoma

(H) mongolian spot

(I) spider angioma

(J) glomus tumor

(K) squamous cell cancer

Match the following descriptions with the correct diagnosis above.

24. Malignant, but does not metastasize beyond the skin (SELECT ONE)

25. Malignant, and may metastasize beyond the skin (SELECT TWO)

26. May be cured with x-ray therapy (SELECT TWO)

27. More common in Asian children than Caucasian children (SELECT ONE)

28. May develop in long-standing scars (SELECT ONE)

DIRECTIONS (Questions 29 through 42): Each of the numbered items in this section is followed by answers. Select the ONE lettered answer that is BEST in each case.

29. A 60-year-old man presents with the skin lesion pictured in Fig. 2–8. Which of the following is the most likely diagnosis?

(A) erythema nodosum

(B) acanthosis nigricans

(C) herpes zoster

(D) alopecia variegata

(E) bullous pemphigoid

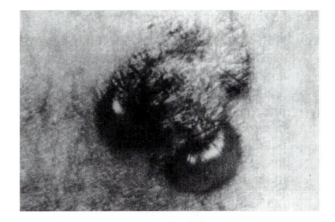

Figure 2–8.

30. An 18-year-old woman has severe acne for many years. She has tried many topical therapies with no lasting benefit. On examination, she has multiple inflammatory papules on her face, with some even larger nodules and cysts. Which of the following is the most appropriate next step in management?

(A) dietary controls

(B) radiotherapy

(C) ultraviolet light

(D) tetracycline

(E) isotretinoin

31. A 70-year-old man comes to the emergency department because of a skin rash and severe itching. He appears ill; there is a generalized skin rash that is scaly, erythematous, and thickened. His palms, soles, and scalp are also involved. Which of the following is the most likely diagnosis?

(A) pemphigus vulgaris

(B) rosacea

(C) erythroderma (exfoliative dermatitis)

(D) dermatitis herpetiformis

(E) disseminated varicella

32. A 32-year-old woman comes to the emergency department because of a generalized erythematous skin rash. She was recently started on trimethoprim-sulfamethoxazole (Septra) for a urinary tract infection. Examination shows the diffuse rash involving her whole body including the palms and soles. Except for generalized lymphadenopathy, the rest of the examination is normal. Which of the following is the most appropriate interpretation of the generalized lymphadenopathy finding?

(A) a viral infection
(B) pyoderma
(C) lymphoma
(D) leukemia
(E) nothing specific

33. A 62-year-old man develops scaling and non-scaling patches, and plaques over his chest and back. They are itchy, but not painful. The rest of the examination is normal, except for lymphadenopathy. Examinations of the blood film and skin biopsy histology, both, reveal unusually large monocytoid cells. Which of the following is the most likely diagnosis? (See Fig. 2–9.)

(A) leukemia
(B) visceral B-cell lymphoma
(C) primary cutaneous T-cell lymphoma
(D) viral infection (usually Epstein-Barr)
(E) paraneoplastic syndrome secondary to lung cancer

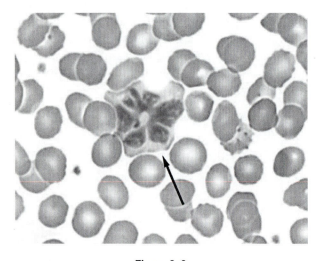

Figure 2–9.

34. Which of the following statements about the prognosis of cutaneous T-cell lymphoma is true?

(A) rapidly downhill
(B) determined by the type of medical care
(C) rarely fatal
(D) remissions and exacerbations, but with eventual progression to a fatal outcome
(E) eventual complete recovery, regardless of treatment

35. Which of the following treatments is used for most patients with cutaneous T-cell lymphoma?

(A) antibiotics
(B) antiviral medication
(C) aggressive systemic chemotherapy to ensure cure
(D) symptomatic treatment
(E) early use of high-dose systemic steroids

36. A 72-year-old man is newly diagnosed with bullous pemphigoid. Which of the following is the most appropriate next step in the management?

(A) plasmapheresis
(B) low-dose prednisone (10–20 mg/day)
(C) high-dose prednisone (50–100 mg/day)
(D) azathioprine 150 mg/day
(E) dapsone (100–150 mg/day)

37. Which of the following features indicates a more negative prognosis for patients with malignant melanoma?

(A) female sex
(B) location on the leg
(C) dark pigmentation of the lesion
(D) nodularity of the lesion
(E) level A invasion

38. A 34-year-old man presents with a chronic and progressive skin rash. He has a history of poorly controlled Crohn's disease and has lost 20 lb in the past 6 months. On examination, there are dry, scaly patches and plaques, which are sharply marginated and bright red around his mouth, and anogenital regions. There is also involvement of the flexural regions of the arms. Which of the following is the most likely diagnosis?

(A) ichthyosis
(B) acquired zinc deficiency
(C) Paget's disease
(D) candidiasis
(E) herpes simplex

39. A 26-year-old woman develops discomfort on her lower legs and notices a skin rash. On examination, there are tender nodules on her shins with an erythematous base. Which of the following conditions is this rash associated with?

(A) caused by aspergillosis
(B) usually occurs in children
(C) more common in males than females
(D) only caused by malignant disease
(E) can occur with streptococcal infection

40. Which of the following differentiates a patch from a macule?

(A) it is more easily palpable
(B) a patch is erythematous
(C) a patch can contain fluid
(D) the etiology is very different
(E) it is larger

41. A 19-year-old man develops a rash in the groin area. On examination, it is a large well-demarcated area of tan-brown discoloration around his left inguinal area. There is some scaling of the lesion when brushed with a tongue depressor. Which of the following is the most appropriate initial diagnostic test? (See Fig. 2–10.)

(A) punch biopsy of skin
(B) Tzanck smear
(C) potassium hydroxide (KOH) preparation of scrapings
(D) blood culture for fungi
(E) diascopy

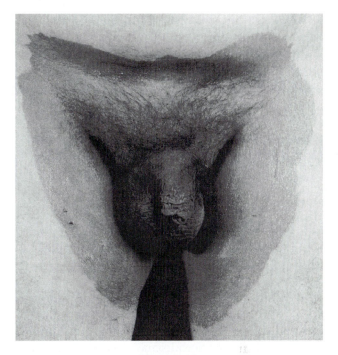

Figure 2–10.
(Reproduced, with permission, from Wolff K and Johnson RA, *Fitzpatrick's Color Atlas & Synopsis of Clinical Dermatology*, 5th ed. New York: McGraw-Hill, 2005:699.)

42. A 7-year-old boy develops a skin rash in the right axillary area. On examination, there are superficial small pustules, with some that have ruptured and formed golden-yellow crusts. The area is itchy, but not painful, and he has no systemic symptoms. Treatment with oral antibiotics is started. Which of the following statements about this condition is most likely correct?

(A) caused by fungi of the *Microsporum* species
(B) caused exclusively by staphylococcal infections
(C) characterized by premalignant changes
(D) treated by improved hygiene
(E) characterized by papulosquamous lesions

DIRECTIONS (Questions 43 through 53): Each set of matching questions in this section consists of a list of lettered options followed by several numbered items. For each numbered item, select the appropriate lettered option(s). Each lettered option may be selected once, more than once, or not at all. EACH ITEM WILL STATE THE NUMBER OF OPTIONS TO SELECT. CHOOSE EXACTLY THIS NUMBER.

Questions 43 through 48

    (A) generalized vitiligo
    (B) localized vitiligo
    (C) telangiectasia
    (D) erythroderma
    (E) tuberculoid leprosy
    (F) sarcoid
    (G) limited scleroderma
    (H) dermatomyositis
    (I) secondary syphilis
    (J) diabetes
    (K) eruptive xanthoma

For each patient with the skin lesion, select the most likely diagnosis or associated condition.

43. A 20-year-old man who recently emigrated from Southeast Asia has chronic skin lesions on his back and chest. On examination, there are multiple well-defined hypopigmented macules with raised edges. They vary in size from 1.0 to 5.0 cm, and some have lost sensation to touch and pinprick. (SELECT ONE)

44. A 47-year-old woman has symptoms of heartburn and skin changes in her hands. She notices pain and discomfort in her hands while washing dishes with cold water, and that the fingers sometimes become pale and colorless when they are painful. The fingers then change color to blue, and red after warming. On examination, there are areas of telangiectasias on her face. (SELECT ONE)

45. A 25-year-old woman presents with a diffuse skin rash, starting a few days after starting antibiotics for a urinary tract infection. On examination, her skin was warm to touch, and red in color. (SELECT ONE)

46. A 32-year-old man notices the sudden eruption of tiny nodules on his lower arms and knees. On examination, he has multiple crops of papules on his lower arms and knees. They are dome shaped, discrete, and have a yellow center with surrounding areas of redness. (SELECT ONE)

47. A 24-year-old man presents with malaise, fever, and a new rash on his abdomen. Eight weeks ago he had a painless 1-cm ulcer on his penis that resolved spontaneously. On examination, there are faint pink brownish-red macules on his abdomen ranging in size from 0.5 to 1.0 cm. (SELECT ONE)

48. A 51-year-old man with obesity (body mass index [BMI] >30) presents with skin changes in his right axilla. On examination, there is increased pigmentation and the skin appears dirty. The area feels velvety and the skin folds are accentuated. (SELECT ONE)

Questions 49 through 53

    (A) dystrophic nail changes
    (B) may mottle teeth
    (C) black pigmentation of face
    (D) erythema nodosum
    (E) morbilliform eruption in patients with acquired immune deficiency syndrome (AIDS)
    (F) gingival hyperplasia
    (G) reactions in patients with nasal polyps

For the following medications, select the most appropriate skin manifestations.

49. Bleomycin (SELECT ONE)

50. Chloroquine (SELECT ONE)

51. Birth control pills (SELECT ONE)

52. Tetracycline (SELECT ONE)

53. Sulfamethoxazole and trimethoprim (SELECT TWO)

Answers and Explanations

1. **(A)** Koebner phenomenon is typically seen in psoriasis. The kind of injury eliciting the phenomenon is usually mechanical, but ultraviolet light or allergic damage to the skin may be provocative. Koebner phenomenon can also occur in lichen planus, lichen nitidus, keratosis follicularis, and pemphigoid. The Koebner phenomenon has been used to study early skin changes in these diseases. *(Wolff, p. 54)*

2. **(G)** Kaposi sarcoma often manifests as multiple blue dermal plaques. Lesions have two prominent features: accumulation of spindle cells and presence of vascular elements. Classical Kaposi sarcoma is an indolent disease of later life and is much more common in men than women. Kaposi sarcoma in association with HIV infection is a much more aggressive disorder. In all types of Kaposi the deoxyribonucleic acid (DNA) of human herpes virus 8 has been identified. *(Wolff, p. 536)*

3. **(F, K, L)** Psoriasis does not present a progression of lesions unless therapy is applied. Lesions vary in size and configuration from patient to patient and in the same patient from time to time and vary from drop-shaped lesions to large plaques. Nail changes are characteristic. *(Wolff, p. 54)*

4. **(B, C, G)** In dermatomyositis, the dermatitis may be the most striking feature of the illness or so minor as to be easily overlooked. The classic manifestation is a purplish-red heliotrope erythema of the eyelids, upper cheeks, forehead, and temples, often with edema of the eyelids and of the periorbital tissue. Telangiectasia and skin atrophy can also occur. The typical hand changes involve scaly, bluish-red plaques around the base of the nails and backs of the joints of the fingers. These are most frequently found in elderly patients and are called Gottron's papules. There is an association with malignancy in those over 55 years of age. *(Wolff, p. 372)*

5. **(E)** The history should not reveal worsening eruption during the weekend. Allergy, acne, diabetes, psoriasis, xeroderma, or seborrheic dermatitis may all be mistaken for occupational disorders. The list of possible occupational skin hazards is long. At times, a site visit to the workplace is required to confirm the diagnosis. First aid in the workplace often involves sensitizing agents that worsen the situation. Skin problems can be severe and permanent. Relatively few patients are malingerers. *(Wolff, p. 24)*

6. **(D)** A change of environment is among the best treatments for atopic dermatitis. The patient should be kept in as dust-free an environment as possible and should not wear rough garments. Maintenance of adequate humidity is also important. *(Wolff, p. 33)*

7. **(A)** This tumor as a rule occurs on exposed, hairy skin. It grows rapidly but involutes slowly, occasionally up to 1 year. It is more common in white-skinned males. The lesion starts as a small, rounded, flesh-colored or reddish papule. It grows rapidly and may reach 10–20 mm in a few weeks. There are telangiectasias just below the surface and the center contains a horny plug or is covered by a crust concealing a keratin-filled crater. Histology can

be difficult to differentiate from squamous cell cancer. *(Wolff, p. 208)*

8. **(C)** There are antibodies to skin basement membrane, but unlike pemphigus, antibody levels do not correlate with disease activity. Bullous pemphigoid is most common in the elderly, and the disease often starts with urticaria-like and pruritic erythematous lesions, before classic blisters occur. The blisters arise from inflamed and normal skin, unlike in pemphigus where they arise from normal skin. As well, unlike pemphigus, mucosal lesions are minimal or absent. *(Wolff, p. 106)*

9. **(A)** Patients with acanthosis nigricans should be studied for a visceral carcinoma. There are hereditary, drug-induced, and benign forms of acanthosis nigricans as well. Given this patient's symptoms a gastric malignancy should be ruled out. Diabetics get a benign form of the disorder. Other dermatoses associated with malignancy include dermatomyositis, flushing, acquired ichthyosis, and thrombophlebitis migrans. *(Wolff, p. 86)*

10. **(A)** Ointments are not used, but wet dressings are applied several times a day, using Burow's solution or boric acid, and baths are also included in the treatment. The key aspect of care is prevention. When contamination does occur, washing the affected area is the first mode of treatment. Oral corticosteroids are only used in severe cases. In less severe cases, topical class I glucocorticoid preparations can be helpful. *(Wolff, p. 23)*

11. **(A)** Ringworm of the skin is most common in children because of their intimacy with animals and other children. The lesions are round or oval scaly patches. Secondary bacterial infection is common with certain fungi. *(Wolff, p. 707)*

12. **(A)** Verrucae are viral in etiology. The human papillomavirus is a DNA-containing virus of the papovavirus group that includes animal tumor viruses. Although most warts are not felt to be premalignant; there is evidence to show that genital warts are correlated with malignancy. *(Wolff, p. 776)*

13. **(C)** This is likely a case of primary syphilis. Serology is the most appropriate test; it can remain negative for a period up to 1 month after the infection is contracted. The serologic test for syphilis usually is positive within 1 week after the chancre appears. With therapy the chancre heals rapidly, but will heal in 4–6 weeks even without treatment. Genital chancres are usually painless, unless superinfected, but extragenital chancres (e.g., fingers) can be quite painful. Biopsy is usually not necessary for diagnosis, and the spirochetes are seen with dark-field examination, not with Gram stain. *(Wolff, p. 915)*

14. **(D)** In bullous pemphigoid, biopsy reveals immunoglobulin G (IgG) deposits in the basement membrane area. In pemphigus vulgaris, the immune deposition and damage is within the lower zone of the epidermis. IgA deposits are seen in dermatitis herpetiformis. *(Wolff, p. 106)*

15. **(C)** About 15% of patients with ulcerative colitis will develop skin manifestations. Typical lesions include erythema nodosum, pyoderma gangrenosum (painless, but can heal with scarring), aphthous ulcers, and ocular inflammation (episcleritis, iritis, uveitis). The activity of the skin manifestations typically parallels the severity of the colonic disease. *(Wolff, p. 148)*

16. **(C)** Mycosis fungoides is best described as a cutaneous T-cell lymphoma. Lesions may remain confined to the skin for years, and internal organ involvement occurs when the disease advances into late stages. It is a disorder involving T lymphocytes. Treatment is usually palliative rather than curative. *(Wolff, p. 528)*

17. **(C)** Rhinophyma is a complication of rosacea. It can be treated surgically by shaving off the excessive tissue with a scalpel, but regrowth occurs in time. There is very little evidence to support the association between alcoholism and rhinophyma. The other conditions do not cause flushing or blushing-type appearance. Psoriasis and seborrheic dermatitis have lesions that have white dry scales. *(Wolff, pp. 8–10)*

18. **(D)** Glossitis and cheilitis result from the vitamin deficiency affecting rapidly turning over tissues. Patients may complain of a "burning" tongue, and examination reveals atrophy of papillae, a deep red mucosa, and a "cobblestone" appearance. Vitamin B_{12} administration rapidly relieves these symptoms. The vitiligo is caused by an associated autoimmune disorder. *(Kasper, pp. 603–604)*

19. **(C)** The description and age range (60–80) is typical of bullous pemphigoid. PV is usually associated with a positive Nikolsky's sign (pressure on blister leads to lateral extension), and very severe oral lesions. Cicatricial pemphigoid is also a disease of the elderly, but is rare and usually involves the eyes as well. EB is an inherited disorder that usually presents in earlier life. DH does not usually affect mucous membranes, and the lesions are grouped in clusters. However, it can mimic early bullous pemphigoid, and biopsy is needed for confirmation. Permanent remission is frequent, and continued therapy would not be required. *(Wolff, pp. 106–108)*

20. **(D)** PV is most common from 40 to 60 years of age, whereas bullous pemphigoid is seen most frequently after the age of 80. Dermatitis herpetiformis is most common in the age group from 30 to 40, but has a wide age range. *(Wolff, p. 100).*

21. **(B)** Captopril and other drugs can cause PV, but D-penicillamine is the most likely to cause the disease. Drug-induced PV usually, but not invariably, remits when the offending agent is withdrawn. *(Wolff, p. 103)*

22. **(A, C, H)** Neurofibromatosis is inherited in an autosomal manner. Incomplete forms are frequent. The skin manifestations include café au lait spots (more than six required for diagnosis), axillary freckles, cutaneous neurofibromas, and pigmented iris hamartomas (Lisch nodules). There are numerous other manifestations as well including neural tumors. *(Wolff, p. 464)*

23. **(A, B, D)** Early recognition of acanthosis nigricans warrants a thorough search for underlying pathology such as malignancy or insulin resistance. The earliest changes are usually pigmentation, dryness, and roughness of the skin. The skin is gray brown or black, palpably thickened, and covered by small papillomatous elevations, which give it a velvety texture. The most common sites are axillae, back, neck, anogenital region, and the groin. *(Wolff, p. 86)*

24. **(A)** Basal cell tumors have a substantial capacity for local destruction but metastasize very rarely. *(Wolff, p. 282)*

25. **(C, K)** Both squamous cell cancer and melanoma can spread beyond the skin. Only about 3–4% of squamous cell cancers metastasize, but metastasis is quite common in melanoma. Melanoma is the most dangerous primary skin cancer. *(Wolff, pp. 278, 303)*

26. **(A, K)** In both squamous and basal cell carcinomas, early detection may lead to cure by surgical removal. Radiotherapy may be curative, but is usually reserved for cases where surgery is not feasible, or likely to be disfiguring.*(Wolff, pp. 278, 282)*

27. **(H)** Mongolian spots are congenital gray blue macular lesions, characteristically located on the lumbosacral area, although they can occur anywhere on the skin. They are almost always (99–100%) in infants of Asiatic or Amerindian origin, although reports in Black, and rarely, White infants have occurred. They usually disappear in early childhood, and generally the lesions are solitary. *(Wolff, p. 176)*

28. **(K)** Squamous cell carcinoma of the skin can arise in areas of inflammation such as burn scars, chronic ulcers, radiation dermatitis, and chronic cutaneous lupus erythematosis. Other early lesions include solar keratoses, cutaneous horns, arsenical keratoses, and Bowen's disease. *(Wolff, p. 276)*

29. **(E)** Bullous pemphigoid is most common in older adults. It is not as severe as pemphigus vulgaris, and histology reveals an absence of acantholysis, and immunofluorescence reveals

specific antibodies in the basement membrane area. *(Wolff, p. 106)*

30. **(E)** Tetracyclines are commonly used in the treatment of moderate acne, but may be associated with risk of dental discoloration or photosensitivity. Isotretinoin is the most effective drug for severe acne, but is teratogenic, and may cause lipid abnormalities, hepatoxicity, and night blindness. It cannot be combined with tetracycline because of the risk of pseudo-tumor cerebri. *(Wolff, p. 6)*

31. **(C)** Exfoliative dermatitis is a rare skin condition, but because of its severity, patients with this syndrome are often admitted to a hospital. The syndrome can be primary, appearing in otherwise healthy individuals, or secondary to malignancy, contact dermatitis, drugs, or other dermatologic diseases (e.g., psoriasis). Even mild cases require systemic treatment for the severe itching. Antihistamines are usually the first choice. *(Wolff, pp. 158–163)*

32. **(E)** Most cases of exfoliative dermatitis will have widespread lymphadenopathy, whether they are primary or secondary forms. Biopsy will usually reveal nonspecific changes and is only warranted if there is a suspicion of lymphoma. *(Wolff, p. 160)*

33. **(C)** These large cells are typical of Sézary syndrome, a leukemic form of cutaneus T-cell lymphoma (CTCL). This is frequently an early presentation of mycosis fungoides or CTCL. There may be a relationship to human T-cell lymphotropic virus (HTLV) I and II, but it is not universal. CTCL is a malignancy of helper T cells (CD^{4+}). *(Wolff, p. 528)*

34. **(D)** The typical course of mycosis fungoides is an initial erythematous stage (which might become diffuse and cause an exfoliative dermatitis as in this case), a plaque stage, and a tumor stage. The course is usually progressive through these stages, but all stages can be bypassed. The early stages may progress slowly with remissions or exacerbations. The disease can be rapidly progressive, particularly

when the tumor stage is reached. The disease is invariably fatal. *(Wolff, p. 530)*

35. **(D)** There is no curative therapy, and most experts provide treatment only when symptoms occur. Therapy includes topical treatments such as tar cream plus ultraviolet light or local nitrogen mustard, and systemic treatment with steroids and radiation therapy.

    Chemotherapy regimens are used but not with great success. *(Wolff, pp. 530–531)*

36. **(C)** Severe cases require systemic steroids, often with the addition of azathioprine. Dapsone is useful in mild cases, and occasionally in very mild cases (or for local recurrences) topical glucocorticoid therapy will suffice.

37. **(D)** Nodular melanoma is invasive from the start. Women do better than men; trunk lesions and depigmented lesions carry a worse prognosis. Prognosis is directly related to depth of the lesion. *(Wolff, pp. 289, 305)*

38. **(B)** It is a persistent dermatitis around the mouth, with acral involvement that begins as vesicles but is soon crusted. Later it goes on to involve the scalp, hands and trunk, and feet. Treatment is zinc replacement in the diet. It has been described after prolonged parenteral alimentation, malabsorption states, intestinal bypass surgery, and chronic alcoholism. There is an inherited form (autosomal recessive) of the syndrome called acrodermatitis enteropathica. The inherited form occurs in infants and is also treated with zinc. *(Wolff, p. 454)*

39. **(E)** Erythema nodosum is a hypersensitivity vasculitis associated with many infections, drugs, malignancies, and inflammatory conditions (sarcoidosis). The peak age is 20–30 and it occurs more commonly in females. The lesions are rare in children. It is a nodular erythematous eruption, usually on the extensor aspects of the legs, less commonly on the thighs and forearms. It regresses by bruise-like color changes in 3–6 weeks without scarring. *(Wolff, pp. 148–149)*

40. **(E)** A macule is a flat, colored lesion not raised above the surface of the surrounding skin. It is less than 1 cm in diameter. A patch differs from a macule only in size, being greater than 1 cm in diameter. *(Kasper, p. 283)*

41. **(C)** A KOH preparation is useful when performed on scaling skin lesions, when a fungal etiology is suspected. The scraped scales are placed on a microscope slide, treated with one or two drops of KOH solution, and examined for hyphae, pseudohyphae, or budding yeast. A Tzanck smear is a cytologic technique for the diagnosis of herpes virus infection from vesicles, and diascopy is to assess whether a skin lesion will blanch with pressure. *(Kasper, p. 286)*

42. **(D)** Impetigo is a superficial bacterial infection of skin caused by group A beta-hemolytic streptococci or *Staphylococcus aureus.*

    It is characterized by superficial pustules that rupture, resulting in a honey-colored crust. The bullous variant is more likely staphylococcal in origin. Treatment requires improving hygiene and soaking the crust, as well as oral antibiotics. *(Wolff, pp. 588–589)*

43. **(E)** Localized areas of vitiligo can be seen in numerous primary skin disorders. It can also be caused by systemic disorders such as sarcoidosis and tuberculoid leprosy. In the latter disorder, there is associated anesthesia, anhidrosis, and alopecia of the lesions. Biopsy of the palpable border will reveal granulomas. *(Wolff, p. 658)*

44. **(G)** Scleroderma is characterized by typical fibrotic and vascular lesions. These lesions may be periungual telangiectasias that are found in lupus erythematosus and dermatomyositis. Another form of telangiectasia, mat telangiectasia, is seen only in scleroderma. These lesions are broad macules 2–7 mm in diameter. They are found on the face, oral mucosa, and hands. The nail beds of scleroderma patients often reveal loss of capillary loops, with dilatation of the remaining loops when examined under magnification. *(Wolff, p. 398)*

45. **(D)** Drug reactions most frequently result in papulosquamous reactions or diffuse erythroderma. Sulfa drugs frequently cause erythroderma. Other drugs commonly implicated include penicillins, gold, allopurinol, captopril, phenytoin, and carbamazepine. Fever, eosinophilia, and interstitial nephritis frequently accompany the erythroderma. *(Kasper, pp. 158–160)*

46. **(K)** Hyperlipoproteinemia is frequently associated with xanthomas, yellow-colored cutaneous papules or plaques. Xanthomas associated with hypertriglyceridemia are frequently eruptive; these yellow papules have an erythematous halo and are most frequently found on extensor surfaces of the extremities and buttocks. *(Wolff, p. 450)*

47. **(I)** The first exanthem of secondary syphilis is always macular and faint. Later eruptions may be papulosquamous and often involve the palms and soles. Associated findings that help make the diagnosis include annular plaques on the face, nonscarring alopecia, condylomata lata, mucous patches, lymphadenopathy, malaise, fever, headache, and myalgia. *(Wolff, p. 917)*

48. **(J)** Obesity is the most common cause of acanthosis nigricans—a velvety, localized hyperpigmentation. Other causes include gastrointestinal malignancy and endocrinopathy such as acromegaly, Cushing's syndrome, Stein-Leventhal syndrome, or insulin-resistant diabetes. *(Wolff, p. 86)*

49. **(A)** Cancer chemotherapy most frequently involves rapidly proliferating elements of the skin, resulting in stomatitis and alopecia. Bleomycin, hydroxyurea, and 5-fluorouracil can cause dystrophic nail changes. Other skin manifestations of cancer drugs include sterile cellulitis, phlebitis, ulceration of pressure areas, urticaria, angioedema, and exfoliative dermatitis. The underlying malignancy often makes diagnosis of skin disease more difficult. *(Wolff, p. 1011)*

50. **(C)** Chloroquine is used for certain skin diseases such as lupus and polymorphous light eruption, but can also cause skin reactions and exacerbate porphyria cutanea tarda. Black pigmentation can involve the face, mucous membrane, and pretibial and subungual areas. *(Kasper, pp. 302, 322)*

51. **(D)** Birth control pills, sulfonamides, and penicillins are common drugs that can cause erythema nodosum. This is a panniculitis characterized by tender, subcutaneous, erythematous nodules characteristically found on the anterior portion of the legs. *(Wolff, pp. 148–149)*

52. **(B)** The only common skin reaction with tetracyclines is photosensitivity. However, the drug is contraindicated in children under 8 years of age because of the risk of discoloring permanent teeth. *(Kasper, p. 802)*

53. **(D, E)** The combination of sulfamethoxazole and trimethoprim causes two distinct cutaneous reactions: an urticarial eruption in the first few days of therapy and a morbilliform eruption occurring a week or more after therapy has begun. This latter reaction is particularly common in patients with AIDS. Sulfonamides cause numerous skin lesions, including erythema nodosum. *(Wolff, pp. 148–149)*

CHAPTER 3

Endocrinology
Questions

DIRECTIONS (Questions 1 through 34): Each of the numbered items in this section is followed by answers. Select the ONE lettered answer that is BEST in each case.

1. A 42-year-old woman has noticed dry skin, fatigue, and weight gain over the past 3 months. Her blood pressure is 110/70 mm Hg, pulse 60/min, and heart and lungs are normal. Her skin feels rough and dry, but the rest of the examination is normal. Her biochemistry is normal but the thyroid-stimulating hormone (TSH) is 39 mU/L (0.5–5 mU/L). Which of the following is the most likely cause for her elevated TSH?

   (A) trauma
   (B) radioactive iodine ingestion
   (C) primary hypothyroidism
   (D) parathyroid surgery
   (E) antithyroid chemicals

2. A 53-year-old man has had gout for many years, and usually experiences 4–5 attacks a year. He is not on any medications for gout prophylaxis, and takes an over-the-counter nonsteroidal anti-inflammatory drug (NSAID) to treat his flares. On examination, there are no active joints presently, but he does have some tophaceous deposits on his left hand. As part of his complete evaluation, screening for renal complications is performed. Which of the following findings is most likely compatible with chronic gouty nephropathy?

   (A) nephrotic syndrome
   (B) decrease urinary concentrating ability and proteinuria
   (C) acute renal failure
   (D) acute tubular necrosis (ATN)
   (E) malignant hypertension

3. Which of the following is the most common presentation of anterior pituitary hyposecretion in a 26-year-old woman?

   (A) occurrence of myxedema
   (B) decreased melanin pigmentation
   (C) emaciation and cachexia
   (D) loss of axillary and pubic hairs
   (E) amenorrhea

4. A 19-year-old woman presents with primary amenorrhea. Her physical examination is normal, and she has female sex characteristics and breast development. The only abnormality is the absence of body hair. Genetic testing reveals an XY chromosome pattern. Which of the following mechanisms is most likely to explain her phenotypic pattern and amenorrhea?

   (A) estrogen receptor defect
   (B) excess hormone production
   (C) androgen receptor defect
   (D) decreased hormone production
   (E) abnormal hormone production

5. A 17-year-old woman has skin photosensitivity since childhood but has gotten worse recently. Her skin appears fine indoors, but within a short period of sun exposure, she develops burning, redness, and itching. A diagnosis of erythropoietic protoporphyria is made by a dermatologist. Which of the following treatments is most likely to be helpful? (See Fig. 3–1.)

(A) phenobarbital

(B) corticosteroids

(C) high carbohydrate diet

(D) beta-carotene

(E) chlorpromazine

6. A 23-year-old woman presents for evaluation of irregular periods and infertility. Her clinical examination is entirely normal. Biochemical tests show a reduced estradiol and follicle-stimulating hormone (FSH) levels. She is diagnosed with central hypogonadism. Which of the following is the most important function of FSH?

(A) causes ovulation

(B) encourages progesterone secretion

(C) causes the secretory phase of the uterine mucosa

(D) inhibits estrogen secretion

(E) encourages maturation of the follicle

7. A healthy 42-year-old woman is found on routine blood testing to have a calcium level of 12 mg/dL. She feels well, and her physical examination is normal. Further investigations reveal a parathormone (PTH) level of 750 pg/mL (230–630 pg/mL). Which of the following findings is also associated with this disorder?

(A) osteoblastic lesions of bone

(B) polycythemia

(C) prolonged QT interval on electrocardiogram (ECG)

(D) orthostatic hypotension

(E) cystic bone lesions

8. A 32-year-old woman is feeling unwell because of muscle cramps and generalized fatigue. Her blood pressure is 120/70 mm Hg, pulse 100/min, and the heart and lungs are normal. Muscle strength and bulk are normal but the reflexes are increased symmetrically. She had a previous thyroidectomy for a goiter 3 years ago. Her serum calcium level is 7 mg/dL (8.4–10.2 mg/dL), TSH 3 mU/L (0.5–5 mU/L)

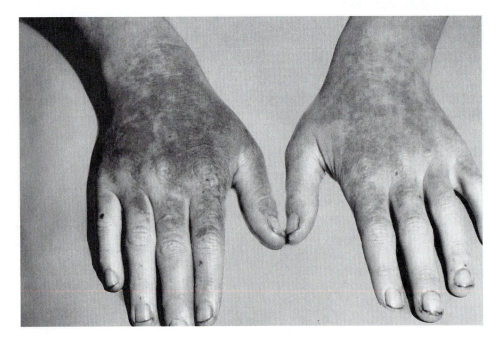

Figure 3–1.
(Reproduced, with permission, from Wolff K and Johnson RA, *Fitzpatrick's Color Atlas & Synopsis of Clinical Dermatology*, 5th ed. New York: McGraw-Hill, 2005:257.)

and albumin 4 g/dL (3.5–5.5 g/dL). Which of the following is the most likely explanation for her low calcium?

(A) idiopathic
(B) familial
(C) postradiation
(D) end-organ resistance
(E) surgical removal

9. A 27-year-old woman presents with weight loss, fatigue, and weakness. She also experiences nausea and vomiting but no dysphagia. Her physical examination is normal except for increased generalized skin pigmentation. Her serum sodium is low and potassium is high. Which of the following features is also most likely to be present? (See Fig. 3–2.)

(A) the skin is shiny and pale
(B) a diabetic glucose tolerance is characteristic
(C) water diuresis is impaired
(D) the urinary steroids are high
(E) the serum calcium is elevated

10. A patient with polyuria and polydipsia is newly diagnosed with central diabetes insipidus (DI). Which of the following is the most likely finding on magnetic resonance imaging (MRI) of the brain?

(A) hypothalamic tumor
(B) hyperintense signals in the cerebral cortex
(C) agenesis of the corpus callosum
(D) lack of hyperintense signals from the posterior pituitary
(E) communicating hydrocephalus

11. A 17-year-old man is 5′7″ tall and weighs 370 lb. No medical cause for this "essential obesity" is found. Which of the following abnormalities can he also be expected to have?

(A) normal mortality risk
(B) hypothyroidism
(C) low P_{CO_2} values
(D) hypertriglyceridemia
(E) hyperadrenocorticalism

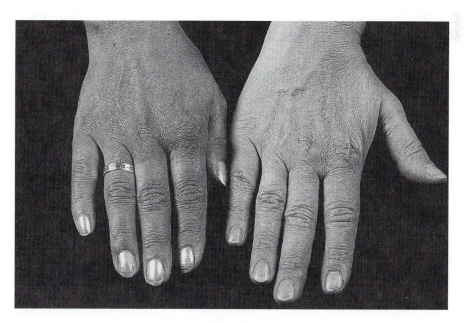

Figure 3–2.
(Reproduced, with permission, from Wolff K and Johnson RA, *Fitzpatrick's Color Atlas & Synopsis of Clinical Dermatology*, 5th ed. New York: McGraw-Hill, 2005:445.)

12. A 56-year-old man presents with a change in skin color, fatigue, and abdominal pain. He has also noticed increased urine output and thirst. On examination, his skin appears bronze in color, his liver span is 16 cm, and there is loss of body hair, and testicular atrophy. His ferritin is 600 ng/mL (15–200 ng/mL), aspartate amino transferase (AST) 130 U/L (8–20 U/L), alanine amino transferase (ALT) 150 U/L (8–20 U/L), and total bilirubin 0.5mg/dL (0.1–1 mg/dL). Coagulation tests and albumin level are normal but the random glucose is elevated at 250 mg/dL. Which of the following is the most likely diagnosis?

    (A) diabetes mellitus (DM)
    (B) amyloidosis
    (C) Wilson's disease
    (D) hemochromatosis
    (E) Addison's disease

13. A 35-year-old man has had recurrent attacks of abdominal pain and proximal motor neuropathy since puberty. The episodes are precipitated by infections and certain medications. During one of the attacks, the plasma porphobilinogen levels were increased. Which of the following medications is not considered safe in patients with this condition?

    (A) chlorpromazine
    (B) sulfonamide antibiotics
    (C) penicillin and derivatives
    (D) narcotics
    (E) glucocorticoids

14. A 43-year-old man weighs 85 kg and is 1.8 m tall. His calculated body mass index (BMI) is 23 kg/m^2. Which of the following conditions is he most likely at risk for?

    (A) DM
    (B) hyperlipoproteinemia
    (C) abnormal growth hormone response
    (D) atherosclerosis
    (E) no increased risk for mortality

15. A 47-year-old woman with bipolar disorder develops new symptoms of polyuria and polydipsia. She has been on lithium for a long time to control her illness. Which of the following is the most likely explanation for this complication of lithium treatment?

    (A) impairing glucose absorption at the cellular level
    (B) decreasing production of vasopressin
    (C) increasing production of vasopressin
    (D) causing a solute diuresis
    (E) impairing vasopressin action at the tubular level

16. The 2-year-old daughter of a Jewish couple, whose parents emigrated from Russia, develops progressive loss of motor skills. There is macular pallor on ophthalmic examination, and she has a short stature, thin limbs, but full cheeks. She is also prone to developing hypoglycemia and lactic acidosis. Which of the following metabolic abnormalities is most likely associated with this disorder?

    (A) glycogen storage
    (B) ganglioside accumulation
    (C) amyloid accumulation
    (D) corneal deposits
    (E) cholesterol accumulation

17. A 63-year-old man develops edema, and dyspnea on exertion. He has no prior cardiac or renal conditions, and his examination is significant for macroglossia, elevated jugular venous pressure (JVP), hepatomegaly, and 3+ pedal edema. His investigations reveal 3.5 g/d of protein in the urine, anemia, normal fasting glucose, and serum immunoelectrophoresis is positive for a monoclonal immunoglobulin. Which of the following is the most characteristic neurologic finding associated with this condition? (See Fig. 3–3.)

    (A) peripheral motor and sensory neuropathy
    (B) spinal cord compression in the lumbar region
    (C) spinal cord compression in the thoracic region
    (D) a peripheral neuropathy associated with cerebral manifestations
    (E) a Guillain-Barré-type syndrome

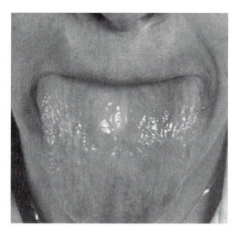

Figure 3–3.

18. A 30-year-old man presents with recurrent flushing, diarrhea, and weight loss. His examination is normal. Lab investigations reveal an elevated urinary 5-hydroxyindoleacetic acid. Which of the following is the most likely diagnosis?

    (A) phenylketonuria
    (B) alkaptonuria
    (C) malignant melanoma
    (D) carcinoid syndrome
    (E) disseminated carcinomatosis

19. A 25-year-old woman presents with symptoms of polyuria and polydipsia. So far investigations have ruled out psychogenic causes and diabetes. A fluid deprivation test is performed. At the end of the test, the urine osmolality is 240 mOsm/kg and the serum antidiuretic hormone (ADH) level is elevated. Which of the following is the most likely diagnosis?

    (A) adrenal cortex defect
    (B) nephrogenic diabetes insipidus
    (C) central (posterior pituitary) diabetes insipidus
    (D) acute tubular necrosis (ATN)
    (E) Addison's disease

20. A 40-year-old man has lipid investigations suggesting familial hypercholesterolemia (increased cholesterol, increased low-density lipoprotein [LDL], and normal triglycerides). This condition is characterized by increased risk for premature atherosclerosis and by the occurrence of tuberous and tendon xanthomas. Before making the assumption of familial hypercholesterolemia, secondary causes need to be considered. Which of the following conditions is most likely to cause secondary hyperlipidemia?

    (A) cholestatic liver disease
    (B) alcoholism
    (C) estrogen replacement
    (D) malabsorption syndromes
    (E) chronic lung disease

21. A 61-year-old woman with poorly controlled Type II diabetes is seen in follow-up. Her blood sugars are persistently elevated to levels greater than 200 mg/dL. On examination, she is obese, blood pressure 165/90 mm Hg, pulse 80/min, and there is sensory loss in the feet. Which of the following fasting lipid profiles is most likely to be consistent with her values?

    (A) high total cholesterol, low LDL, and normal triglycerides
    (B) high total cholesterol, high LDL, low triglycerides
    (C) high total cholesterol, normal LDL, high triglycerides
    (D) high total cholesterol, low LDL, and low triglycerides
    (E) high total cholesterol, high LDL, and high triglycerides

22. A 26-year-old man is evaluated for back pain and fatigue. He was previously healthy. On examination, he is pale, there is lumber spine tenderness, and an enlarged liver (18 cm). He is pancytopenic, and there is a vertebral fracture on lumbar x-rays. A bone marrow biopsy reveals infiltration with lipid-laden macrophages (Gaucher cells). Which of the following is the most likely diagnosis?

    (A) metachromatic leukodystrophy
    (B) inherited Gaucher's disease
    (C) acquired Gaucher's disease
    (D) glycogen storage disease
    (E) familial hyperchylomicronemia

23. A 19-year-old man has early fatigue and muscle cramps while playing sports. He is fine when walking or doing light levels of work. On examination, he appears well and the muscle strength in the proximal muscles is normal. There is no muscle fatigue with repetitive arm grip exercises. After an exercise stress test, his serum creatine kinase (CK) is elevated and lactate level is normal. Which of the following is the most likely diagnosis?

(A) Gaucher's disease
(B) Tay-Sachs disease
(C) McArdle's disease (glycogen storage disease)
(D) hemochromatosis
(E) myasthenia gravis

24. A 33-year-old man develops severe left flank pain that radiates to the front inguinal region. The pain eventually subsides after the passage of "sand-like" urine. A urinalysis reveals flat hexagonal plate like crystals (cystine). Which of the following statements about this condition is most likely true?

(A) commonest cause of renal stones
(B) stones are radiolucent on x-ray
(C) increased cystine concentration in the urine
(D) decreased cystine concentration in the urine
(E) acquired disorder of cystine metabolism

25. A 50-year-old man presents with feeling tired and unsteady on his feet. He has a poor appetite and has lost 10 lb. On examination, he appears cachectic, his heart and lungs are normal, but his liver span is 18 cm. His lab tests show a very low magnesium level (0.7 mEq/L). On further questioning, he reports drinking heavily since losing his job. Which of the following is the most likely explanation for his low magnesium level?

(A) alcoholism
(B) chronic malabsorption
(C) DM
(D) kwashiorkor
(E) hypervitaminosis E

26. A 27-year-old woman presents with feeling unwell ever since going on a high vitamin diet. She has dry skin, vomiting, headaches, and amenorrhea. Her examination and lab data are positive for hepatomegaly, splenomegaly, leukopenia, anemia, periosteal changes, sparse and coarse hair, and increased serum lipids. Which of the following is the most likely diagnosis?

(A) vitamin D intoxication
(B) vitamin D deficiency
(C) vitamin A deficiency
(D) vitamin A intoxication
(E) carotenemia

27. The patient whose hands are shown in Fig. 3–4 is developmentally delayed with a short, stocky build. Which of the following is the most likely diagnosis?

(A) achondroplastic dwarf
(B) Down syndrome
(C) Klinefelter's syndrome
(D) pseudohypoparathyroidism
(E) Turner's syndrome

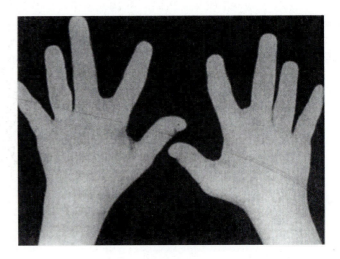

Figure 3–4.

28. Which of the following laboratory values is consistent with the patient shown in Fig. 3–4?

(A) hypercalcemia, hypophosphatemia
(B) hypocalcemia, low PTH

(C) hypocalcemia, high PTH

(D) hypocalcemia, hypophosphatemia

(E) hyperphosphatemia, low PTH

29. A 25-year-old man requests cholesterol screening because of a family history of premature coronary artery disease (CAD). His lipid levels reveal an elevated total and LDL cholesterol. The high-density lipoprotein (HDL) and triglyceride values are normal. His physical examination is completely normal. Which of the following is the most common cause of genetic dyslipidemia?

(A) familial combined hyperlipidemia

(B) familial hypercholesterolemia

(C) familial defective Apo B

(D) Apo C-II deficiency

(E) lipoprotein lipase deficiency

30. A 28-year-old woman with diabetes presents with lesions on her leg. They are not painful, and have a central depression and raised irregular margin. They are shown in Fig. 3–5. Which of the following is the most likely diagnosis?

(A) eruptive xanthomas

(B) necrobiosis lipoidica diabeticorum

(C) gangrene

(D) staphylococcal infection

(E) erythema nodosum

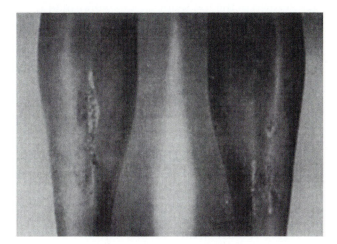

Figure 3–5.

31. A 54-year-old man comes to the emergency room with severe pain in his right toe. He has had less severe episodes in the past, which he always treated with pain medications. The toe is red, inflamed, and exquisitely sensitive to movement. Needle aspiration of the toe confirms uric acid crystals, and he is treated with oral indomethacin (NSAID). One month later, he remains symptom free, and allopurinol is recommended for prevention of this condition. Which of the following is the most likely mechanism of action of allopurinol?

(A) inhibition of xanthine oxidase

(B) solubilization of uric acid

(C) reactivity with hypoxanthine

(D) anti-inflammatory effect on joint tissue

(E) increased renal tubular secretion of uric acid

32. A 53-year-old woman with chronic renal failure develops hyperphosphatemia and hypocalcemia. Which of the following findings is most likely associated with this electrolyte disturbance?

(A) lethargy

(B) neuromuscular irritability

(C) anorexia

(D) tachyarrhythmias

(E) hyperkalemia

33. A 22-year-old man has features of arm span greater than height, subluxed lenses, flattened corneas, and dilation of the aortic ring. Which of the following is the most likely diagnosis?

(A) Ehlers-Danlos syndrome

(B) Marfan syndrome

(C) Werner's syndrome

(D) Laurence-Moon-Biedl syndrome

(E) Hunter's syndrome

34. A 33-year-old man is complaining of feeling thirsty all the time and passing more urine than usual. His physical examination is normal, except for a JVP at the sternal angle. His serum sodium is 150 mEq/L, glucose 120 mg/dL, and osmolality 315 mOsm/kg. The urine sodium is 20 mE/L and osmolality 260 mOsm/kg. Which of the following drugs is most likely to cause this disorder?

    (A) lithium
    (B) cyclophosphamide
    (C) barbiturates
    (D) nicotine
    (E) morphine

DIRECTIONS (Questions 35 through 39): The group of matching questions in this section consists of a list of lettered options followed by several numbered items. For each numbered item, select the appropriate lettered option(s). Each lettered option may be selected once, more than once, or not at all. EACH ITEM WILL STATE THE NUMBER OF OPTIONS TO SELECT. CHOOSE EXACTLY THIS NUMBER.

Questions 35 through 39

    (A) palmar plane xanthomas
    (B) triglycerides >1000
    (C) subcutaneous extensor tendon xanthomas
    (D) low serum cholesterol
    (E) normal cholesterol levels
    (F) xanthelasma after age 50 only

For each of the following dyslipidemias, select the most characteristic finding.

35. Hyperchylomicronemia (SELECT ONE)

36. Hyperbetalipoproteinemia (SELECT ONE)

37. Type III hyperlipoproteinemia (SELECT ONE)

38. Hyperprebetalipoproteinemia (SELECT ONE)

39. Hypertriglyceridemia (SELECT ONE)

DIRECTIONS (Questions 40 through 73): Each of the numbered items in this section is followed by answers. Select the ONE lettered answer that is BEST in each case.

40. A 20-year-old woman is complaining of passing large amounts of urine. She is otherwise well and her physical examination is normal. The serum sodium is 140 mEq/L and the urinalysis is negative for protein and glucose. The urine sodium is 33 mEq/L, and urine osmolality is 268 mOsm/kg. She weighs 60 kg, and her 24-hour urine output is over 4 l. Which of the following is the most likely diagnosis?

    (A) diabetes mellitus (DM)
    (B) psychogenic polydipsia
    (C) diabetes insipidus (DI)
    (D) contracted bladder
    (E) solute diureses

41. A 62-year-old man is seen in the office. Routine blood testing reveals elevated LDL cholesterol. Which of the following is the most likely cause for the elevated LDL?

    (A) an autosomal dominant disease
    (B) an X-linked recessive disease
    (C) a polygenic disease
    (D) a poor diet
    (E) DM

42. Which of the following dietary abnormalities is most commonly associated with elevated cholesterol levels?

    (A) inadequate fiber
    (B) excess calories resulting in obesity
    (C) excess dietary cholesterol
    (D) excess total fat intake
    (E) excess trans-fatty acid intake

43. A 63-year-old asymptomatic woman is investigated for a high alkaline phosphatase (ALP) level. X-rays of the pelvis show multiple porotic and sclerotic lesions with characteristic whorls of trabeculation. Her excretion of urinary hydroxyproline is also elevated. Which of the following is the most likely diagnosis?

(A) rickets and osteomalacia

(B) osteogenic sarcoma

(C) vitamin D deficiency

(D) Paget's disease of bone

(E) metastatic cancer

44. A 20-year-old man develops symptoms of weakness with numbness and tingling in his hands. The physical examination is normal, but his calcium is 7.4 mg/dL (8.4–10.2 mg/dL). Which of the following additional serum values is most consistent with the diagnosis of vitamin D deficiency?

(A) low vitamin D, low phosphate, high PTH

(B) low vitamin D, low phosphate, low PTH

(C) low vitamin D, high phosphate, low PTH

(D) normal vitamin D, low phosphate, high PTH

(E) normal vitamin D, high phosphate, high PTH

45. A 19-year-old woman develops weight loss, tremor, and heat intolerance. On examination, she has goiter, warm skin, and a fine tremor of her hands. Her TSH is low and her free T4 and T3 are elevated. Which of the following cardiac findings is most likely to occur in her?

(A) atrial fibrillation

(B) sinus tachycardia

(C) bradycardia

(D) increase in heart size

(E) pericardial effusion

46. A thyroid nodule is found on a 40-year-old woman on routine evaluation. She has no prior history of thyroid disease and clinically feels well. There is a 15-mm nontender nodule on the right lobe of the thyroid with no associated lymphadenopathy. Thyroid function tests are normal. Which of the following is the most appropriate next step in management?

(A) thyroid scan

(B) fine needle aspiration (FNA) biopsy

(C) repeat assessment in 6 months

(D) partial thyroidectomy

(E) complete thyroidectomy

47. Which of the following mechanisms is responsible for the release of vasopressin (antidiuretic hormone)?

(A) toxicity of the blood perfusing the liver

(B) phosphate levels in the renal plasma

(C) cerebrospinal fluid pressure

(D) calcium levels in the cerebral inflow

(E) volume receptors in the left atrium

48. A 40-year-old woman develops light-headed episodes associated with sweating, palpitations, and hunger whenever she misses a meal. Her physical examination is normal, and she is not taking any medications. On one such episode, while in hospital, her blood glucose level was 30 mg/dL and the symptoms resolved with giving her juice. Which of the following is the most likely diagnosis?

(A) excess growth hormone

(B) Cushing's disease

(C) thyrotoxicosis

(D) tumor of the pancreatic beta-cells

(E) gastrin deficiency

49. A 63-year-old has newly diagnosed light-chain amyloidosis (AL). In which of the following organs, is deposition of amyloid protein most likely to cause symptoms?

(A) heart

(B) red cells

(C) thyroid

(D) pancreas

(E) liver

50. A 25-year-old woman presents with intermittent symptoms of sweating, palpitations, and hunger. During each episode, her glucose level is less than 40 mg/dL. Her insulin level is low and glucagon level is high. Which of the following best describes the hormone function of glucagon?

    (A) promotes glycogenolysis and gluconeogenesis
    (B) a carbohydrate in structure
    (C) effective in lowering blood sugar levels
    (D) antigenically similar to insulin
    (E) effective in decreasing cyclic adenosine monophosphate (cAMP) in target cells

51. A 34-year-old woman notices lumps on her elbows and yellow patches below her eyelids. On examination, she has tendon xanthomas on her elbows and xanthelasma under the eyelids. Her lipid profile is consistent with a diagnosis of familial hypercholesterolemia (increased LDL). Which of the following statements regarding the treatment of this condition is correct?

    (A) dietary therapy is usually sufficient
    (B) cholestyramine is as effective as hepatic hydroxymethylglutaryl-coenzyme A (HMG-CoA) reductase inhibitors (statins)
    (C) ninety percent of patients can be controlled with a statin
    (D) a statin is the only type of medication suitable for monotherapy
    (E) combined therapy is frequently required

52. Which of the following is the most common manifestation of multiple endocrine neoplasia, type I (MEN I)?

    (A) Zollinger-Ellison syndrome
    (B) an adrenal adenoma
    (C) primary hyperparathyroidism
    (D) acromegaly
    (E) testicular cancer

53. A 51-year-old woman is experiencing irregular periods for the past 6 months as well as symptoms of hot flashes and night sweats. Her physical examination is normal. Hormone replacement therapy (HRT) is prescribed for her symptoms. Which of the following is the most likely additional benefit of HRT?

    (A) decreased CAD
    (B) a decreased risk of Alzheimer's disease
    (C) reduced venothromboemolism
    (D) decreased breast cancer risk
    (E) decreased osteoporosis-related fractures

54. A 37-year-old woman presents with symptoms of fatigue, muscle weakness, and weight gain. She has no past medical history and is not taking any medications. On examination, her blood pressure is 164/92 mm Hg and pulse 84/min. She has multiple skin bruises, facial fullness, and trunkal obesity with red "stretch marks." Muscle strength in the proximal muscles is 4+/5 and reflexes are normal. Which of the following is the most appropriate initial diagnostic test?

    (A) computerized tomography (CT) scan of the abdomen
    (B) fasting glucose
    (C) overnight dexamethasone suppression test
    (D) electromyogram (EMG) studies
    (E) MR of the brain

55. A 43-year-old woman develops increased hand and foot size. On examination, she has spade-like hands, coarsened facial features, and a gap between her incisors. Her blood pressure is 155/85 mm Hg and pulse 80/min, cardiac apical beat is sustained with normal heart sounds. Which of the following is the most likely effect of this syndrome on the muscles?

    (A) enlargement
    (B) spasm
    (C) increased strength
    (D) myositis
    (E) rhythmic contraction

56. A 7-year-old boy has demineralized bones with pseudofractures. Physiologic doses of vitamin D do not result in improvement. Which of the following is most likely to be associated with this syndrome?

   (A) hyperphosphatemia
   (B) low 1,25(OH)2 vitamin D levels
   (C) alopecia
   (D) osteoporosis
   (E) mental retardation

57. An 18-year-old girl is brought to hospital because of weakness. She feels well, but is under a lot of stress at school. Most of her time is spent studying, dieting, and exercising. She is 5'8", weighs 78 lb, and appears unwell. Her blood pressure is 85/70 mm Hg, pulse 50/min, and there is muscle wasting. Which of the following is this patient most likely at risk for?

   (A) renal failure
   (B) ventricular tachyarrhythmias
   (C) DM
   (D) hyperthermia
   (E) pernicious anemia

58. A 53-year-old man develops severe pain, redness, and swelling in his left big toe. Which of the following conditions is most likely associated with this condition?

   (A) pernicious anemia
   (B) DI
   (C) Alzheimer's disease
   (D) anorexia
   (E) renal disease

59. A 27-year-old woman complains of pain in her left shin. X-rays of the leg reveal a stress fracture of the tibia, decreased cortical bone density, and increased radiolucency. She is suspected of

having osteomalacia (impaired mineralization of bone matrix). Which of the following is the most common biochemical manifestation of osteomalacia?

   (A) hyperphosphatemia
   (B) hypoparathyroidism
   (C) decreased vitamin D
   (D) hypercalcemia
   (E) low alkaline phosphatase (ALP)

60. A 44-year-old man presents with worsening abdominal distension, edema, and jaundice. He has chronic viral hepatitis B and cirrhosis. Recently he has noticed decreased urine output despite adequate fluid intake. On examination he is icteric, the blood pressure is 110/70 mm Hg, pulse 74/min, JVP is 4 cm, heart sounds are normal, and there are tense ascites and pedal edema. Which of the following is an early manifestation of hepatorenal syndrome?

   (A) intrarenal vasodilatation
   (B) sodium retention
   (C) potassium retention
   (D) severe jaundice
   (E) polyuria

61. Which of the following is the most appropriate management for phenylketonuria?

   (A) a gluten-free diet from age 6 months to 12 years
   (B) supplemental insulin
   (C) enteral feeding
   (D) tyrosine supplements
   (E) a low carbohydrate diet

62. A 21-year-old woman on no medications develops rigidity, tremor, and incoordination. She has a history of unexplained hepatitis 2 years ago and depression 1 year ago. Her examination is pertinent for increased tone, normal muscle strength, and coarse tremor of the hands. An ophthalmologic examination is positive for a brownish pigmented ring at the corneal margin. Which of the following findings is most likely to be present in this patient? (See Fig. 3–6.)

(A) renal failure

(B) cirrhosis of the liver

(C) elevated ceruloplasmin

(D) sensory loss

(E) increased plasma copper

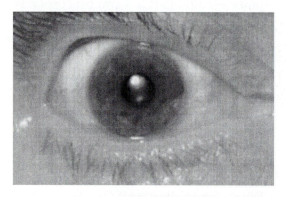

Figure 3–6.

63. A 57-year-old man complains of increased thirst and urination. His examination is normal except for obesity (BMI>30). Which of the following is the most appropriate initial diagnostic test?

(A) a urine osmolality

(B) hemoglobin A1C level

(C) a fasting blood sugar (FBS)

(D) a glucose tolerance test (GTT)

(E) random glucose

64. Which of the following is the most likely effect of insulin at the cellular receptor level?

(A) stimulating tyrosine kinase

(B) binding to ion channels

(C) binding to intracellular erb A receptors

(D) stimulating guanylate cyclase

(E) activating G-proteins

65. Which of the following is the most likely metabolic effect of insulin on adipose tissue?

(A) decrease of glucose transport

(B) decrease in glucose phosphorylation

(C) decrease in lipolysis

(D) decrease in lipoprotein lipase

(E) enhancement of glucagon effect

66. A 32-year-old woman presents with heat intolerance, palpitations, diarrhea, weakness, and weight loss. Her blood pressure is 90/60 mm Hg, pulse 110/min, and she has a fine tremor in her hands. The TSH level is suppressed and T3 and T4 are elevated. Which of the following is most likely to precipitate this condition?

(A) propylthiouracil administration

(B) high-dose prednisone therapy

(C) beta-adrenergic blockade

(D) pneumonia

(E) salicylate administration

67. A 15-year-old youth has not gone through puberty. Which of the following is the most likely diagnosis?

(A) inadequate diet

(B) normal variation

(C) pituitary tumor

(D) Leydig cell dysfunction

(E) drug side effects

68. A 44-year-old woman is recently diagnosed with breast cancer and undergoes a mastectomy. Which of the following features is most likely to be important in determining response to tamoxifen therapy?

(A) metastases confined to liver

(B) patient more than 5 years premenopausal

(C) androgen receptors on the tumor cell membrane

(D) tumor has progesterone receptors (PR)

(E) metastases confined to brain

69. Which of the following increases a woman's risk of breast cancer?

   (A) castration before age 40 years

   (B) late first pregnancy

   (C) long-term nursing

   (D) history of breast cancer in an aunt

   (E) multiparity

70. Which of the following statements is correct?

   (A) resting metabolic rate (RMR) is identical in men and women when corrected for weight and height

   (B) virtually all nitrogen loss is through urine in the form of urea

   (C) increasing the proportion of protein in the diet increases the efficiency of protein production in the body

   (D) generally, physical activity accounts for only 15% of total energy expenditure over most conditions

   (E) recommended levels of adult protein ingestion should be decreased by 30% for the very elderly

71. A 35-year-old woman, on hemodialysis for chronic renal disease, complains of pain in the hands. On examination, the joints are normal with no inflammation or tenderness on palpation. Lab values reveal a low calcium, high phosphate, and high PTH level. What is the most likely diagnosis? (See Fig. 3–7.)

   (A) scleroderma

   (B) gout

   (C) secondary hyperparathyroidism

   (D) pseudogout

   (E) Paget's disease

72. A 35-year-old woman presents with fatigue, weakness, and weight gain. Her blood pressure is 155/90 mm Hg, pulse 80/min, and there is central obesity with skin striae. Investigations are shown in Table 3–1. Which of the following is the most likely diagnosis?

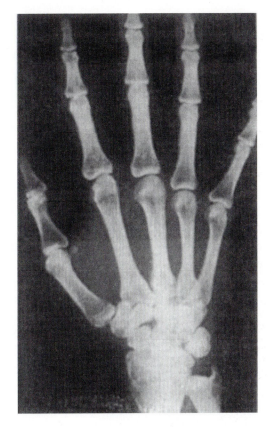

Figure 3–7.

   (A) adrenal hyperplasia secondary to hypothalamic dysfunction

   (B) adrenal adenoma with complete autonomy

   (C) exogenous steroids, iatrogenic

   (D) pituitary tumor

   (E) carcinoma of the adrenal

TABLE 3–1. CASE WORK-UP

	Normal	Patient
Plasma ACTH pg/mL	< 150	< 50
Plasma cortisol u/dL	17	35
Urine 17-OH mg/24 h	2 to 10	25
Urine 17-Ks mg/24 h	5 to 15	10
Urine 17-OH response to:		
ACTH IV	Increase × 5	No response
Dexamethasone 0.5 mg	< 3.0	No response
2.0 mg	< 3.0	No response
Metyrapone 750 mg	Increase × 2	No response

Abbreviation: ACTH—adrenocorticotropic hormone

73. A 55-year-old obese woman complains of vulvar pruritus, recent weight loss in spite of a large appetite, and waking up frequently at night to urinate. Which of the following is the most likely diagnosis?

(A) DM

(B) DI

(C) vaginitis and cystitis

(D) myxedema

(E) pheochromocytoma

DIRECTIONS: (Questions 74 through 84): Each set of matching questions in this section consists of a list of lettered options followed by several numbered items. For each numbered item, select the appropriate lettered option(s). Each lettered option may be selected once, more than once, or not at all. EACH ITEM WILL STATE THE NUMBER OF OPTIONS TO SELECT. CHOOSE EXACTLY THIS NUMBER.

Questions 74 through 76

(A) microaneurysms

(B) vitreal hemorrhage

(C) dilated veins

(D) retinal detachment

(E) hemorrhage (dot and blot)

(F) open-angle glaucoma

(G) erythema multiforme

(H) pyoderma gangrenosum

(I) necrobiosis lipoidica

(J) candidiasis

For each patient with a complication of diabetes, select the most likely diagnosis or findings.

74. A 72-year-old man with Type II diabetes notices painless skin lesions on his legs. They have an irregular raised border with a flat depressed center that is hyperpigmented brown in color. (SELECT ONE)

75. A 59-year-old man with Type II diabetes goes for a screening eye examination. The ophthalmologist reports that the patient has developed nonproliferative retinopathy. (List the findings.) (SELECT THREE)

76. A 35-year-old woman with Type I diabetes develops progressive vision loss in her left eye. The ophthalmologist reports the development of proliferative retinopathy. (List the findings.) (SELECT TWO)

Questions 77 through 80

(A) loss of sexual desire

(B) failure of erection with absent nocturnal penile tumescence (NPT)

(C) absence of emission

(D) absence of orgasm with normal libido and erectile function

(E) failure of detumescence

For each of the following causes of sexual dysfunction, select the most likely clinical feature.

77. Can be caused by high prolactin level (SELECT ONE)

78. Rarely indicates organic disease (SELECT ONE)

79. Can be caused by hematologic disease (SELECT ONE)

80. Can be caused by vascular disease (SELECT ONE)

Questions 81 through 84

(A) drugs

(B) adrenal tumor

(C) polycystic ovarian disease (PCOD)

(D) adrenal hyperplasia

(E) idiopathic hirsutism

(F) ovarian tumor

For each of the following explanations for hirsutism, select the most likely cause.

81. Slight elevation of plasma testosterone and androstenedione (SELECT ONE)

82. Can be associated with anovulation, obesity, and amenorrhea (SELECT ONE)

83. May stimulate surrounding tissue to secrete androgens (SELECT ONE)

84. Often associated with elevated 17-hydroxyprogesterone levels (SELECT ONE)

DIRECTIONS (Questions 85 through 91): Each of the numbered items in this section is followed by answers. Select the ONE lettered answer that is BEST in each case.

Questions 85 through 91

85. A 15-year-old girl has been losing weight and exercising vigorously. She feels overweight and wants to lose more weight. On examination, she is thin with muscle wasting. Which of the following physical signs is also suggestive of the diagnosis?

    (A) salivary gland enlargement
    (B) coarse body hair
    (C) diarrhea
    (D) tachycardia
    (E) hypertension

86. A 17-year-old man is brought to the emergency room because of weakness and weight loss. He is diagnosed with an eating disorder and admitted to the hospital. Which of the following lab values is not consistent with this diagnosis?

    (A) hypokalemia
    (B) hypochloremia
    (C) metabolic alkalosis
    (D) hyperglycemia
    (E) low blood urea nitrogen (BUN)

87. A 22-year-old woman is brought to hospital because of syncope. There were no warning symptoms, and she was fine after the event. Recently she has lost 40 lb because of an eating disorder. She weighs 70 lb, looks unwell, and has little muscle bulk. The blood pressure is 80/60 mm Hg and pulse 50/min. Which of the

following is the most likely abnormality on her ECG?

    (A) resting sinus tachycardia
    (B) increased QRS voltages
    (C) short QT interval
    (D) increased T waves
    (E) prolonged QT interval

88. Which of the following indications for hospitalization is the most appropriate for patients with eating disorders?

    (A) when body weight is less than 90% of expected
    (B) when body weight is less than 75% of expected
    (C) when electrolyte disturbances occur
    (D) when body weight is less than 60% of expected
    (E) when vomiting is being induced

89. Which of the following is the most likely explanation for the dental abnormalities in bulimia nervosa (BN)?

    (A) self-induced physical trauma
    (B) self-induced vomiting
    (C) excess cortisol levels
    (D) osteoporotic changes
    (E) estrogen deficiency

90. A 64-year woman with Type II diabetes for 10 years now develops increasing fatigue, dyspnea, and pedal edema. On examination, her blood pressure is 165/90 mm Hg, pulse 90/min, JVP is 4 cm, heart sounds are normal, lungs are clear, and there is 3+ pedal edema. Her urinalysis is positive for 3 gm/L of protein and no casts. Which of the following renal diseases is the most likely diagnosis in this patient?

    (A) acute glomerulonephritis
    (B) obstructive uropathy
    (C) glomerulosclerosis with mesangial thickening
    (D) renal infarction
    (E) polycystic kidneys

91. Which of the following statements concerning the prognosis of anorexia nervosa (AN) and bulimia nervosa (BN) is correct?

    (A) both have an excellent prognosis with mortality not different from age matched controls
    (B) AN has significant mortality (5% per decade), but BN does not
    (C) BN has significant mortality (5% per decade), but AN does not
    (D) both diseases have a high recovery rate
    (E) both BN and AN have significant mortality (3–5% per decade)

DIRECTIONS: (Questions 92 through 97): Each set of matching questions in this section consists of a list of lettered options followed by several numbered items. For each numbered item, select the appropriate lettered option(s). Each lettered option may be selected once, more than once, or not at all. EACH ITEM WILL STATE THE NUMBER OF OPTIONS TO SELECT. CHOOSE EXACTLY THIS NUMBER.

    (A) diabetes
    (B) obesity
    (C) hypertension
    (D) anorexia nervosa (AN)
    (E) gastroesophageal reflux (GERD)
    (F) postgastrectomy
    (G) Parkinson's disease
    (H) cirrhosis
    (I) Crohn's disease
    (J) osteoporosis
    (K) celiac disease
    (L) irritable bowel syndrome
    (M) hyperlipidemia

For each patient placed on a dietary restriction, select the most likely diagnosis.

92. A 24-year-old female is placed on a low residue and low fiber diet. She has a long history of right lower quadrant pain, cramps, and diarrhea. (SELECT ONE)

93. A 56-year-old man is started on a low caloric and weight loss diet. He recently started feeling unwell, had vision changes, and noticed numbness in his feet. (SELECT ONE)

94. A 52-year-old woman is started on a low sodium diet. She feels well and is experiencing no symptoms. Her physical examination is normal except for a sustained cardiac apical impulse. (SELECT ONE)

95. A 64-year-old man is placed on a low simple sugar diet. He is experiencing symptoms of crampy abdominal discomfort, nausea, diarrhea, and diaphoresis 15–30 minutes after eating. (SELECT ONE)

96. A 45-year-old woman is placed on a protein restriction diet and a daily laxative regimen. She recently had a hospital admission for confusion related to a chronic illness. (SELECT ONE)

97. A 38-year-old woman is told to limit chocolate and caffeine intake for worsening symptoms. She is also told that weight loss is helpful in improving the symptoms for her condition. (SELECT ONE)

DIRECTIONS (Questions 98 through 102): Each lettered heading below describes an essential vitamin. Each numbered phrase describes a syndrome of vitamin deficiency or excess. For each numbered phrase, select the ONE lettered heading that is most closely associated with it. Each lettered heading may be selected once, more than once, or not at all.

    (A) niacin
    (B) thiamine
    (C) pyridoxine
    (D) vitamin C
    (E) vitamin A
    (F) vitamin E
    (G) vitamin K

For each patient with vitamin deficiency or excess, select the most likely diagnosis.

98. An 83-year-old man with poor nutrition notices easy bruising and bleeding gums. On examination, he has inflamed bleeding gums, multiple areas of ecchymoses, and perifollicular hemorrhages. His coagulation profile and liver function is normal.

99. A 26-year-old woman started developing frequent headaches, dizziness, and double vision after starting a "megavitamin" program. Her examination is normal except for papilledema.

100. A 57-year-old man has dyslipidemia with a low HDL and high triglyceride pattern. Recently the dose of one of his medications was increased and he started experiencing flushing and pruritus secondary to histamine release.

101. A 43-year-old woman with chronic alcoholism presents with shortness of breath and edema. On examination, her blood pressure is 100/60 mm Hg, pulse 110/min, JVP is 8 cm, the cardiac apex is displaced and enlarged, there are bilateral inspiratory crackles, and there is pedal edema.

102. A 52-year-old alcoholic notices a skin rash on his chest, and also has symptoms of diarrhea and abdominal pain. On examination, he has a scaly and pigmented rash on the sun-exposed areas of his skin, the abdomen is soft, and his short-term memory is impaired. He has dermatitis, diarrhea, and dementia syndrome.

Answers and Explanations

1. **(C)** Primary hypothyroidism is the most common cause of hypothyroidism in adults. Primary hypothyroidism is several times more common in women than in men and occurs most often between the ages of 40 and 60. Postablative hypothyroidism (radiation or surgery induced) is also very common. *(Felig, p. 316)*

2. **(B)** Diminished concentrating ability and proteinuria occur even when the glomerular filtration rate is near normal. The severity of renal involvement correlates with the duration and magnitude of serum uric acid elevation. Uric acid and monosodium urate deposit in the renal parenchyma. These deposits can cause intrarenal obstruction and elicit an inflammatory response as well. Hypertension, nephrolithiasis, and pyelonephritis can also contribute to the nephropathy of gout. *(Kasper, p. 1704)*

3. **(E)** With pituitary hypofunctioning, gonadotropin deficiency is the most common early manifestation in both men and women. Growth hormone secretion is also impaired early on, but is less clinically apparent. *(Felig, p. 681)*

4. **(C)** Disease states, due to abnormal intracellular receptors, include androgen insensitivity; cortisol resistance; vitamin D-dependent rickets, type II; thyroid hormone resistance; and pseudohypoaldosteronism. Androgen insensitivity syndrome is caused by a mutation in the androgen receptor, and it affects 1 in 100,000 chromosomal males. Because the androgen receptor is X-linked, it only affects males. The phenotypic presentation can vary from complete androgen insensitivity (female external features) to partial insensitivity causing ambiguous or normal male features and infertility. There are several different types of cell membrane receptors. *(Kasper, pp. 2217–2218)*

5. **(D)** Beta-carotene increases the patient's tolerance for sunlight, apparently by quenching active intermediates. Beta-carotene is an effective scavenger of free radicals. Although many affected individuals can tolerate sun exposure while taking beta-carotene, it has no effect on the basic metabolic defect in porphyrin-heme synthesis. *(Kasper, p. 2308)*

6. **(E)** FSH is said to encourage maturation of a follicle in the human menstrual cycle. The cardinal hormonal change in phase I is a rise in FSH caused by a decrease in the level of estrogens and a waning activity of the corpus luteum. In men, FSH stimulates Sertoli cells, which have an important role in spermatogenesis. *(Kasper, p. 2094)*

7. **(E)** In hyperparathyroidism, bony lesions are lytic and can cause pain. The cortical surfaces are thinned and much of the bone is demineralized. The fibrotic bulging lesions within bone are termed *brown tumors*. Fluid-filled cysts can also occur (osteitis fibrosa cystica). Anemia is common, and the QT interval can be shortened if the calcium is high enough. Hypertension is common. Most patients with hyperparathyroidism have a simple adenoma that functions autonomously, so that hormone is secreted with high calcium. In about 10–15% of cases, hyperplasia of all the parathyroid glands (chief cell hyperplasia) is the cause. Differentiation from adenoma is important to determine the

correct surgical approach but is, unfortunately, very difficult. *(Kasper, p. 2254)*

8. **(E)** Surgical removal is the most common cause of hypoparathyroidism. When the glands, or their blood vessels, have merely been damaged and not removed, tissue often regenerates. Hypoparathyroidism can frequently follow thyroid surgery. The incidence varies and depends on the extent of resection, the skill of the surgeon, and the degree of diligence in diagnosing hypocalcemia. *(Kasper, p. 2264)*

9. **(C)** Water diuresis is impaired in adrenocortical insufficiency. Lack of aldosterone also favors the development of hyperkalemia and mild acidosis. The decreased circulating volume, secondary to aldosterone deficiency, is one of the factors resulting in elevated basal antidiuretic hormone (ADH) levels and thus hyponatremia. *(Kasper, p. 2141)*

10. **(D)** Because DI is usually caused by destruction, or agenesis, of the posterior pituitary, its normal signaling is lost. Pituitary DI can also result from trauma, tumors (both primary and secondary), granulomas, infections, inflammatory diseases, chemical toxins, congenital malformations, and genetic disorders.

    Depending on the cause, the MRI may demonstrate other associated findings. *(Kasper, p. 3100)*

11. **(D)** Hypertriglyceridemia may result in part from hyperinsulinism, because insulin is one of the factors involved in lipoprotein secretion by the liver. With massive obesity, there is an increased prevalence of cardiovascular disease, hypertension, diabetes, pulmonary disorders, and gallstones. Young men with morbid obesity have a 12-fold higher mortality risk than the general population. Even in old age (65–74 years), the mortality is doubled in obese men. Cardiovascular disease is the most important factor. *(Felig, pp. 954–958)*

12. **(D)** High ferritin, hepatomegaly, skin changes, and diabetes suggest hemochromatosis. The arthritis is characterized by chondrocalcinosis, but, unlike idiopathic chondrocalcinosis, the hands are usually involved first. The arthropathy often progresses despite phlebotomy. Liver disease is usually the presenting feature. Skin pigmentation is predominantly by melanin. Heart failure is the most common cardiac problem. Addison's does not involve the liver, and Wilson's usually presents at an earlier age and does not cause diabetes. In amyloidosis, skin pigmentation is not a feature. *(Kasper, p. 2301)*

13. **(B)** In patients with acute intermittent porphyria, oral phenothiazines may be used for abdominal or muscle pains, and narcotics may also be used, but barbiturates should be avoided. Sulfonamides are unsafe, but penicillin and its derivatives are safe. Other unsafe medications include alcohol, carbamazepine, valproic acid, and synthetic estrogens and progestogens. Most heterozygotes remain asymptomatic unless a precipitating factor such as a drug or weight loss is present. Poorly localized abdominal pain is the most common symptom. *(Kasper, pp. 2305–2306)*

14. **(E)** One of the most efficient ways to define obesity is by BMI, which is calculated by weight/height^2, calculated using kilograms for weight and meters for height. This man's BMI is between 23 and 24 kg/m^2 and confers no special risk. (The acceptable range is 20–25.) *(Kasper, p. 422)*

15. **(E)** Nephrogenic diabetes insipidus is caused by a defect in the action of vasopressin on the renal tubules. This can be genetic, and variants include X-linked recessive, autosomal dominant, and autosomal recessive. Numerous drugs can cause the syndrome, as can many forms of renal disease. Hypercalcemia and hypokalemia can also cause the syndrome. *(Felig, p. 233)*

16. **(B)** Glycogen storage is not characteristic of Tay-Sachs disease. Ganglioside accumulation can now be diagnosed by decreased hexosaminidase in peripheral leukocytes. Tay-Sachs is characterized as a lysosomal storage disease. Mental retardation, seizures, blindness, and a retinal cherry red spot are characteristic.

It is most common in Ashkenazi Jews and is inherited in an autosomal recessive manner. *(Kasper, pp. 2319–2320)*

17. **(A)** In addition to peripheral motor and sensory neuropathy, cardiac involvement, tongue enlargement, gastrointestinal (GI) manifestations, and carpal tunnel syndrome are also seen in amyloidosis. The specific diagnosis requires tissue biopsy with presence of amyloid with specific stains. In primary amyloidosis and myeloma, the amyloid protein is of the AL type. In reactive amyloidosis, the protein is of the amyloid A protein (AA) type. *(Kasper, p. 2027)*

18. **(D)** Carcinoid syndrome is characterized by increased levels of 5-hydroxyindolacetic acid. The syndrome occurs in relation to malignant tumors that have metastasized, usually with hepatic implants. Gastrointestinal carcinoids are most commonly found in the appendix. These are very slow growing, thus the 5-year survival rate is 99%. Many carcinoids are discovered as incidental findings on autopsy. *(Kasper, pp. 2224–2225)*

19. **(B)** Central diabetes insipidus is most commonly caused by a primary deficit in the secretion of vasopressin by the posterior pituitary. It is usually caused by agenesis or destruction of vasopressin-producing neurons by either a developmental, acquired, genetic, or idiopathic disorder. Nephrogenic diabetes insipidus is the failure of the kidney to respond to ADH. It can be acquired, genetic, or medication related. *(Kasper, pp. 2098–2099)*

20. **(A)** In familial hypercholesterolemia, there is an increased incidence of CAD, and hypercholesterolemia occurs along with tuberous xanthomas, arcus senilis, and atheromas. Most affected individuals are heterozygous for the mutant gene. Important secondary causes include DM, obesity/dietary intake, hypothyroidism, renal disease (nephritic syndrome), and cholestatic liver disease. Alcohol usually improves lipid profiles in small amounts and in excess causes increases in triglycerides. Estrogen as well improves lipid profiles. The

other choices are not important in affecting lipid levels. *(Kasper, pp. 2288–2294)*

21. **(E)** In Type II diabetes, high levels of insulin and insulin resistance have multiple effects on lipid metabolism. These include increases in triglycerides, low HDL, and normal to high LDL. The high triglycerides respond to insulin therapy and to weight loss, while the low HDL responds to exercise. *(Kasper, p. 2294)*

22. **(B)** The diagnosis is inherited Gaucher's disease since it is an autosomal recessive disorder. There is no acquired form of the disease. The glucocerebrosides are derived from lipid catabolites, from the membranes of senescent leukocytes and erythrocytes. Although the juvenile form may have severe neurologic symptoms (mental retardation, spasticity, ataxia), the adult form usually has no neurologic symptoms. Like Tay-Sachs, it is a lysosomal storage disease with a predilection for Ashkenazi Jews. *(Kasper, p. 2318)*

23. **(C)** There are many types of glycogen storage diseases, each caused by a different enzymatic abnormality. The best known types of glycogen storage disease are those that have hepatic-hypoglycemic pathophysiology (e.g., von Gierke's disease) or those that have muscle energy pathophysiology (McArdle's disease). In McArdle's symptoms usually develop in adulthood, and it is marked by cramps and muscle injury with strenuous exercise, but not with usual activities. Gaucher's and Tay-Sachs disease are lysosomal storage diseases. *(Kasper, p. 2322)*

24. **(C)** Cystinuria is commonly associated with hexagonal crystals in the urine. Cystine, lysine, arginine, and ornithine are excreted in great excess by patients homozygous for the disease. The tissues manifesting the transport defect of cystinuria are the proximal renal tubule and the jejunal mucosa. It is inherited as an autosomal recessive trait. Cystine kidney stones (1% of all renal stones) are the major clinical manifestation, and they are radiopaque. *(Kasper, p. 1714)*

25. **(A)** Magnesium deficiency is most commonly due to alcoholism. Renal loss and malabsorption are also common causes. Magnesium deficiency is not seen in hypervitaminosis E. Causes of magnesium deficiency also include milk diets in infants, the diuretic phase of acute tubular necrosis, chronic diuretic therapy, acute pancreatitis, and inappropriate antidiuretic hormone. The symptoms of hypomagnesemia include anorexia, nausea, tremor, and mood alteration. Symptoms can also be caused by the associated hypocalcemia or hypokalemia. *(Kasper, pp. 2244–2245)*

26. **(D)** Symptoms of vitamin A intoxication occur in infants or adults ingesting over 50,000 IU of vitamin A daily. The prognosis is good when vitamin A intake ceases. Rare occurrences of hypercalcemia with vitamin A intoxication have been reported. *(Kasper, pp. 407–408)*

27. **(D)** The deformity of the hands is due to short metacarpals. Other deformities include short metatarsals, round facies, and thickening of the calvarium. The syndrome is caused by target organ unresponsiveness to PTH, and was the first hormone resistance syndrome described. *(Felig, pp. 1143–1145)*

28. **(C)** The findings of hypocalcemia and hyperphosphatemia are the same as in hypoparathyroidism, but the serum PTH levels are appropriately increased. The normal urinary rise in cAMP does not occur when these patients are injected with exogenous (normal) PTH. *(Felig, pp. 1143–1145)*

29. **(A)** Familial combined hyperlipidemia has an incidence of 1/100. It is an autosomal dominant disorder and different affected family members may display different dyslipidemic phenotypes. Familial hypercholesterolemia (1/500) and familial defective Apo B (1/1000) are also common. The other two disorders (Apo C-II deficiency and lipoprotein lipase deficiency) are extremely rare. *(Felig, p. 1010)*

30. **(B)** This lesion is more frequent in females and may antedate other clinical signs and symptoms of diabetes. The plaques are round, firm,

and reddish-brown to yellow in color. They most commonly involve the legs but can also involve the hands, arms, abdomen, and head. *(Kasper, p. 2169)*

31. **(A)** Allopurinol inhibits the enzyme xanthine oxidase, resulting in decreased uric acid production. Allopurinol is particularly useful in the treatment of uric acid nephrolithiasis in gouty individuals. Even if the gouty individual has calcium oxalate stones, allopurinol may be helpful. *(Kasper, p. 2047)*

32. **(B)** Hyperphosphatemia rarely causes any symptoms directly. Its secondary effects on calcium can result in hypocalcemic tetany or metastatic calcification. The usual cause of hyperphosphatemia is uremia. *(Felig, pp. 1156–1157)*

33. **(B)** The severe form of Marfan syndrome is caused by a mutation in a single allele of the fibrillin gene (FBN1). The gene product is a major component of elastin-associated microfibrils. Long, thin extremities; ectopia lentis; and aortic aneurysms are the classical triad. Milder forms of the disease probably also occur but are hard to classify. Mutations in the FBN2 gene can also cause Marfan syndrome, but without aneurysms. *(Kasper, pp. 2329–2330)*

34. **(A)** Nephrogenic DI can be caused by drugs such as lithium, metabolic factors, vascular disease, ureteral obstruction, and genetic factors. *(Kasper, p. 2099)*

35. **(B)** In the familial type 1 form, the defect is believed to be a deficiency of lipoprotein lipase activity. It is a rare autosomal recessive syndrome, and usually presents in childhood with typical eruptive xanthoma and abdominal pain secondary to acute pancreatitis. Secondary hyperchylomicronemia (diabetes, hypothyroidism, uremia) is a much more common syndrome. *(Felig, p. 1027)*

36. **(C)** Subcutaneous xanthomas begin to appear at about age 20 and may involve Achillis tendons, elbows, and tibial tuberosities. Familial hypercholesterolemia may be monogenic or

polygenic in its inheritance. The disorder is common, and heterozygous familial hypercholesterolemia is felt to affect 1 in 500 individuals. It can be secondary to other diseases such as hypothyroidism, nephrotic syndrome, or even porphyria. Xanthelasmas after the age of 50 are often not related to any dyslipidemia at all. *(Felig, p. 1016)*

37. **(A)** In the rare familial form, raised yellow plaques appear on palms and fingers, and reddish-yellow xanthomas occur on the elbows. This disorder is felt to be secondary to accumulation of abnormal chylomicron and very low-density lipoprotein (VLDL) remnants. It is probably due to inherited homozygous defects in Apo E-II structure. *(Felig, pp. 1024–1025)*

38. **(E)** Triglycerides are over 150 and are raised by alcohol intake, estrogens, stress, insulin, and physical activity. Cholesterol levels are average or mildly elevated. HDL is usually low. Dietary therapy and the maintenance of ideal weight is the cornerstone of therapy. *(Felig, pp. 1029–1030)*

39. **(B)** Hypertriglyceridemia is usually secondary to DM or drugs, rather than a genetic disorder. It can be a normal response to caloric excess or alcohol ingestion and is common in the third trimester of pregnancy. *(Felig, p. 1027)*

40. **(C)** In DM, there is an obligatory osmotic diuresis, but in DI there is lack of water resorption in the tubules. Both result in polyuria, but in DM, there will be substantial glucosuria as well. The large amount of urine output (usually >50 mL/kg/day) is characteristic of polyuric states, such as DI, not a bladder problem. Psychogenic polydipsia is commonly seen in patients with psychiatric problems on medications. *(Kasper, pp. 2098–2099)*

41. **(D)** In Western societies, most dyslipidemias are secondary. The most common predisposing cause is diet, and the second common is DM. Hypothyroidism, renal disease, alcoholism, and anorexia nervosa are also associated with secondary dyslipidemias. Many drugs (e.g.,

estrogen, glucocorticoids) can also cause secondary dyslipidemias. *(Felig, pp. 1009–1015)*

42. **(D)** The most important factors in diet-induced cholesterol elevation are the amount of total fat and saturated fat consumed. Cholesterol intake is next in importance. Obesity and caloric excess usually result in high triglyceride levels. *(Felig, p. 1010)*

43. **(D)** The elevated ALP and hydroxyproline are diagnostic for Paget's disease. The bony lesions are blastic and the sacrum and pelvis are most frequently involved, followed closely by the tibia and femur. Hypercalcemia can complicate immobilization. The etiology is unknown, but a viral agent has been postulated. Symptoms may be absent or severe (pain, deformity). In metastatic cancers of most types the lesion are lytic, and the other metabolic abnormalities do not have an elevation in hydroxyproline. *(Kasper, pp. 2279–2281)*

44. **(A)** Many affected persons with vitamin D deficiency have no demonstrable abnormality except for hypocalcemia, hypophosphatemia, and increased PTH levels. Decreased calcium absorption, which is vitamin D dependent, results in mild hypocalcemia that leads to the secondary hyperparathyroidism. This in turn results in increased renal phosphate excretion and hypophosphatemia. *(Kasper, p. 2248)*

45. **(B)** Atrial fibrillation and cardiomegaly are common cardiac manifestations, but are more common in the elderly. Other symptoms include palpitations, tachycardia, nervousness, sweating, and dyspnea. Sinus tachycardia is the most common cardiac manifestation in a young individual with hyperthyroidism. *(Kasper, p. 2113)*

46. **(B)** Needle biopsy can be used in numerous diseases, but the main rationale is to differentiate benign from malignant nodules. A thyroid scan is appropriate if the TSH is suppressed suggesting a possible "hot" nodule (hyperfunctioning nodules are very rarely malignant). The specimen must be read by an experienced cytologist. It is difficult to diagnose differentiated follicular carcinoma or to differentiate lymphoma from

Hashimoto's thyroiditis. Papillary carcinoma is the easiest diagnosis to make by needle biopsy. *(Kasper, pp. 2126–2127)*

47. **(E)** Regulation of vasopressin is by osmotic and nonosmotic stimuli such as volume and neural stimuli arising outside the hypothalamus. As little as 15% of cells remaining in the posterior hypothalamus are sufficient to prevent permanent DI. *(Kasper, p. 2097)*

48. **(D)** Classification of hypoglycemia includes spontaneous causes such as reactive or fasting hypoglycemia and pharmacologic or toxic causes. The diagnosis of insulinoma is most certain when Whipple's triad is fulfilled: symptoms consistent with hypoglycemia, low plasma glucose, and relief of symptoms with elevation of plasma glucose to normal. *(Kasper, p. 2227)*

49. **(A)** Cardiac failure and arrhythmias frequently occur in cardiac amyloid. The ECG reveals low-voltage QRS complexes and conduction disturbances. Red cells are not involved, and involvement of the thyroid, liver, and pancreas is usually asymptomatic. The precursors of the AL, amyloid protein found in primary AL and myeloma, are kappa and lambda light chains. Serum amyloid A protein (SAA) is the precursor for the AA amyloid found in secondary AL. *(Kasper, pp. 2024–2029)*

50. **(A)** This person has either fasting or reactive hypoglycemia. Glucagon exerts a marked effect on carbohydrate, fat, and lipid metabolism, and increases cAMP in many tissues. It is the first counterregulatory hormone to respond to hypoglycemia, and it does this by increasing glycogenolysis and gluconeogenesis. Glucagonomas of the pancreas present with features such as mild DM, psychiatric disturbances, diarrhea, venous thromboses, and skin findings (necrolytic migratory erythema). *(Kasper, p. 2180)*

51. **(E)** In mild cases, dietary therapy may suffice, but the vast majority of patients require drug therapy. Statins are clearly the most effective medications available, but the majority of patients will not have optimal cholesterol control, even with maximum doses of a statin.

Homozygous patients always require combination therapy. *(Felig, pp. 1019–1021)*

52. **(C)** Primary hyperparathyroidism develops in over 87% of those with MEN I. Polyendocrine adenomatosis, type I, frequently includes islet cell tumors of the pancreas, leading to the Zollinger-Ellison syndrome, insulinomas, and glucagonomas. Inheritance is via an autosomal dominant pattern. Hypercalcemia does not usually occur until after the first decade. *(Felig, p. 1356)*

53. **(E)** HRT can reduce osteoporosis related fractures. Estrogens cause thickening of vaginal mucosa and can improve urogenital symptoms, and postmenopausal symptoms. The evidence for protection against CAD and dementia is epidemiologic. Randomized trials have failed to show a reduction in CAD risk with HRT. The risk of venothromboembolism and breast cancer is increased not decreased. *(Kasper, pp. 2210–2212)*

54. **(C)** This patient has Cushing's syndrome. The diagnosis is established by demonstrating increased cortisol secretion (24-hour urine cortisol collection) or by failure to suppress AM cortisol levels after overnight dexamethasone administration. Investigations for either adrenal tumor or pituitary adenoma (with CT or MR) are only considered once the diagnosis of Cushing's syndrome is established. *(Kasper, pp. 2134–2135)*

55. **(A)** Growth hormone excess in acromegaly produces hypertrophy of muscle. Initially, strength may be increased, but this is transient, and a third of patients will experience weakness, likely secondary to myopathy. *(Kasper, p. 2090)*

56. **(C)** Vitamin D-resistant rickets is a familial disorder, with an X-linked recessive pattern, treated with pharmacologic doses of vitamin D. Half the affected individuals have alopecia, and this tends to correlate with severity.

Rickets and osteomalacia are characterized by impaired mineralization of bone. Osteoporosis is a disorder with a diminished amount of normally mineralized bone. *(Felig, p. 1186)*

57. (B) Risk of death in anorexia nervosa is also associated with hypothermia, suicide, or pneumonia with emaciation. Because of the danger of ventricular tachyarrhythmias, patients should be followed with ECGs. A prolonged QT interval is a sign of danger. In addition, severe weight loss can lead to both systolic and diastolic dysfunction of the ventricles. *(Kasper, pp. 430–431)*

58. (E) In gouty patients, nephrolithiasis and uric acid nephropathy may occur. The association of cardiovascular disease, hypertension, pyelonephritis, and hyperlipoproteinemia with gout contributes to the high prevalence of renal disease in these individuals. *(Kasper, p. 2046)*

59. (C) Vitamin D levels are decreased in osteomalacia. In severe osteomalacia, there is bowing of the long bones, inward deformity of the long bones, and wide osteoid borders on bone surfaces. Hypocalcemia is characteristic of osteomalacia; however, secondary hyperparathyroidism often raises the serum calcium to low normal levels. The PTH-mediated increase in phosphate clearance often produces hypophosphatemia. *(Kasper, p. 2248)*

60. (B) Hepatorenal syndrome frequently complicates hepatic failure. Although it can develop gradually, acute renal failure can also be precipitated by hemodynamic stresses (bleeding, diuresis). The earliest manifestations are intrarenal vasoconstriction and avid sodium retention. *(Kasper, p. 1867)*

61. (D) In phenylketonuria, a low phenylalanine diet with relentless attention to details of diet is required for a good outcome. The diet should be started by 3 weeks of age. Children of mothers with phenylketonuria can be affected if exposed to phenylalanine in utero. Therefore, women with the disorder should stay on a restricted diet until they complete childbearing. In phenylalanine hydroxylase deficiency, tyrosine becomes an essential amino acid and dietary supplements must be provided. *(Kasper, p. 2333)*

62. (B) Wilson's disease includes cirrhosis of the liver, signs of basal ganglia disease, and a brownish pigmented ring at the corneal margin (Kayser-Fleischer ring). Ceruloplasmin levels are low. The gene for Wilson's disease is located on the long arm of chromosome 13. In some cases, it is possible to identify carrier states and make prenatal diagnoses. The relationship between the abnormal gene and the metabolic defect (inability to regulate copper balance) is unclear. *(Kasper, p. 2314)*

63. (C) The gold standard is still a fasting plasma glucose = 7 mmol/L (126 mg/dL) on two separate occasions. GTTs are rarely required. With typical symptoms even an elevated random sugar is diagnostic. *(Felig, p. 857)*

64. (A) Other stimulators of protein kinases include platelet-derived growth factor and epidermal growth factor. Tyrosine phosphorylation results from this interaction. Insulin-resistant states can be caused by prereceptor resistance (mutated insulin, anti-insulin antibodies) or receptor and postreceptor resistance. *(Kasper, p. 2155)*

65. (C) The action of insulin involves all three major metabolic fuels (carbohydrate, protein, fat). It is active in liver, muscle, and adipose tissue. In each there are anticatabolic as well as anabolic effects. These tend to reinforce each other. *(Felig, p. 835)*

66. (D) Infection or other acute medical condition is the usual precipitant for thyroid storm. Radioactive iodine treatment or abrupt withdrawal of antithyroid medications is also implicated. The key diagnostic features are fever, tachycardia, and central nervous system dysfunction. *(Felig, pp. 309–310)*

67. (B) All the causes listed may delay puberty, but the most common cause by far is normal variation in growth pattern. There is often a family history of delayed puberty in parents or siblings. In these individuals, bone age often correlates better with the onset and progression of puberty than does chronologic age. *(Felig, p. 678)*

68. **(D)** Approximately, one-third of unselected women with metastatic breast cancer will respond to tamoxifen. Presence of estrogen receptors (ER) or PR improves the likelihood of response. If the tumor is both ER and PR positive, the response rate is 70%. *(Felig, p. 1441)*

69. **(B)** A generally increased risk of breast cancer is associated with nulliparity, late first pregnancy, and, especially, a history of maternal breast cancer. Prior history of breast cancer is of course a powerful risk factor. *(Felig, p. 1439)*

70. **(D)** Although the variation is great depending on occupation, hobbies, and so forth, generally only one-third of energy is utilized for physical activity. Height is not used at all in calculating RMR, and RMR is higher in men than in women of identical weight. Amino acids ingested without other energy sources are inefficiently incorporated into protein. Current recommendations are to encourage full adult levels of protein, vitamins, and minerals in the elderly. *(Kasper, pp. 399–403)*

71. **(C)** The diagnosis is secondary hyperparathyroidism as a consequence of the chronic renal disease. Calcium deposits are seen in the periarticular areas of the fourth and fifth metacarpophalangeal, third proximal interphalangeal, and fourth distal interphalangeal joints. There is slight soft tissue swelling, especially, of the fourth and fifth metacarpophalangeal joints. Calcification in scleroderma is subcutaneous in location. In gout, if monosodium urate is deposited it could appear as a soft tissue mass. *(Kasper, p. 1656)*

72. **(B)** Autonomous adrenal tumors are adrenocorticotropic hormone (ACTH) insensitive and fail to demonstrate a brisk rise in urinary 17-hydroxycorticoids. Androgenic effects, such as hirsutism, are usually absent. In Cushing's syndrome, secondary to an autonomous adrenal tumor, onset is usually gradual, and hirsutism,

other androgenic effects, and hyperpigmentation are absent. *(Felig, pp. 2135–2136)*

73. **(A)** DM is a syndrome consisting of hyperglycemia, large vessel disease, microvascular disease, and neuropathy. The classic presenting symptoms are increased thirst, polyuria, polyphagia, and weight loss. In Type II diabetes, the presentation can be more subtle and is often made when the patient is asymptomatic. *(Felig, p. 856)*

74. **(I)** Pyoderma gangrenosum is not a cutaneous manifestation of diabetes. Perineal pruritus in a diabetic is almost always associated with *Candida albicans*. A severe external otitis can occur in older patients. It is caused by *Pseudomonas aeruginosa* and is characterized by ear pain, drainage, fever, and leukocytosis. Facial nerve paralysis can occur and is a poor prognostic sign. Necrobiosis lipoidica is a plaque-like lesion with a brown border and yellow center usually found on the anterior leg surface. *(Kasper, p. 2169)*

75. **(A, C, E)** Background retinopathy is present in about 90% of diabetes after 25–30 years of disease. Microaneurysms, dilated veins, dot and blot hemorrhages, cotton wool spots, and hard exudates are common findings. *(Kasper, p. 2163)*

76. **(B, D)** Proliferative retinopathy carries a high risk of vitreous hemorrhage, scarring, retinal detachment, and blindness. Proliferative retinopathy is associated with nephropathy and CAD, and is associated with a poor prognosis, for life as well as for vision. *(Kasper, pp. 2163–2164)*

77. **(B)** High prolactin level suppresses luteinizing hormone-releasing hormone (LH-RH), and can result in low plasma gonadotropin and testosterone levels. It may not be obvious on physical examination. Therapy with a dopamine agonist may lower prolactin levels and reverse impotence. *(Kasper, pp. 271–274)*

78. **(D)** An absent orgasm, when libido and erectile function are normal, invariably indicates that organic disease is absent. Loss of desire can

also be caused by psychologic disturbance, but may indicate androgen deficiency or drug effect. *(Kasper, pp. 271–274)*

79. **(E)** Failure of detumescence—priapism—can be caused by sickle cell anemia or chronic granulocytic leukemia. Priapism must be treated promptly to preserve future erectile functioning. *(Kasper, p. 272)*

80. **(B)** Vascular disease, by itself or in conjunction with peripheral neuropathy in DM, is a common cause of erectile dysfunction. The lesions can be in large vessels (aortic occlusion, Leriche syndrome), small arteries, or even in the sinusoidal spaces. *(Kasper, pp. 271–274)*

81. **(E)** Idiopathic hirsutism may simply represent an extreme of normal androgen production. It is diagnosed by demonstrating minimal elevation of androgens and exclusion of other causes. Management is primarily by cosmetic therapy, although drugs to suppress androgen production and/or androgen effects on the hair follicle can be used. *(Kasper, pp. 275–278)*

82. **(C)** The most severe form of PCOD, Stein-Leventhal syndrome, is associated with chronic anovulation, hirsutism, enlarged cystic ovaries, obesity, and amenorrhea. The spectrum of disease, however, is quite wide, and some patients have only mild hirsutism. *(Kasper, pp. 275–277)*

83. **(F)** Krukenberg's tumors of the ovary stimulate surrounding ovarian stromal tissue to produce excess androgen. When onset of hair growth (with or without frank virilization) is very rapid, a neoplastic source of androgen is suggested. As well as ovarian tumors, the potential neoplasms include adenomas and carcinomas of the adrenal gland. *(Kasper, pp. 275–278)*

84. **(D)** Attenuated forms of adrenal hyperplasia can present with hirsutism at puberty or in adulthood. Elevated levels of a precursor of cortisol biosynthesis such as 17-hydroxyprogesterone, 17-hydroxypregnenolone, or 11-deoxycortisol can present. ACTH infusion will increase the precursor level, and dexamethasone will suppress it. *(Kasper, pp. 275–278)*

85. **(A)** Salivary gland enlargement occurs both in anorexia nervosa (AN) and bulimia (BN). Other common findings in AN include constipation, bradycardia, hypotension, hypercarotinemia, and soft downy hair growth (lanugo). Menses are usually absent. *(Kasper, p. 430)*

86. **(D)** Hyperglycemia is not seen in eating disorders, and would suggest an alternate diagnosis for the weight loss such as diabetes. Hypoglycemia and low estrogens and gonadotropins are frequently seen in anorexia nervosa (AN). BUN and creatinine may be elevated. Hypochloremia, hypokalemia, and alkalosis are frequently seen in BN. *(Kasper, p. 430)*

87. **(E)** Low QRS voltages, sinus bradycardia, and ST-T changes are common. However, the presence of a prolonged QT interval is most suggestive of serious cardiac arrhythmias. *(Kasper, p. 431)*

88. **(B)** Hospitalization should be considered when the body weight dips below 75% of the expected. The goal is to achieve a weight of 90% of that expected. Vomiting is more characteristic of bulimia than anorexia nervosa (AN). *(Kasper, p. 432)*

89. **(B)** Recurrent vomiting and exposure of the teeth to stomach acid leads to loss of dental enamel and eventual chipping and erosion of the teeth. The vomiting may be manually induced, but eventually most patients with bulimia (BN) are able to trigger vomiting at will. *(Kasper, p. 433)*

90. **(C)** The patient is most likely to develop glomerulosclerosis. This can be diffuse or nodular (Kimmelstiel-Wilson nodules). Poor metabolic control is probably a major factor in the progression of diabetic nephropathy. *(Felig, pp. 900–901)*

91. **(B)** AN has one of the highest mortality rates of any psychiatric illness at 5% per decade. The mortality for BN is very low, and 50% have a full recovery within 10 years. Only 25% have persistent symptoms of BN over many years,

and the disease does not usually progress to AN. *(Kasper, pp. 431–433)*

92. **(I)** Low fiber diets are frequently prescribed during flares of inflammatory bowel disease to reduce diarrhea and pain. There is no level 1 evidence to support this practice. Similar diets are often prescribed for diverticulitis or other conditions associated with a narrowed or stenosed colon. It may be prescribed for patients with a new ostomy. When acute symptoms subside, however, restrictions concerning dietary fiber should be stopped. *(Kasper, p. 1786)*

93. **(A)** Restricting caloric intake and weight reduction are important components of the medical nutrition therapy for patients with diabetes. Most patients should be referred to a dietician to help construct a diet appropriate in caloric intake. *(Kasper, p. 2171)*

94. **(C)** Some patients with hypertension are salt sensitive, and will lower their blood pressure with salt restriction. Low sodium diets are also recommended in patients with congestive heart failure (CHF), ascites, or chronic renal failure. *(Kasper, p. 1472)*

95. **(F)** After gastrectomy, avoiding simple sugars and limiting liquids can ameliorate symptoms of dumping. Early dumping occurs within 30 minutes of eating and is characterized by vasomotor symptoms such as palpitations, tachycardia, lightheadedness, and diaphoresis. Late dumping includes similar symptoms plus dizziness, confusion, and even syncope. It occurs 1.2–3 hours after eating. *(Kasper, p. 1757)*

96. **(H)** The symptoms of hepatic encephalopathy are improved with protein restriction and a bowel elimination routine with lactulose. It is presumed that this results in lower levels of serum ammonia, but other substances in the serum may be implicated. These include mercaptans, short-chain fatty acids, and phenol. Gamma-aminobutyric acid (GABA) levels in the brain are also increased. Chronic encephalopathy can be controlled with restricting protein intake and taking lactulose (osmotic laxative).

Restricting daytime protein intake in patients with Parkinson's disease may improve the efficacy of levodopa therapy. *(Kasper, p. 1868)*

97. **(E)** Chocolate, ethanol, caffeine, and tobacco decrease lower esophageal sphincter pressure. Other effective treatments for GERD include low fat diet, weight loss, avoiding bedtime snacks, and elevating the head of the bed while sleeping. *(Kasper, pp. 1742–1743)*

98. **(D)** Scurvy is characterized by a tendency to hemorrhage and perifollicular hyperkeratotic papules in which hairs become fragmented and buried. Gums are involved only if teeth are present. It can occur in infants 6–12 months of age who are on processed milk formulas, without citrus fruit or vegetable supplementation. The peak incidence in the United States is in poor and elderly people and alcoholics. It is frequently associated with other nutritional deficiencies (e.g., folic acid). *(Kasper, pp. 406–407)*

99. **(E)** Excessive vitamin A ingestion can cause abdominal pain, nausea, vomiting, headache, dizziness, and papilledema. Deficiency of vitamin A can cause night blindness and progress to visual loss. It is common in children in developing countries and is a major cause of blindness. *(Kasper, p. 408)*

100. **(A)** Pharmacologic doses of niacin for hypercholesterolemia may cause histamine release, which results in flushing, pruritus, and GI disturbance. Asthma may be aggravated, acanthosis nigricans can occur, and in high doses, elevation of uric acid and fasting blood sugar can occur. Hepatic toxicity, including cholestatic jaundice, has been described with large doses. *(Kasper, p. 405)*

101. **(B)** Thiamine deficiency can cause high-output cardiac failure (wet beriberi) or neurologic symptoms (dry beriberi). In North America, thiamine deficiency occurs in alcoholics or those with chronic disease. In alcoholics, deficiency is secondary to low intake, impaired absorption and storage, and accelerated destruction. Genetic factors are important as clinical manifestations

occur only in a small proportion of chronically malnourished individuals. Beriberi heart disease is characterized by peripheral vasodilatation, sodium and water retention, and high-output CHF. *(Kasper, p. 403)*

102. **(A)** Diarrhea, dementia, and dermatitis are the classic triad for pellagra (niacin deficiency).

The diagnosis is based on clinical suspicion and response to therapy, and can be confirmed by demonstrating low levels of the urinary metabolites 2-methylnicotinamide and 2-pyridone. Small doses of niacin (10 mg/day) with adequate dietary tryptophan will cure pellagra secondary to nutritional deficiency. *(Kasper, p. 405)*

Gastroenterology
Questions

Questions 1 through 6

    (A) polypoid adenoma
    (B) leiomyoma
    (C) lipoma
    (D) adenocarcinoma
    (E) primary gastrointestinal (GI) lymphoma
    (F) carcinoid tumor

For each patient with a small bowel tumor, select the most likely diagnosis.

1. A 56-year-old woman presents with weight loss and watery diarrhea. She also notices periumbilical pain and bloating after eating. A small bowel x-ray reveals an area of narrowing and the lesion is surgically resected. The pathology report shows this to be the most common endocrine tumor of the GI tract. (SELECT ONE)

2. A 72-year-old man is investigated for iron deficiency anemia. There is no clinical history of upper or lower GI bleeding, but his stools are fecal occult blood positive. His colonoscopy is negative for any obvious sources of bleeding, but upper endoscopy reveals ulceration in the distal duodenum that is biopsied. The pathology report shows this to be the most common primary malignancy of the small bowel. (SELECT ONE)

3. A 23-year-old man of Middle Eastern decent is investigated for symptoms of chronic diarrhea, vomiting, and abdominal cramps. He has lost 20 lb and appears unwell. A small bowel x-ray shows diffuse nonspecific mucosal abnormality. Upper endoscopy is performed to visualize the small bowel and obtain biopsies. The pathology report identifies the mucosal abnormality as "immunoproliferative small intestinal disease" (IPSID). This form of small bowel tumor can be treated with antibiotics in its early stages. (SELECT ONE)

4. A 21-year-old woman develops acute periumbilical pain that localizes to the right lower quadrant. She appears unwell, and on examination, there is tenderness and guarding in the right lower quadrant. A pregnancy test is negative and a pelvic examination rules out pelvic inflammatory disease. A clinical diagnosis of acute appendicitis is made and she has an uncomplicated laparoscopic appendectomy. The pathology report notes acute inflammation and a tumor for which the appendix is a very common site of involvement. (SELECT ONE)

5. A 57-year-old woman with a 20-year history of celiac disease now presents with weight loss, cramps, and abdominal discomfort. She is adherent to her gluten-free diet, and is not taking any new medications. On examination, her abdomen is soft and there is fullness in the right lower quadrant. A small bowel x-ray reveals an area of narrowing in the distal ileum, and there is thickening and nodularity of the mucosal folds. She undergoes surgical resection of the lesion, and the pathology report confirms a tumor that is more common in patients with celiac disease, Crohn's disease, or depressed immune function such as human immunodeficiency virus (HIV). (SELECT ONE)

6. A 48-year-old man presents with periumbilical pain made worse by eating and weight loss. A small bowel x-ray reveals an area of narrowing in the distal ileum. The differential diagnosis includes tumors that most commonly involve the distal part of the small bowel. (SELECT TWO)

Questions 7 through 10

(A) celiac sprue
(B) gastrinoma
(C) associated with decrease in pancreatic enzymes
(D) hyperthyroidism
(E) regional enteritis
(F) associated arthritis
(G) associated with skin pigmentation
(H) increase in pancreatic enzymes
(I) hypersensitivity reaction
(J) an infectious agent
(K) may present with iron deficiency
(L) associated with skin disease

For each patient with GI symptoms, select the possible diagnoses and associated findings.

7. A 29-year-old woman has recently developed milk intolerance. (SELECT TWO)

8. A 19-year-old man has a long history of weight loss, abdominal distention, bloating, and diarrhea. Investigation reveals steatorrhea, and a small bowel biopsy reveals blunting and flattening of villi. (SELECT FOUR)

9. A 53-year-old man presents with weight loss, low-grade fever, and peripheral lymphadenopathy. Steatorrhea is documented, and small bowel biopsy reveals para-aminosalicylic acid (PAS) positive macrophages. (SELECT TWO)

10. A 43-year-old woman has had a 10-year history of severe and recurrent peptic ulcer disease (PUD) that is refractory to medical therapy. She has had ulcers at multiple sites of the small bowel including the distal duodenum and jejunum. She also has chronic diarrhea, but not enough fat to make the diagnosis of steatorrhea. Evaluation for *Helicobacter pylori* infection is negative. (SELECT ONE)

DIRECTIONS (Questions 11 through 37): Each of the numbered items in this section is followed by answers. Select the ONE lettered answer that is BEST in each case.

11. A 79-year-old woman with severe constipation is found to have multiple diverticuli on colonoscopy. Which of the following is the most appropriate next step in management?

(A) stool softeners
(B) prophylactic surgery
(C) phenolphthalein laxatives
(D) increasing dietary fiber
(E) psychotherapy

12. A 77-year-old woman is brought to the emergency room because of nonspecific abdominal discomfort. She has no anorexia, fever, chills, or weight loss. Her abdomen is soft and nontender on physical examination. Abdominal x-rays show lots of stool in the colon, but no free air or air-fluid levels. The amylase is 150 U/L (25–125 U/L), and the rest of her biochemistry and complete blood count are normal. Which of the following conditions can cause a false-positive elevation in the serum amylase?

(A) maturity-onset diabetes mellitus (DM)
(B) gastric ulcer

(C) renal failure

(D) sulfonamide therapy

(E) gastric carcinoma

13. A 71-year-old man develops progressive weight loss and dysphagia over a 3-month period. Upper endoscopy and biopsy of the lesion confirm esophageal cancer. Which of the following statements regarding this cancer is most likely correct?

(A) is very responsive to chemotherapy

(B) is more common in females

(C) has a 5-year cure rate of 20%

(D) may be either adenocarcinoma or squamous cell carcinoma

(E) is characterized by significant complications from hemorrhage

14. A 23-year-old woman presents with weight loss and chronic diarrhea. She appears unwell and cachectic. Routine laboratory tests reveal a low hemoglobin level and an increased international normalized ratio (INR) even though she is not taking any anticoagulants. The liver enzymes are normal, but the albumin and calcium levels are low, suggesting generalized malnutrition. Which of the following is the most appropriate initial diagnostic test for malabsorption?

(A) xylose absorption

(B) Schilling test

(C) x-ray studies

(D) stool fat quantitation

(E) small intestinal biopsy

15. A 33-year-old man has never been vaccinated for hepatitis B. Serologic tests reveal negative hepatitis B surface antigen (HBsAg) and positive antibody to surface antigen. Which of the following conditions does this serologic pattern best fit with?

(A) previous hepatitis B infection

(B) chronic active hepatitis

(C) acute hepatitis B infection

(D) poor prognosis

(E) need for vaccine to hepatitis B

16. A 29-year-old woman is found, on routine annual blood testing, to have an increase in unconjugated bilirubin. There is no evidence of hemolysis and liver tests are otherwise normal. Which of the following is the most likely diagnosis?

(A) Crigler-Najjar syndrome

(B) Dubin-Johnson syndrome

(C) Rotor's syndrome

(D) Gilbert's syndrome

(E) pregnanediol therapy

17. An 18-year-old woman was diagnosed 7 years earlier with precocious pseudopuberty secondary to ovarian tumor. Physical examination reveals oral and lingual dark pigmentation. Which of the following is the most likely diagnosis?

(A) Peutz-Jeghers syndrome

(B) Gardner's syndrome

(C) Lynch syndrome

(D) juvenile polyposis

(E) Turcot's syndrome

18. A 63-year-old man has stools positive for occult blood. Which of the following is the most likely location of bowel cancer?

(A) cecum

(B) sigmoid

(C) transverse colon

(D) appendix

(E) ascending colon

19. A 74-year-old man underwent some type of peptic ulcer surgery years ago. He has symptoms that include abdominal pain and bloating about 30–40 minutes after eating, accompanied by nausea. If he vomits, the symptoms are relieved. Which of the following is the most likely cause for his symptoms?

(A) early dumping syndrome

(B) late dumping syndrome

(C) bile reflux gastropathy

(D) retained gastric antrum

(E) afferent loop syndrome

20. A 29-year-old man with acquired immune deficiency syndrome (AIDS) comes to the emergency department because of progressively increasing abdominal discomfort. Examination shows voluntary guarding in the upper abdomen. His biochemistry is normal except for an elevated amylase at 370 U/L (25–125 U/L). Which of the following infections can trigger this disorder in AIDS patients?

(A) toxoplasmosis
(B) *Mycobacterium avium* complex
(C) *Mycobacterium tuberculosis*
(D) *Pneumocystis carinii*
(E) herpes virus

21. A 55-year-old man from China is known to have chronic liver disease, secondary to hepatitis B infection. He has recently felt unwell, and his hemoglobin level has increased from 130 g/L, 1 year ago, to 195 g/L. Which of the following is the most appropriate initial diagnostic test?

(A) alkaline phosphatase
(B) alpha-fetoprotein (AFP)
(C) aspartate transaminase (AST)
(D) alanine transaminase (ALT)
(E) unconjugated bilirubin

22. A 63-year-old man with a long history of alcohol abuse presents with ascites. He is experiencing mild abdominal discomfort and nausea. Examination reveals tense ascites and generalized tenderness but no rigidity. A diagnostic paracentesis of the fluid is performed. Which of the following ascitic fluid results is most likely to suggest an uncomplicated ascites due to portal hypertension from cirrhosis?

(A) hemorrhage
(B) protein >25 g/L
(C) bilirubin level twice that of serum
(D) serum to ascites albumin gradient >1.1 g/dL
(E) more than 1000 white cells/mm^3

23. A 64-year-old woman develops sudden-onset abdominal discomfort after eating a large meal. The pain is constant, localizes to the epigastric area with radiation to her right scapula. She also has nausea and vomiting. It eventual subsides 1 hour later. An ultrasound of the abdomen reveals a dilated common bile duct secondary to stones. Which of the following statements regarding common bile duct stones is most likely true?

(A) all originate in the gallbladder
(B) always produce jaundice
(C) produce constant level of jaundice
(D) can be painless
(E) indicate anomalies of the bile duct

24. A 53-year-old man presents with diarrhea. He also complains of facial flushing lasting minutes at a time. Physical examination reveals facial telangiectasias and a heart murmur not present 2 years before. This murmur is accentuated by deep breathing. Which of the following is the most appropriate initial diagnostic test?

(A) urinary vanillylmandelic acid (VMA)
(B) serum noradrenaline levels
(C) barium enema
(D) serum serotonin levels
(E) urinary 5-hydroxyindolacetic acid (5-HIAA)

25. A 29-year-old woman complains of dysphagia with both solids and liquids, worse when she is eating quickly or is anxious. Manometry reveals normal basal esophageal sphincter pressure, with no relaxation of the sphincter on swallowing. Which of the following is the most appropriate next step in management?

(A) beta-blocker therapy
(B) partial esophagectomy
(C) anticholinergic drugs
(D) calcium channel blockers
(E) dietary modification

26. A 34-year-old woman complains bitterly of heartburn. Physical examination reveals healing lesions of the fingertips that she says were small ulcers, and there are small areas of telangiectasias on her face. Esophageal manometry reveals a decrease in the expected amplitude of smooth muscle contraction. Lower esophageal sphincter tone is subnormal, but relaxes normally with swallowing. Which of the following statements regarding this condition is most likely correct?

(A) characterized by systemic signs of inflammation

(B) predominantly treated symptomatically

(C) characterized by a poor prognosis

(D) usually more frequent in men

(E) characterized by death secondary to a renal crisis

27. A 59-year-old man presents with abdominal pain, anorexia, and nausea. He has lost weight and started to develop pedal edema. Endoscopy reveals large gastric mucosal folds. Which of the following explanations for the edema is most likely correct?

(A) hypoalbuminemia secondary to malnutrition

(B) hypoalbuminemia secondary to protein loss

(C) impaired hepatic synthesis of albumin

(D) humorally mediated cardiac disease

(E) constrictive pericarditis

28. A 35-year-old White man has a long past history of diarrhea, rectal bleeding, crampy abdominal pain, and the passage of mucus. He now presents with a worsening of his symptoms despite taking his medications. A barium enema is performed and is shown in Fig. 4–1. Which of the following is the most likely diagnosis of this new complication?

(A) toxic megacolon

(B) amoebic colitis

(C) appendicitis

(D) ischemic colitis

(E) annular carcinoma

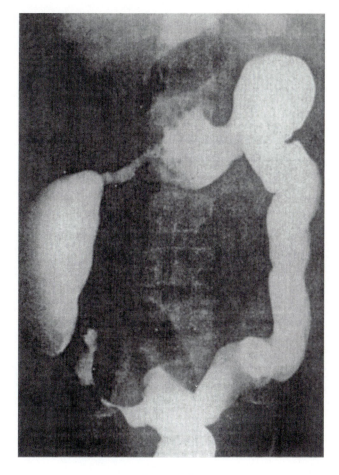

Figure 4–1.

29. A 45-year-old man with a long history of alcohol intake comes into the emergency room with upper gastrointestinal (UGI) bleeding. Urgent endoscopy reveals the following findings (Fig. 4–2). Which of the following is the most likely diagnosis?

    (A) esophageal varices
    (B) esophageal carcinoma
    (C) foreign body
    (D) tertiary waves
    (E) Barrett's esophagus

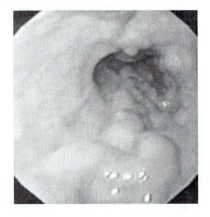

Figure 4–2.

30. A 33-year-old woman develops mild epigastric abdominal pain with nausea and vomiting of 2 days duration. Her abdomen is tender on palpation in the epigastric region, and the remaining examination is normal. Her white count is 13,000/mL, and amylase is 300 U/L (25–125 U/L). Which of the following is the most common predisposing factor for this disorder?

    (A) drugs
    (B) gallstones
    (C) malignancy
    (D) alcohol
    (E) hypertriglyceridemia

31. A 40-year-old taxicab driver presents with worsening epigastric pain (Fig. 4–3). Which of the following is the most likely diagnosis?

    (A) gastric ulcer
    (B) achalasia

    (C) duodenal ulcer
    (D) normal
    (E) hiatus hernia

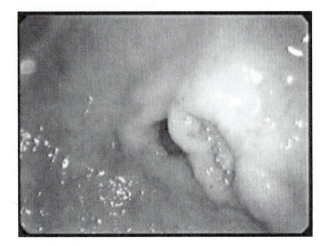

Figure 4–3.

32. A 54-year-old man complains of burning epigastric pain that usually improves after a meal, and is occasionally relieved with antacids. On examination, he appears well and besides some epigastric tenderness on palpation, the rest of the examination is normal. Upper endoscopy confirms a duodenal ulcer. Which of the following statements concerning PUD is most likely correct?

    (A) duodenal ulcer is seen more often in older people than is gastric ulcer
    (B) clinically, gastric ulcers are more common than duodenal ulcers
    (C) duodenal ulcers can frequently be malignant
    (D) infection can cause both types of peptic ulcer
    (E) peptic gastric ulcers are usually quite proximal in the stomach

33. A 30-year-old man complains of chronic diarrhea for the past 6 months. There is no weight loss, fever, or abdominal pain. He takes no medications and feels fine. His physical examination is completely normal. Further history reveals that this man does not take laxatives; however, in an effort to stay slim he eats a lot of sugar-free

gum and sugarless candy. Which of the following explanations is the most likely cause of his diarrhea?

(A) direct stimulant effect of chemicals in the candies
(B) lack of fiber in his diet
(C) pancreatic insufficiency secondary to chronic protein-calorie malnutrition
(D) secondary intestinal mucosal atrophy
(E) nonabsorbed carbohydrates

34. Which of the following is a risk factor for *Helicobacter pylori* infection?

(A) excess exposure to antibiotics
(B) female sex
(C) alpha1-antitrypsin deficiency
(D) low socioeconomic indicators
(E) proton pump inhibitor therapy

35. Which of the following is an established risk factor for nonsteroidal anti-inflammatory disease (NSAID)-induced gastric or duodenal ulceration?

(A) *Helicobacter pylori* infection
(B) cigarette smoking
(C) alcohol consumption
(D) glucocorticoids
(E) age under 30

36. A 73-year-old woman presents to the emergency room with black tarry stools and symptoms of presyncope when standing up. Digital rectal examination confirms the presence of melena. She recently started using ibuprofen for hip discomfort. Upper endoscopy confirms the diagnosis of a gastric ulcer. Which of the following is the most likely explanation for the gastric ulcer?

(A) increasing acid production
(B) causing direct epithelial cell death
(C) promoting replication of *Helicobacter pylori*
(D) an antiplatelet effect
(E) inhibiting mucosal repair

37. A 52-year-old woman is experiencing abdominal discomfort after meals as well as early in the morning. There is no weight loss or constitutional symptoms, and she has tried antacids but experienced minimal relief. Upper endoscopy reveals a duodenal ulcer and the biopsy is negative for malignancy. Which of the following is the most appropriate next step in management?

(A) 6–8 weeks of omeprazole or ranitidine
(B) long-term acid suppression with omeprazole
(C) antibiotic therapy
(D) antibiotic therapy with omeprazole
(E) bismuth citrate therapy

DIRECTIONS (Questions 38 through 45): Each set of matching questions in this section consists of a list of lettered options followed by several numbered items. For each numbered item, select the appropriate lettered option(s). Each lettered option may be selected once, more than once, or not at all. EACH ITEM WILL STATE THE NUMBER OF OPTIONS TO SELECT. CHOOSE EXACTLY THIS NUMBER.

(A) hepatitis A virus
(B) hepatitis B virus
(C) hepatitis C virus
(D) hepatitis D virus
(E) hepatitis E virus

For each patient with viral hepatitis, select the most likely viral agents.

38. A 24-year-old man develops acute onset of anorexia, nausea, and vomiting. This is followed by clinical jaundice and right upper quadrant discomfort 1 week later. Four weeks ago, he was traveling in South America, where he ate food from street vendors. He also had unprotected sex with a new partner while there. On examination, he is icteric with right upper quadrant tenderness but the rest of the examination is normal. His hepatitis serology is positive for an agent that could have been prevented with vaccination. (SELECT TWO)

39. A couple returns from a trip to Central America and develops nonspecific abdominal symptoms followed by clinical jaundice. They stayed at a resort, and ate fresh fruits and salads. Serology for hepatitis virus spread by the fecal-oral route is positive. (SELECT TWO)

40. A 23-year old sex trade worker develops acute-onset jaundice and seeks medical attention. There is no history of intravenous drug use or travel. On examination, she is icteric, there is no lymphadenopathy, and the heart and lungs are normal. Her liver span is 14 cm and the liver edge is smooth but tender. Her pelvic examination is normal. Serology for viral hepatitis transmitted via the sexual route is positive. (SELECT TWO)

41. A 34-year-old man is seen for asymptomatic elevations in his AST and ALT. He appears well and the physical examination is normal. There is no prior history of intravenous drug use, blood transfusions, or multiple sex partners. His hepatitis serology is positive for the virus, most likely to lead to chronic infection. (SELECT ONE)

42. A 45-year-old woman is evaluated for chronic elevations in her liver enzymes (AST and ALT). She feels well and her physical examination is normal. Nonviral etiologies, such as medications and autoimmune conditions, are ruled out. Her serology is positive for the hepatitis virus that can respond to specific antiviral therapy. (SELECT TWO)

43. A 24-year-old woman is pregnant with her first baby at 14 weeks. She feels well and the pregnancy is noncomplicated. Routine screening is positive for chronic viral hepatitis for which perinatal transmission is of major epidemiologic significance. (SELECT ONE)

44. A 38-year-old woman is worried about a recent potential exposure to an individual with active viral hepatitis. She is seeking treatment for viral hepatitis for which passive immunotherapy can provide some protection. (SELECT TWO)

45. A 28-year-old man, who emigrated from North Africa, is evaluated for chronic elevations in liver enzymes (AST and ALT). He has no symptoms of acute hepatitis, and his physical examination is normal with no characteristics of chronic liver disease. His hepatitis serology is positive for a virus that requires presence of another infectious agent before becoming clinically apparent. (SELECT ONE)

DIRECTIONS (Questions 46 through 71): Each of the numbered items or incomplete statements in this section is followed by answers or by completions of the statement. Select the ONE lettered answer or completion that is BEST in each case.

46. A 53-year-old man presents to the emergency department with severe epigastric abdominal pain. His temperature is 37.2°C, blood pressure 110/70 mm Hg, pulse 110/min, and respirations 20/min. Examination of the heart and lungs is normal, and his abdomen is tender in the epigastric region. His white count is 15,000/mL and amylase is 450 U/L (25–125 U/L). Which of the following laboratory abnormalities is also most likely to be present?

    (A) hypoglycemia
    (B) hypercholesterolemia
    (C) hyperglycemia
    (D) hypercalcemia
    (E) hypercarbia

47. A 43-year-old man feels vaguely unwell. Physical examination is unremarkable except for evidence of scleral icterus. The skin appears normal. Which of the following is the most likely explanation for why early jaundice is visible in the eyes but not the skin?

    (A) the high type II collagen content of scleral tissue
    (B) the high elastin content of scleral tissue
    (C) the high blood flow to the head with consequent increased bilirubin delivery
    (D) secretion via the lacrimal glands
    (E) the lighter color of the sclera

48. A 25-year-old previously healthy man experiences fatigue and malaise. One week ago he had a "viral"-type illness consisting of a sore throat, fever, and myalgias. He now appears jaundiced, but the rest of the physical examination is normal. His investigations reveal a total bilirubin of 4 mg/dL (0.1–1.0 mg/dL) and a direct bilirubin of 0.3 mg/dL (0.0–0.3 mg/dL). Which of the following is the most likely diagnosis?

    (A) hemolysis
    (B) gallstones
    (C) alcoholic liver disease
    (D) pancreatic carcinoma
    (E) Dubin-Johnson syndrome

49. Which of the following is most likely to cause protein-losing enteropathy?

    (A) scleroderma
    (B) amyloidosis
    (C) disaccharidase deficiency
    (D) ischemic colitis
    (E) Ménétrier's disease

50. A 28-year-old man presents with symptoms of frequent bowel movements, crampy abdominal pain, and the passage of mucus. There is no history of any bloody diarrhea, but recently, he developed joint discomfort in his hands, knees, and back. On examination he is thin, and his abdomen is soft with voluntary guarding in the left lower quadrant. His joints are not actively inflamed and there is an asymmetric distribution. Which of the following is the most likely diagnosis?

    (A) lymphoma of the bowel
    (B) amyloid infiltration
    (C) chronic pancreatitis
    (D) ulcerative colitis
    (E) tropical sprue

51. A 57-year-old man, recently discharged from the hospital, develops severe diarrhea and abdominal pain. Sigmoidoscopy reveals a granular friable mucosa. Which of the following is the most common cause of this syndrome?

    (A) ischemic colitis
    (B) rotavirus
    (C) *Clostridium perfringens* infection
    (D) cephalosporin therapy
    (E) bacterial invasion of the bowel wall

52. A 42-year-old previously well woman presents with pruritus. She is not taking any medications, and only drinks alcohol on a social basis. Her physical examination is entirely normal with no signs of chronic liver disease or jaundice. Laboratory evaluation reveals an alkaline phosphatase level of three times normal, and an ultrasound of the liver and gallbladder is normal. Which of the following is the most appropriate next step in diagnosis?

    (A) INR or prothrombin time
    (B) antinuclear antibodies
    (C) protein immunoelectrophoresis
    (D) abdominal ultrasound
    (E) antimitochondrial antibodies

53. A 53-year-old man has weight loss, chronic diarrhea, and steatorrhea. He undergoes diagnostic investigations including small bowel biopsies. The biopsy report reveals normal small bowel mucosa. Which of the following is the most likely diagnosis?

    (A) tropical sprue
    (B) postgastrectomy steatorrhea
    (C) Whipple's disease
    (D) nontropical sprue
    (E) abetalipoproteinemia

54. A 22-year-old man with inflammatory bowel disease is noted to have a "string sign" in the ileal area on barium enema. In which of the following conditions is this sign most often seen? (See Fig. 4–4.)

    (A) in the stenotic or nonstenotic phase of the disease
    (B) in the stenotic phase only
    (C) as a rigid, nondistensible phenomenon
    (D) with gastric involvement
    (E) with rectal involvement

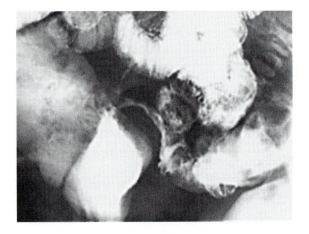

Figure 4–4.

55. A 22-year-old woman presents with chronic diarrhea. She has no abdominal discomfort, feels well, and reports no weight loss or systemic symptoms. Physical examination reveals a healthy young woman who is 5'7" tall and weighs 150 lb. The complete physical examination is normal. Which of the following is the most likely cause of a secretory diarrhea in this young woman?

    (A) surreptitious use of stimulant laxatives
    (B) carcinoid tumor
    (C) ulcerative colitis
    (D) lactose deficiency
    (E) celiac disease

56. A 59-year-old man presents with abdominal distention and a decrease in bowel movements. He has had previous abdominal surgery. Which of the following findings is most likely to favor large bowel obstruction over small bowel obstruction?

    (A) milder degree of pain
    (B) temperature 103.1°F
    (C) stepladder pattern and air-fluid levels on abdominal films
    (D) bile in the vomitus
    (E) hiccups

57. A 57-year old man comes to the office with a complaint of food "sticking on the way down." Which of the following characteristics suggests a benign problem is causing the dysphagia?

    (A) severe weight loss in comparison to the degree of dysphagia
    (B) hoarseness following the onset of dysphagia
    (C) episodic dysphagia for several years
    (D) difficulty only with solids
    (E) hiccups

58. A 70-year-old man is investigated for symptoms of dysphagia with solids, but not with liquids. There is no history of weight loss, and his physical examination is normal. Investigations reveal a Zenker's diverticulum of the esophagus. Which of the following historical characteristics suggests a Zenker's diverticulum?

    (A) severe weight loss
    (B) greater problems with liquids than solids
    (C) hoarseness
    (D) worse in semirecumbent position
    (E) aspiration unrelated to swallowing

59. A 27-year-old man with HIV complains of pain every time he swallows (odynophagia). He is not on any antiretroviral therapy and otherwise feels well. Examination of the mouth and pharynx are normal. Which of the following is the most likely diagnosis?

    (A) midesophageal cancer
    (B) distal esophageal cancer
    (C) peptic stricture
    (D) candida infection
    (E) bacterial esophagitis

60. A 33-year-old woman is recently diagnosed with primary biliary cirrhosis (PBC). She is inquiring about available treatments for this condition, including if there is a cure for the disease. Which of the following treatments is most likely to "cure" her PBC?

(A) ursodiol
(B) methotrexate
(C) azathioprine
(D) liver transplantation
(E) glucocorticoids

61. A 47-year-old woman complains of food sticking every time she eats anything solid. She has lost 10 lb since the symptoms started, and points to her midthorax as the site where she feels the food is sticking. If this is due to mechanical obstruction, this historical information suggests which of the following locations?

(A) at the location the patient points to
(B) at or above the location the patient points to
(C) below the location the patient points to
(D) at or below the location the patient points to
(E) the historical information is unhelpful in suggesting a location

62. A 52-year-old man has episodes of severe chest pain associated with dysphagia. He has been seen twice in the emergency room, and both times the symptoms responded to sublingual nitroglycerin. He then had a full cardiac evaluation including electrocardiogram (ECG), cardiac biomarkers, and an exercise stress test, which were all normal. Which of the following is the most likely diagnosis?

(A) herpetic infection
(B) a motor disorder
(C) midesophageal cancer
(D) peptic stricture
(E) external esophageal compression

63. A 16-year old girl has recently been referred to your family practice. She is a recent immigrant from Southeast Asia, and has been taking isoniazid (INH) and rifampin for uncomplicated tuberculosis. Routine blood tests are unremarkable, except for an elevated direct bilirubin. Other liver enzymes and function tests are completely normal. Which of the following is the most likely diagnosis?

(A) hemolytic anemia
(B) INH toxicity
(C) Crigler-Najjar syndrome type I
(D) rifampin toxicity
(E) Rotor's syndrome

64. A 45-year-old woman presents with a 1-week history of jaundice, anorexia, and right upper quadrant discomfort. On examination she is icteric, with a tender right upper quadrant and liver span of 14 cm. There is no shifting dullness or pedal edema and the heart and lungs are normal. On further inquiry, she reports consuming one bottle of wine a day for the past 6 months. Which of the following laboratory tests is most likely to be characteristic of a patient with jaundice secondary to alcoholic hepatitis?

(A) ratio of AST:ALT is 3:1 and the AST is 500 U/L
(B) ratio of AST:ALT is 2:1 and the AST is 250 U/L
(C) ratio of AST:ALT is 1:1 and the AST is 500 U/L
(D) ratio of AST:ALT is 1:1 and the AST is 250 U/L
(E) ratio of AST:ALT is 1:3 and the AST is 750

65. Which of the following medications causes predictable, dose-dependent hepatocellular injury?

(A) morphine
(B) INH
(C) gold
(D) acetaminophen
(E) acetylsalicyclic acid (ASA)

66. Which of the following is the mostly likely mechanism of acetaminophen hepatotoxicity toxicity?

    (A) an allergic mechanism
    (B) an active metabolite
    (C) a reaction with hepatic glycogen stores
    (D) direct toxicity of the parent compound
    (E) circulating immune complexes

67. Blood-filled lesions in the liver (peliosis hepatis) are most likely to be seen with which of the following medications?

    (A) methyltestosterone
    (B) oral contraceptives
    (C) trimethoprim-sulfamethoxazole
    (D) chlorpromazine
    (E) erythromycin

68. A 24-year-old man with a history of depression is brought to the emergency room because of a drug overdose. He is experiencing some nausea and vomiting, but no other symptoms. Physical examination and vital signs are normal. Six hours prior to presentation, he intentionally took 40 tablets of acetaminophen (500 mg/tablet). Which of the following is the most appropriate next step in management?

    (A) give ethanol to compete with the parent drug for metabolism, therefore preventing formation of toxic metabolites
    (B) give Narcan to block its actions directly
    (C) give intravenous prostacyclins to maintain cellular integrity
    (D) give N-acetylcysteine to allow binding of the toxic metabolite
    (E) give glucocorticoids to block the immune cascade

69. A 16-year-old girl is referred to the office because of chronic diarrhea and weight loss. She is experiencing large-volume watery diarrhea that is painless. The symptoms persist even when she is fasting, and there is no relationship to foods or liquids. She is not on any medications, and there is no travel history or other constitutional symptoms. Her physical examination is normal. Which of the following is the most likely diagnosis?

    (A) partial small bowel obstruction
    (B) partial large bowel obstruction
    (C) osmotic diarrhea
    (D) secretory diarrhea
    (E) inflammatory bowel disease

70. A 52-year-old man has suffered with chronic diarrhea for several years, but has refused to see a doctor. He finally comes because he is having trouble driving at night, because of difficulty seeing. Physical examination reveals a slender, pale, unwell-looking man. He has a microcytic anemia, low calcium, and albumin levels. Which of the following is the most likely cause for his diarrhea?

    (A) malabsorption
    (B) osmotic diarrhea
    (C) secretory diarrhea
    (D) inflammatory bowel disease
    (E) colonic tumor

71. A 49-year-old woman is being investigated for chronic diarrhea and weight loss. Malabsorption is suspected. Which of the following investigations is most likely to make a definitive diagnosis?

    (A) presence of fecal osmotic gap
    (B) D-xylose test
    (C) stool fat measurements
    (D) Schilling test
    (E) mucosal biopsy

DIRECTIONS (Questions 72 through 76): Each set of matching questions in this section consists of a list of lettered options followed by several numbered items. For each numbered item, select the appropriate lettered option(s). Each lettered option may be selected once, more than once, or not at all. EACH ITEM WILL STATE THE NUMBER OF OPTIONS TO SELECT. CHOOSE EXACTLY THIS NUMBER.

    (A) bile acid reflux implicated in pathogenesis
    (B) immune or autoimmune pathogenesis suspected

(C) ischemia of the gastric mucosa implicated in the pathogenesis

(D) associated with *Helicobacter pylori* infection

(E) unknown mechanism

(F) interruption of prostaglandin synthesis

For each patient with gastritis, select the most likely mechanism of injury.

72. A 67-year-old man is admitted to the intensive care unit (ICU) because of respiratory failure from pneumonia. He requires artificial ventilation and inotropic support. On the third day in the ICU, he develops melena and a drop in his hemoglobin. Urgent upper endoscopy is performed and it reveals three gastric ulcers in the fundus and body of the stomach. Appropriate treatment is started. (SELECT ONE)

73. A 70-year-old man has a long history of heartburn and dyspepsia. He has tried many medications but the symptoms always return. His upper endoscopy is normal with no ulcers. Routine biopsies of the gastric mucosa report "gastritis." (SELECT ONE)

74. A 57-year-old woman experiences frequent symptoms of heartburn. She reports no weight loss, diarrhea, or dysphagia symptoms. Past medical history is significant for B_{12} deficiency treated with monthly injections. She appears well, and the examination is normal, except for some patches on her arms where she has lost all the skin pigmentation. Her upper endoscopy is normal, except for gastric biopsies commenting on gastritis. (SELECT ONE)

75. A 54-year-old man is investigated for weight loss, epigastric pain, nausea, and vomiting. He appears ill; on examination, there is epigastric tenderness and marked peripheral edema. Upper endoscopy reveals large mucosal folds in the body and fundus of the stomach. Biopsies are consistent with a diagnosis of Ménétrier's disease. (SELECT ONE)

76. A 65-year-old man has developed abdominal pain, early satiety, nausea, and vomiting. He reports no weight loss or change in bowel habits. He had a partial gastrectomy 30 years ago for a bleeding gastric ulcer. Upper endoscopy finds erythema of the gastric remnant, and biopsies report epithelial injury and minimal inflammation (gastritis). (SELECT ONE)

Answers and Explanations

1. **(F)** Carcinoid tumors account for up to 75% of all GI endocrine tumors. They are frequently multiple. Primary carcinoid tumors of the appendix are common but rarely metastasize. Those in the large colon may metastasize but do not function. Carcinoids are the most common GI endocrine tumors. They arise from neuroendocrine cells most commonly in the GI tract, pancreas, or bronchi. GI carcinoids cause abdominal pain, bleeding, or even obstruction (usually via intussusception). Carcinoid syndrome is characterized by flushing, diarrhea, and valvular heart disease. *(Kasper, p. 532)*

2. **(D)** Adenocarcinoma of the small bowel accounts for about 50% of malignant tumors of the small bowel. They are most commonly found in the distal duodenum and proximal jejunum. Hemorrhage, or obstruction, is the most common presenting symptom. X-ray findings can mimic chronic duodenal ulcer disease or Crohn's disease. *(Kasper, p. 532)*

3. **(E)** There is one unique form of lymphoma called IPSID or Mediterranean lymphoma. It diffusely involves the small intestine and usually presents with diarrhea and steatorrhea. Oral antibiotics, early in the disease, provide some benefit, suggesting a possible infectious component to the disorder. Antibiotics and chemotherapy are frequently combined. *(Kasper, p. 532)*

4. **(F)** Appendiceal tumors make up nearly half of all carcinoid tumors and are a frequent finding in routine appendectomy specimens. They are usually small, solitary, and benign. Even if they invade locally, they rarely metastasize. *(Kasper, p. 532)*

5. **(E)** Primary small bowel lymphoma is more common in the settings of celiac disease, regional enteritis, congenital immune disorders, prior organ transplantation, autoimmune disorders, and AIDS. *(Kasper, p. 532)*

6. **(C, F)** Lipomas and carcinoid tumors are most frequently found in the distal ileum. Adenocarcinomas are characteristically more proximal. The ileum has more lymphatic tissue, than the rest of the small bowel, so lymphoma is more common here than in the jejunum or duodenum. However, there is not as strong a predilection for the distal ileum as there is for lipomas and carcinoids. *(Kasper, p. 532)*

7. **(A, E)** Acquired lactase deficiency is very common in GI diseases with evidence of mucosal damage. Examples include celiac and tropical sprue, viral and bacterial infections, giardiasis, cystic fibrosis, ulcerative colitis, and regional enteritis. It is not caused by a hypersensitivity reaction. *(Kasper, p. 228)*

8. **(A, C, K, L)** This syndrome is likely celiac sprue, but a clinical and histologic improvement with a gluten-free diet would be required for confirmation. The decrease in pancreatic enzyme production is secondary to decreased intestinal secretion of hormones that stimulate the pancreas. Dermatitis herpetiformis might be related to celiac disease. Although gross malabsorption is the classical description of celiac sprue, it can present with isolated deficiencies such as iron deficiency anemia. *(Kasper, pp. 1770–1773)*

9. **(F, J)** Whipple's disease is caused by infection with a Gram-positive bacillus called *Tropheryma whippelii*. The disease, previously invariably fatal, can be controlled with long-term antibiotic therapy (at least 1 year), and some patients seem to be cured. Arthritis and central nervous system (CNS) involvement are other manifestations of this rare disease. *(Kasper, pp. 1774–1775)*

10. **(B)** Zollinger-Ellison syndrome is caused by a nonbeta islet cell tumor of the pancreas. It may be associated with the syndrome of multiple endocrine neoplasia, type I (MEN I). The syndrome should be suspected in patients with multiple ulcers, ulcers resistant to therapy, ulcers in unusual locations, strong family history of ulcers, unexplained diarrhea, or evidence of MEN I. *(Kasper, p. 1758)*

11. **(D)** Diverticula are present in over 50% of octogenarians. Most patients remain asymptomatic. They are most common in the sigmoid colon and decrease in frequency in the proximal colon. The relative scarcity of diverticula in underdeveloped nations has led to the hypothesis that low fiber diets result in decreased fecal bulk, narrowing of the colon, and an increased intraluminal pressure to move the small fecal mass. This results in thickening of the muscular coat, and eventually herniations or diverticula of the mucosa at the points where nutrient arteries penetrate the muscularis. *(Kasper, p. 1798)*

12. **(C)** Amylase accumulates in the setting of renal failure and thus becomes a less-valuable diagnostic test. Numerous other conditions involving the pancreas, the gut, and the salivary glands can raise amylase levels. Sulfonamides cause pancreatitis; therefore, an elevated amylase is not confusing, but rather a useful test for pancreatitis in patients taking the drug. Morphine can elevate amylase levels in the absence of pancreatitis. *(Kasper, p. 1893, 1897)*

13. **(D)** This presentation is typical of esophageal cancer. Lesions in the upper two-thirds of the esophagus are squamous, but in the distal esophagus, most are adenocarcinomas. The adenocarcinomas develop more commonly from columnar epithelium in the distal esophagus (Barrett's esophagus). Adenocarcinomas of the esophagus have the biologic behavior of gastric cancers. The incidence of squamous cell cancer of the esophagus is decreasing while adenocarcinoma is increasing. Currently, over 50% of esophageal cancer is adenocarcinoma. The 5-year survival for esophageal cancer is <5%. Combination therapy seems to be more effective than surgery alone. *(Kasper, pp. 523–524)*

14. **(D)** Fat malabsorption demonstrated on stool collection for 72 hours is the gold standard, but does not indicate the exact cause. The Schilling test is useful in testing for vitamin B_{12} absorption. X-rays can be helpful in diagnosing underlying disorders, but are nonspecific. Small intestinal biopsy is useful in determining the cause of malabsorption. *(Kasper, p. 1768)*

15. **(A)** The antibody can be demonstrated in 80–90% of patients, usually late in convalescence, and indicates relative or absolute immunity. In contrast, HBsAg occurs very early and disappears in <6 months. Persistence of HBsAg indicates chronic infection. The pattern in this patient is also seen postvaccination, and perhaps as a consequence of remote infection. *(Kasper, p. 1834)*

16. **(D)** Gilbert's syndrome may be associated with impaired hepatic uptake of bilirubin. It is caused by hereditary decrease in the activity of glucoronosyltransferase in the uridine diphosphate glycosyltransferase 1 (UGT1) family. More severe enzyme deficits are the cause of the two variants of Crigler-Najjar syndrome. *(Kasper, pp. 1819–1820)*

17. **(A)** Intestinal polyposis is a possible indication of Peutz-Jeghers syndrome associated with dark brown spots on the lips and palate. There is characteristic distribution of pigment around lips, nose, eyes, and hands. Tumors of the ovary, breast, pancreas, and endometrium are associated with this syndrome. *(Kasper, pp. 198, 553)*

18. **(B)** Despite some decline, distal tumors are still the most common. The fact that up to 60% of tumors are located in the rectosigmoid is the rationale for screening via flexible, fiberoptic sigmoidoscopes. Occult blood testing and colonoscopy are other possible screening techniques. *(Kasper, p. 529)*

19. **(E)** This pattern of symptoms is characteristic of afferent loop syndrome. It is caused by distention and incomplete drainage of the afferent loop and requires surgical correction. Bacterial overgrowth of the afferent loop is more common. Its clinical presentation includes postprandial abdominal pain, bloating, and diarrhea. Fat and vitamin B$_{12}$ malabsorption can occur. *(Kasper, p. 1757)*

20. **(B)** Pancreatitis in AIDS patients can be caused by cytomegalovirus and cryptosporidium as well as *M. avium* complex. Drugs are another cause of AIDS-related pancreatitis. *(Kasper, p. 1899)*

21. **(B)** Hepatoma is the most likely diagnosis in this man. In China, it is estimated that the lifetime risk of hepatoma in people with chronic hepatitis B is close to 40%. AFP elevations, over 500–1000 mg/L in the absence of a colonic tumor (or pregnancy), suggest hepatoma. Paraneoplastic syndromes are not common but include erythrocytosis, hypercalcemia, and acquired porphyria. *(Kasper, p. 534)*

22. **(D)** Ascitic fluid in uncomplicated cirrhosis of the liver shows a specific gravity <1.016. Protein is <25 g/L, and the gross appearance is straw-colored. In spontaneous bacterial peritonitis, the fluid may be cloudy and the number of white cells (neutrophils) increased. In uncomplicated ascites, the difference between plasma albumin and ascitic fluid albumin is >1.1 g/dL. *(Kasper, pp. 244–245)*

23. **(D)** Common duct stones can be painless, or may give rise to severe pain, chills, and fever. The jaundice is generally conjugated hyperbilirubinemia. Partial obstruction of the common duct produces variable amounts of jaundice and is influenced by the presence of concurrent hepatocellular disease or cholangitis. Although most such stones originate in the gallbladder, hemolytic disorders and parasitic infections can result in primary bile duct stones. *(Kasper, p. 1888)*

24. **(E)** The syndrome is characteristic of carcinoid of midgut origin. The cardiac lesions are more common on the right side (hence murmur accentuation on deep inspiration). Foregut carcinoids (bronchus, stomach, duodenum) frequently are associated with wheezing. The most important mediator of the carcinoid syndrome is serotonin. Serotonin is rapidly metabolized to 5-HIAA, which is rapidly cleared by the kidneys. The measurement of 5-HIAA in the urine is thus the most useful diagnostic test. Its specificity is enhanced by an appropriate diet before testing. *(Kasper, p. 2225)*

25. **(D)** These findings are characteristic of achalasia. Anticholinergic medications and dietary changes do not provide much help. Successful therapies include nitroglycerine, nifedipine (a calcium channel blocker), botulinum toxin injected endoscopically, balloon dilatation, and esophageal myotomy (not excision). *(Kasper, pp. 1741–1742)*

26. **(B)** These findings are characteristic of scleroderma. If the disease is limited, the prognosis is not necessarily poor. The limited form is characterized by calcinosis, Raynaud's (often with distal ulceration), esophageal motility disorder, sclerodactyly, and telangiectasia. It has a female preponderance. Renal disease can be severe, but is not the most common cause of death. Esophageal symptoms should be treated aggressively. *(Kasper, pp. 1984–1985)*

27. **(B)** The clinical description suggests Ménétrier's disease; however, biopsy is essential to rule out lymphoma or carcinoma. The edema is usually secondary to protein-losing enteropathy. Treatment consists of a high protein diet, anticholinergic therapy, and H2-blockers. In some cases, gastrectomy is required. *(Kasper, p. 1762)*

28. **(E)** The carcinoma has occurred in a patient with ulcerative colitis. The barium enema shows a long, constricting lesion in the transverse colon, with the whole colon devoid of

haustral markings. Some pressure effects are seen in the ileum due to metastases. The diagnosis of ulcerative colitis is made from the clinical symptoms and proctosigmoidoscopic examination of an abnormally inflamed colonic mucosa. *(Kasper, p. 1788)*

29. **(A)** In esophageal varices, the esophageal folds are thick and tortuous, giving rise to a wormy or worm-eaten appearance. The radiographic picture would vary with the severity of the varices, as well as the distention of the esophagus. When varices are severe, they should be appreciated in any projection. The left anterior oblique projection is most ideal for its demonstration. *(Kasper, pp. 1863–1864)*

30. **(B)** The common causes of acute pancreatitis are alcohol, gallstones, metabolic factors, and drugs. Gallstones still remain the most common cause of pancreatitis. *(Kasper, p. 1896)*

31. **(A)** In benign gastric ulcer, an ulcer niche is present in the prepyloric area, with folds radiating to and extending up to the margin of the niche with a halo around it. The differentiation between benignity and malignancy may be difficult at times, but proper use of radiographic criteria could boost the accuracy to 98%. In the presence of an ulcer niche, a Hampton line, which is an ulcer collar, or a mound should be sought on a profile view. Endoscopy with biopsy is the gold standard of diagnosis. *(Kasper, p. 1752)*

32. **(D)** *Helicobacter pylori* infection is the cause of most peptic ulcers, and the usual route of infection is via the water supply. Duodenal ulcer is clinically more common, although the prevalence on autopsy series is similar. Duodenal ulcer does not represent a malignant potential. Gastric ulcers are seen in an older population and can be malignant. Benign peptic gastric ulcers tend to be more distal. *(Kasper, pp. 1748–1749)*

33. **(E)** Sugarless gums and candy often contain sorbitol, a sugar that is not absorbed in the gut. It thus produces an osmotic diarrhea if present in sufficient quantity. *(Kasper, p. 228)*

34. **(D)** Infection usually occurs early in life and is related to classic socioeconomic indicators such as poverty, domestic crowding, unsanitary living conditions, and unclean water. It is much more common in developing countries. *(Kasper, p. 1749)*

35. **(D)** Concomitant steroid use increases the likelihood of ulceration, as does advanced age. *H. pylori* infection, smoking, and alcohol use are suspected, but not yet established, risk factors. *(Kasper, p. 1751)*

36. **(E)** NSAIDs inhibit prostaglandins, which play an important role in maintaining gastroduodenal mucosal integrity and repair. *(Kasper, p. 1751)*

37. **(D)** Eradication of *H. pylori* is the most effective treatment for duodenal ulcer disease. The most popular regimes include antibiotics and acid suppression medications. *(Kasper, p. 1754)*

38. **(A, B)** Specific vaccines are available for hepatitis A and B. Hepatitis D is most frequently symptomatic in association with hepatitis B infection, so vaccination for hepatitis B will decrease the likelihood of symptomatic hepatitis D infection. *(Kasper, p. 1836)*

39. **(A, E)** Both hepatitis A and E are usually spread by the fecal-oral route. Other forms of transmission are exceedingly uncommon. *(Kasper, p. 1829)*

40. **(B, D)** Only hepatitis B and D are frequently spread by sexual transmission. It does not seem to occur with hepatitis E, and the evidence is equivocal for hepatitis A and C. *(Kasper, p. 1829)*

41. **(C)** Chronic hepatitis C infection occurs in 80–90% of patients. About 50–70% will have evidence of chronic liver disease. In contrast, only 1–10% of adults infected with hepatitis B will go on to chronic infection. *(Kasper, p. 1829)*

42. **(B, C)** Interferon has been used in both hepatitis B and C infection. The response is better in hepatitis B infection. Combination therapy with interferon and ribavirin is more effective in hepatitis C. *(Kasper, p. 1829)*

43. **(B)** In neonates, the transmission of hepatitis B results in a 90% probability of developing chronic infection. The ongoing infection (often resulting in hepatoma) is a major cause of morbidity and mortality in many parts of the world. *(Kasper, p. 1829)*

44. **(A, B)** Immunoglobulin injection can provide prophylaxis against hepatitis A, and it is felt that hepatitis B immune globulin is protective for hepatitis B. *(Kasper, p. 1829)*

45. **(D)** Hepatitis D is a defective ribonucleic acid (RNA) virus that requires the helper function of hepatitis B virus (or other hepadnavirus) for its replication and expression. *(Kasper, p. 1826)*

46. **(C)** Hyperglycemia is very common in pancreatitis and is usually multifactorial in origin. Factors involved include decreased insulin release, increased glucagon release, and elevated adrenal glucocorticoids and catecholamines. *(Kasper, p. 1897)*

47. **(B)** The sclera are high in elastin content, which has an affinity for bilirubin. Therefore, jaundice is usually detected here first. Fluorescent lighting makes recognition more difficult. In some individuals, dark skin color makes jaundice more difficult to detect. *(Kasper, p. 238)*

48. **(A)** Hemolysis results in predominantly unconjugated bilirubin. Unconjugated hyperbilirubinemia is caused by overproduction, decreased uptake, or decreased conjugation. *(Kasper, p. 240)*

49. **(E)** Ménétrier's disease, an uncommon disease involving the stomach, is characterized by large gastric folds. Intravenous administration of radioactive-labeled albumin may show up to a 40% loss in the GI tract in protein-losing enteropathy, but is not available for routine clinical use. Treatment of protein-losing enteropathy is usually directed at the underlying condition. *(Kasper, p. 1762)*

50. **(D)** Joint involvement in inflammatory bowel disease may involve sacroiliitis or specific large joint peripheral arthritis. The latter type of arthritis parallels the course of the bowel disease. The sacroiliitis (spondylitic) variety follows an independent course. *(Kasper, p. 1786)*

51. **(D)** This likely represents diarrhea secondary to *Clostridium difficile* infection. It is mediated by toxins, not by direct bacterial invasion. Cephalosporins, because they are so widely used, are the most common cause of the disease. On a per case basis, however, clindamycin is the most likely antibiotic to cause the disease. *(Kasper, p. 760)*

52. **(E)** The patient with primary biliary cirrhosis (PBC) is typically a middle-aged woman with itching. Patients are often asymptomatic and diagnosed only on routine blood work. The cause of PBC is unknown, but a disordered immune response may be involved. A positive antimitochondrial antibody test is found in over 90% of symptomatic patients. *(Kasper, p. 1861)*

53. **(B)** Postgastrectomy steatorrhea does not result from mucosal abnormality. The mucosa is also normal in pancreatic steatorrhea. Postgastrectomy maldigestion and malabsorption is caused by rapid gastric emptying, reduced dispersion of food in the stomach, reduced luminal levels of bile, rapid transit of food, and impaired pancreatic secretory response. *(Kasper, p. 1770)*

54. **(A)** The string sign represents long areas of circumferential inflammation and fibrosis. It is seen in the stenotic and nonstenotic phase of Crohn's disease. In addition to the string sign, abnormal puddling of barium and fistulous tracts are other helpful x-ray signs of ileitis. Other radiologic findings in Crohn's disease include skip lesions, rectal sparing, small ulcerations, and fistulas. *(Kasper, p. 1781)*

55. **(A)** Although carcinoid tumor can cause diarrhea, it is very uncommon. This young woman is overweight, suggesting an eating disorder, which is associated with laxative abuse. Abuse of stimulant laxatives such as senna can cause a secretory diarrhea. Magnesium-based laxatives will cause an osmotic diarrhea. *(Kasper, p. 228)*

56. **(A)** Colonic obstruction usually causes less pain and vomiting than small bowel obstruction. Fever is usually absent in both. The stepladder pattern is characteristic of small bowel obstruction, as are hiccups. *(Kasper, p. 1804)*

57. **(C)** Episodic dysphagia to solids of several years' duration suggests a benign disease, and is characteristic of a lower esophageal ring. Motor dysphagia presents with dysphagia to solids and liquids. Dysphagia due to obstruction starts with solids and can progress to liquids as well. Hoarseness following the onset of dysphagia can be caused by an esophageal cancer extending to involve the recurrent laryngeal nerve or because of laryngitis secondary to gastroesophageal reflux. Severe weight loss suggests malignancy, and hiccups are a rare occurrence in distal problems of the esophagus. *(Kasper, p. 217)*

58. **(E)** Aspiration, unrelated to swallowing, is seen in a Zenker's diverticulum, achalasia, or gastroesophageal reflex. *(Kasper, p. 217)*

59. **(D)** Painful swallowing can be caused by candida or herpes infection or pill-induced esophagitis. Patients with immunodeficiency states (e.g., AIDS) may have herpetic, candidal, or CMV esophagitis, as well as tumors (lymphoma, Kaposi sarcoma). *(Kasper, p. 219)*

60. **(D)** There is no known effective therapy to prevent progression of liver disease in PBC. In patients with end-stage liver failure, liver transplantation is "curative," since recurrence after transplantation is rare. The other therapies listed have been reported as effective in small case series but not in controlled trials. Ursodeoxycholic acid seems effective in providing at least symptomatic improvement, and may even delay liver transplantation. Replacement of fat-soluble vitamins (e.g., vitamin A to prevent night blindness) is an important part of therapy, as is replacement of calcium and vitamin D to prevent osteoporosis. *(Kasper, p. 1861)*

61. **(D)** The history is helpful. The site of obstruction is usually at or below where the patient says the sticking occurs. *(Kasper, p. 218)*

62. **(B)** Severe chest pain is characteristic of diffuse esophageal spasm and related motor disorders. The symptoms can mimic that of cardiac chest pain and can be difficult to distinguish one from the other, since both conditions respond to nitrates. Cardiac conditions should be ruled out before noncardiac conditions are considered. *(Kasper, p. 1742)*

63. **(E)** Rotor's syndrome is one of the two rare inherited disorders causing elevations in direct bilirubin. The other is Dubin-Johnson syndrome, and both have an excellent prognosis. Hemolytic anemia causes elevation in indirect bilirubin, and hematologic changes would be expected. INH causes elevation in liver enzymes, and although Rifampin can cause isolated hyperbilirubinemia, it is of the indirect kind. Crigler-Najjar type I is a severe disorder of neonates with elevated indirect bilirubin. *(Kasper, p. 240)*

64. **(B)** In alcoholic hepatitis, the AST:ALT ratio is usually >2, and the level of AST is usually <300. When viral hepatitis or toxin-induced hepatitis causes jaundice, the AST:ALT ratio is usually 1 or less, and the transaminases are usually >500. *(Kasper, p. 241)*

65. **(D)** Acetaminophen reliably produces hepatocellular damage when taken in large doses. Daily doses should not exceed 4 g a day, and accidental or intentional overdoses of 10–15 g will result in liver injury. Fatal fulminant disease is usually seen with ingestions over 25 g. *(Kasper, pp. 1840–1841)*

66. **(B)** An active metabolite of acetaminophen is hepatotoxic. It is detoxified by binding to glutathione, and when hepatic glutathione stores are depleted, severe liver damage can occur. *(Kasper, pp. 1840–1841)*

67. **(A)** Anabolic steroids usually cause cholestasis and jaundice without inflammation. Sinusoidal dilatation and peliosis occur less frequently, and there have been deaths linked to peliosis. The other medications also cause various types of liver disease, but not peliosis. *(Kasper, p. 1843)*

68. **(D)** *N*-acetylcysteine probably acts by providing a reservoir of sulfhydryl groups to bind the toxic metabolite of acetaminophen. Narcan is effective for narcotic overdose, and ethanol is the antidote for methanol intoxication. *(Kasper, p. 1841)*

69. **(D)** Secretory diarrhea is caused by a derangement in fluid and electrolyte transport across the gut mucosa. The resultant diarrhea is watery, large volume, painless, and persists even when the patient fasts. *(Kasper, p. 228)*

70. **(A)** His anemia and general appearance are compatible with chronic inflammatory bowel disease as well, but his night blindness suggests vitamin A deficiency, which is much more likely in a malabsorption syndrome. *(Kasper, p. 1768)*

71. **(E)** The osmotic gap is a characteristic of osmotic diarrhea in particular. Stool fat, D-xylose testing, and Schilling tests help establish the diagnosis of malabsorption, but not the etiology. The most common cause of such diffuse malabsorption, celiac disease, has a characteristic biopsy pattern with short or absent villi. Confirmation of the disease requires response to a gluten-free diet. *(Kasper, p. 1770)*

72. **(C)** Acute erosive gastritis is most commonly seen in critically ill hospitalized patients. Ischemia of the gastric mucosa with breakdown of the normal protective barriers of the stomach is a key factor in the syndrome. *(Kasper, p. 1760)*

73. **(D)** Type B chronic gastritis is a more common cause of chronic gastritis. It becomes more common with advancing age and is uniformly associated with *H. pylori* infection. Eradication of *H. pylori* produces histologic improvement, but is not routinely recommended unless peptic ulcer or mucosa-associated lymphoid tissue (MALT) lymphoma occurs. *(Kasper, p. 1761)*

74. **(B)** Type A chronic gastritis may lead to pernicious anemia. Antibodies to parietal cells and to intrinsic factor are frequently seen in the sera, suggesting an immune or autoimmune pathogenesis. These patients can also have autoimmune thyroid disease and vitiligo. *(Kasper, p. 1761)*

75. **(E)** Ménétrier's disease is not a true gastritis, as inflammation is not present on histologic examination. It is characterized by large, tortuous gastric mucosal folds and usually presents with abdominal pain. Protein-losing enteropathy often develops, resulting in hypoalbuminemia and edema. *(Kasper, p.1762)*

76. **(A)** Gastric surgery seems to accelerate the development of asymptomatic gastritis with progressive parietal cell loss. However, some patients develop bile reflux gastritis with symptoms of pain, nausea, and vomiting. *(Kasper, p. 1757)*

CHAPTER 5

Hematology
Questions

DIRECTIONS (Questions 1 through 7): Each of the numbered items in this section is followed by answers. Select the ONE lettered answer that is BEST in each case.

1. During the winter months, a 65-year-old man presents with livedo reticularis and purple fingertips. Other symptoms include arthralgia and weakness. Renal impairment is present on laboratory testing. Which of the following is the most likely diagnosis?

    (A) cold agglutinin disease
    (B) Henoch-Schönlein purpura
    (C) antiphospholipid antibody syndrome
    (D) cryoglobulinemia
    (E) cholesterol embolic disease

2. A 34-year-old woman notices blue toes and a lacey rash on her knees when outside in the winter months. She has chronic hepatitis C virus infection. She has also noticed weakness, joint discomfort, and red spots on her legs. On examination, she has livedo reticularis-type skin on her thighs, and areas of palpable purpura on her toes. She has abnormal proteins detected in her serum. Which of the following is the most likely mechanism for the vessel injury seen in this condition?

    (A) breakdown of erythrocytes
    (B) medium vessel vasculitis
    (C) aggregation of abnormal platelets
    (D) temperature-dependent antibodies
    (E) cold precipitable proteins

3. A 34-year-old man presents with symptoms of fatigue, weakness, nose bleeds, and palpitations with exertion. On examination he is pale, blood pressure 110/70 mm Hg, pulse 100/min, heart sounds are normal, lungs are clear, and he has multiple petechiae and bruises on his legs. His blood count is abnormal: hemoglobin 8.5 g/dL, white blood cells (WBCs) 4000/mL, platelets 50,000/mL, and there are blast cells in the peripheral blood. He is diagnosed with acute promyelocytic leukemia (AML-M3). Which of the following is a characteristic of this acute myelogenous leukemia? (See Fig. 5–1.)

    (A) peak incidence in childhood
    (B) high leukocyte alkaline phosphatase
    (C) Philadelphia chromosome
    (D) Auer bodies in blast cells
    (E) response to vincristine and prednisone

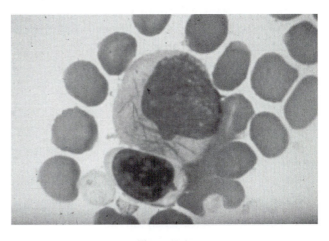

Figure 5–1.
(Reproduced, with permission, from Lichtman MA, et al. *Williams Hematology*, 7th ed. New York: McGraw-Hill, 2006:Plate XVII-2.)

4. A 62-year-old man reports early satiety, fatigue, and generally feeling unwell. On examination he has a large spleen, appears pale, and the rest of the examination is normal. His blood count is abnormal; the WBC is 50,000/mL with increased mature granulocytes, hemoglobin 9.5 g/dL, and platelets 450,000/mL. Which of the following cytogenetic changes is most characteristic of his condition?

   (A) deletion of chromosome 14
   (B) reciprocal translocation of 9 and 22 (Philadelphia chromosome)
   (C) translocation of the renal artery stenosis (RAS) oncogene
   (D) trisomy 21
   (E) translocation of 8–14

5. An 18-year-old man is recently diagnosed with beta-thalassemia minor. His hemoglobin is 10.5 g/dL, and he feels well. Which of the following findings is characteristic of this condition?

   (A) an increased amount of fetal hemoglobin (HbF) or hemoglobin A2 (HbA2)
   (B) increased osmotic fragility of the red cells
   (C) absent bone marrow iron
   (D) increased macroglobulins in the serum
   (E) small amounts of HbS

6. A patient with aplastic anemia receives a bone marrow transplant from a human lymphocyte antigen (HLA)-matched sister. Which of the following is the most likely complication of allogenic bone marrow transplantation?

   (A) graft-versus-host disease
   (B) graft failure
   (C) radiation sickness
   (D) development of leukemia
   (E) secondary skin cancer

7. A 19-year-old man has had recurrent bleeding occur in his knee when playing contact sports. He has no history of spontaneous bleeding, but his brother had similar problems. Consultation with a specialist reveals that he has "mild" hemophilia A. Which of the following factor abnormalities is consistent with this diagnosis?

   (A) abnormal factor VIII function
   (B) decreased levels of functional factor VIII
   (C) decreased factor IX level
   (D) decreased von Willebrand factor
   (E) decreased factor IX level

DIRECTIONS (Questions 8 through 14): Each set of matching questions in this section consists of a list of lettered options followed by several numbered items. For each numbered item, select the appropriate lettered option(s). Each lettered option may be selected once, more than once, or not at all. EACH ITEM WILL STATE THE NUMBER OF OPTIONS TO SELECT. CHOOSE EXACTLY THIS NUMBER.

Questions 8 and 9

   (A) hyperthyroidism
   (B) rectal cancer
   (C) infectious mononucleosis
   (D) acute myelogenous leukemia
   (E) renal cell carcinoma (hypernephroma)
   (F) acute lymphocytic leukemia

For each patient with a hematologic abnormality, select the most likely diagnosis.

8. A 63-year-old man presents with headaches, itching, and feeling unwell. He appears plethoric, and the remaining examination is normal. On laboratory investigations, he is found to have elevated hemoglobin of 20.5 g/dL, normal WBC, and normal platelet count. There is no palpable spleen or lymph nodes. (SELECT ONE)

9. A 19-year-old college student develops a severe sore throat, cervical lymphadenopathy, and atypical lymphocytes on blood film. A heterophil antibody test is positive. (SELECT ONE)

Questions 10 and 11

   (A) increased target cells
   (B) bone pain
   (C) osteoblastic bone lesions
   (D) increased spleen size
   (E) her fertility is impaired

(F) Bence Jones proteinuria

(G) increased osmotic fragility

(H) type III cryoglobulin

(I) marrow hyperplasia

(J) increased plasma cells in bone marrow

For each patient with anemia, select the corresponding clinical and laboratory findings.

10. A 19-year-old woman is found to be anemic with hemoglobin of 10.0 g/dL. She has target cells on the blood film, and is homozygous for HbC. She has no other clinical symptoms. (SELECT THREE)

11. A 74-year-old woman is anemic with hemoglobin of 10.5 g/dL. She has symptoms of tingling in her feet and back discomfort. X-rays of her spine reveal osteopenia and multiple lytic lesions. She has an immunoglobulin G (IgG) spike on serum protein electrophoresis. (SELECT THREE)

Questions 12 through 14

(A) decreased red cell survival

(B) thalassemia

(C) postsplenectomy

(D) increased numbers of reticulocytes

(E) thiamine deficiency

(F) acute hemorrhage

(G) low fecal urobilinogen

(H) pyridoxine deficiency

(I) immediate postoperative period

(J) acute lymphocytic leukemia

(K) iron deficiency

(L) increased urine urobilinogen

For each patient with a blood count anomaly, select the corresponding clinical situation and/or laboratory finding.

12. A 49-year-old woman feels unwell because of fatigue and shortness of breath on exertion. Her hemoglobin is 9.0 g/dL, the direct antiglobulin test (Coombs') is positive, and she is suspected of having a hemolytic anemia. (SELECT THREE)

13. A 69-year-old man presents with increasing symptoms of chest pain on exertion, but never at rest. He has a history of chronic stable coronary artery disease. Repeat evaluation now reveals a hypochromic microcytic anemia as the cause for his increased chest pain symptoms. (SELECT THREE)

14. A 72-year-old woman is admitted to the hospital with an acute illness. Her platelet count is incidentally noted to be 800,000/mL. (SELECT THREE)

DIRECTIONS (Questions 15 through 31): Each of the numbered items in this section is followed by answers. Select the ONE lettered answer that is BEST in each case.

15. A 7-year-old boy has severe microcytic anemia due to beta-thalassemia major (homozygous). He requires frequent blood transfusions (once every 6 weeks) to prevent the skeletal and developmental complications of thalassemia. Which of the following medications is also indicated in the treatment of patients requiring frequent blood transfusions?

    (A) oral calcium supplements

    (B) fresh frozen plasma

    (C) desferrioxamine

    (D) penicillamine

    (E) cryoprecipitate

16. A 45-year-old woman develops symptoms of shortness of breath on exertion, easy fatigue, and jaundice. On examination she is pale, and there is a palpable spleen, but no lymphadenopathy. Her hemoglobin is 9.0 g/dL, the reticulocyte count 9%, and the direct antibody test (Coombs') is positive. Which of the following bone marrow findings is most likely to be seen in this patient?

    (A) megaloblastic changes

    (B) giant metamyelocytes

    (C) increased erythroid-to-myeloid ratio

    (D) increased lymphocytes

    (E) shift to left of the myeloid series

17. A 23-year-old woman of Italian extraction is found to have a hypochromic microcytic anemia of 10 g/dL. In addition, there is a fair degree of anisocytosis, poikilocytosis, and targeting on the blood film. The WBC is 9500/mL, the platelet count is 240,000/mL, and the reticulocyte count is 7%. The spleen is palpated 5 cm below the left costal margin. Which of the following is the most appropriate treatment for her condition?

(A) splenectomy
(B) removal of the abnormal Hb pigment
(C) purely supportive
(D) plasmapheresis
(E) intramuscular iron

18. A 67-year-old man is complaining of fatigue. A routine complete blood count (CBC) reveals a platelet count of 850,000/mL, and the hemoglobin and WBC counts are normal. He reports no other symptoms, and his clinical examination is normal. Which of the following characteristics is most likely to be helpful in differentiating essential (primary) from reactive (secondary) thrombocytosis?

(A) increased megakaryocyte number
(B) increased total platelet mass
(C) increased platelet turnover
(D) normal platelet survival
(E) thromboembolism and hemorrhage

19. A 19-year-old man is found to have a decreased eosinophil count. Which of the following is the most likely cause?

(A) asthma
(B) contact dermatitis
(C) yeast infection
(D) mycobacterial infection
(E) prednisone administration

20. A 68-year-old man with aplastic anemia is due for another blood transfusion. He has had multiple blood transfusions in the past, but with the last transfusion, he developed fever and chills after the transfusion was started. Repeat cross-matching and testing at the time ruled out an acute hemolytic transfusion reaction. The next transfusion is ordered through a "filter" to prevent or minimize the febrile reaction. Which of the following mechanisms is most likely to explain the effect of the filter?

(A) reducing bacterial transmission
(B) reducing viral transmission
(C) reducing parasite transmission
(D) reducing leukocyte transfusion
(E) reducing reticulocyte transfusion

21. A 19-year-old man is found to have low hemoglobin on routine screening. He feels well at the present time, but in the past he has had two presentations to the hospital for severe abdominal and back pain that resolved on its own with no specific diagnosis. His blood film is shown in Fig. 5–2; the hemoglobin is 10 mg/dL, mean corpuscular volume (MCV) 80 fL, and reticulocyte count 0.04 (4%). Which of the following is the most likely explanation for his previous episodes of abdominal pain? (See Fig. 5–2.)

(A) aplastic crisis
(B) sequestration crisis
(C) vaso-occlusive crisis
(D) hemolytic crisis
(E) adrenal crisis

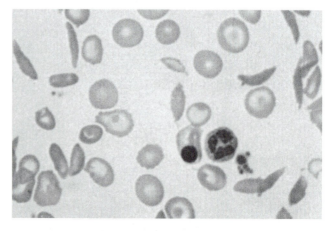

Figure 5–2.
(Reproduced, with permission, from Kasper DL, et al. *Harrison's Principles of Internal Medicine*, 16th ed. New York: McGraw-Hill, 2005:596)

22. A 23-year-old woman has symptoms of fatigue and not feeling well. She appears well and the physical examination is normal, but her hemoglobin is low at 9.8 g/dL with a mean corpuscular volume (MVC) of 76 fL. Her family history is positive for thalassemia. She also mentions a history of heavy menses in the past year. Which of the following would be most helpful in distinguishing thalassemia from one of pure iron deficiency anemia?

(A) peripheral blood smear
(B) osmotic fragility test
(C) Ham's test
(D) Hb electrophoresis on paper
(E) serum ferritin determination

23. A 21-year-old woman is suspected of having mycoplasma pneumonia based on symptoms of a dry cough, fever, normal lung examination but abnormal chest x-ray with bilateral infiltrates. She is also anemic with hemoglobin of 10.5 g/dL, reticulocyte count 7%, and WBC 12,000/mL. Hemolytic anemia from cold agglutinins is suspected as the cause. Which of the following tests will confirm autoimmune causation as the cause of the anemia?

(A) positive antinuclear antibody (ANA)
(B) positive rheumatoid factor
(C) polyclonal gammopathy
(D) presence of Heinz bodies
(E) positive Coombs' test

24. A 59-year-old man presents to the emergency room with left face and arm weakness that lasts for 3 hours. He reports no other symptoms of palpitations, chest pain, or headache. Neurologic examination is now normal. A computerized tomography (CT) head, electrocardiogram (ECG), and laboratory workup are normal. He is started on clopidogrel, and referred for further evaluation as an outpatient. Which of the following is the most likely mechanism of action on platelet function from this medication?

(A) cyclooxygenase-1 inhibition
(B) modulation of cyclic adenosine monophosphate (cAMP) levels

(C) adenosine diphosphate (ADP) receptor blockade
(D) GPIIB-IIIA blocker
(E) cyclooxygenase-2 inhibition

25. A 23-year-old woman has symptoms of leg swelling and discomfort, but no chest pain or shortness of breath. She has no risk factors for a blood clot. On examination, the left leg is swollen when compared to the right. Leg Doppler ultrasound is positive for deep vein thrombosis, and further investigations reveal decreased plasma antithrombin III (AT-III) levels. Which of the following is the most likely clinical effect from the low AT-III levels?

(A) aspirin sensitivity
(B) heparin resistance
(C) warfarin (Coumadin) resistance
(D) platelet dysfunction
(E) disseminated intravascular coagulation

26. A 4-month-old infant is anemic with a hemoglobin level of 9.5 g/dL and MCV 77 fL. The baby looks well, the height and weight growth parameters are normal, and she is breastfeeding well. Which of the following is the most likely cause for her anemia?

(A) inadequate dietary iron
(B) hemolysis
(C) late clamping of cord
(D) iron malabsorption
(E) folate deficiency

27. Which of the following is the most likely effect of increased levels of red blood cell 2,3 diphosphoglycerate (2,3-DPG)?

(A) hemolytic anemia due to sulfa drugs
(B) increased oxygen affinity
(C) decreased oxygen affinity
(D) loss of red cell energy
(E) multiple congenital abnormalities

28. A 63-year-old man is involved in a motor vehicle accident and is brought to the hospital. On examination, his blood pressure is 90/60 mm Hg, pulse 110/min, and his abdomen is distended and rigid. He has internal injuries and bleeding on an abdominal CT scan, and requires emergent blood transfusion on his way to the operating room. His blood group is AB. Which of the following statements is not correct?

(A) he is a universal recipient

(B) he has anti-A and anti-B in his serum

(C) if a cross-match is not available; group O RBCs are universal

(D) if insufficient AB blood is available, type A can be used

(E) if insufficient AB blood is available, type B can be used

29. A 60-year-old man notices right-sided chest pain after sneezing. The pain is made worse with breathing, but he reports no fever, sputum, or cough. Recently, he has been experiencing back discomfort and easy fatigue on exertion. On examination, the heart sounds are normal and lungs are clear. The left 6th rib is tender on palpation. X-rays of his chest are shown in Fig. 5–3 a and b. Which of the following is the most likely diagnosis?

(A) aneurysmal bone cyst

(B) multiple myeloma

(C) lymphosarcoma

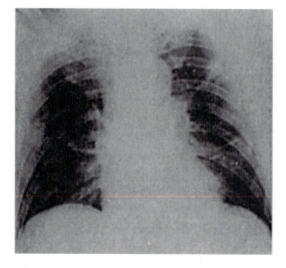

Figure 5–3a.

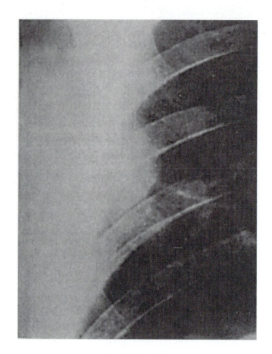

Figure 5–3b.

(D) prostatic metastases

(E) hyperparathyroidism

30. A 36-year-old woman with sickle cell disease presents with increasing pain in her right hip. She has no fever, chills, back or other bone pain, and there is no history of any trauma. On examination, her temperature is 37.3°C, range of motion in the right hip is reduced, she walks with a limp, and the right leg is shorter than the left. Movements of the hip and walking on it are painful. X-rays of the hip are shown in Fig. 5–4. Which of the following is the most likely diagnosis?

(A) avascular necrosis (AVN) of the femoral head

(B) osteomyelitis

(C) hip fracture

(D) septic arthritis

(E) multiple myeloma

31. A 30-year-old woman presents with increasing fatigue, but no other symptoms. On examination the conjunctivae are pale, her sclera are icteric, blood pressure 110/70 mm Hg, pulse 110/min, lungs clear, and heart sounds normal.

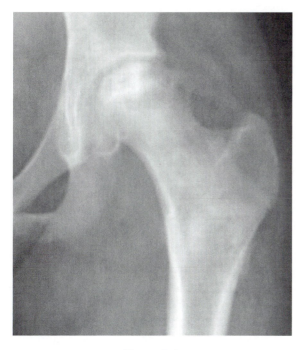

Figure 5–4.

Castell's sign is negative and no spleen is palpable. Her hemoglobin is 6 g/dL, and the rest of the laboratory workup is shown in Table 5–1. Which of the following is the most likely diagnosis?

(A) iron deficiency

(B) congenital spherocytosis

(C) liver failure and hemolysis

(D) splenomegaly and hemolysis

(E) autoimmune hemolytic anemia

TABLE 5–1. CASE WORKUP

Blood film	Polychromatophilia, some spherocytes
Bilirubin	2 mg/100 mL total
	0.3 mg/100 mL direct
Haptoglobin	10 mg/100 mL
Lactate dehydrogenase	200 IU/L
Urine bilirubin	Negative

DIRECTIONS (Questions 32 through 41): Each set of matching questions in this section consists of a list of lettered options followed by several numbered items. For each numbered item, select the appropriate lettered option(s). Each lettered option may be selected once, more than once, or not at all. **EACH ITEM WILL STATE THE NUMBER OF OPTIONS TO SELECT. CHOOSE EXACTLY THIS NUMBER.**

Questions 32 through 33

(A) aspirin

(B) naproxen

(C) tirofiban

(D) trimethoprim-sulfamethoxazole

(E) clopidogrel

(F) fish oils

(G) systemic lupus

(H) uremia

For each mechanism of a prolonged bleeding time, select the most likely cause.

32. Inhibits platelet activation induced by ADP (SELECT ONE)

33. Depletes platelet arachidonic acid (SELECT ONE)

Questions 34 through 41

(A) beta-thalassemia major

(B) HbH disease

(C) sickle cell disease

(D) HbC disease

(E) HbM disease

For each patient with a hemoglobin abnormality, select the most likely diagnosis.

34. A 23-year-old man has recurrent episodes of mild back and chest pain, whenever he is ill. His physical examination is normal. The hemoglobin level is 9 g/dL, MCV 85 fL, and platelets 250,000/mL. His blood film shows characteristic red cell morphologic changes that have hemoglobin units polymerizing in long chains under hypoxic stress as the underlying mechanism. (SELECT ONE)

35. A 32-year-old man has a mild anemia diagnosed on routine testing. He has no symptoms and feels fine. His clinical examination is normal, and a blood film reveals some target cells with some red cells having intraerythrocytic crystals. (SELECT ONE)

36. A 4-month-old baby has developed feeding problems and diarrhea. Laboratory evaluation reveals severe anemia with hemoglobin of 7 g/dL. The blood film shows hypochromic microcytic cells and target cells. In this disorder, decreased beta-chain production leads to excess alpha-chain production and destruction of red cell precursors. (SELECT ONE)

37. A 4-year-old boy has a chronic microcytic anemia, but no other symptoms. His physical examination is normal except for splenomegaly. His condition is due to decreased alpha-chain production, which leads to four beta-chain tetramer formation (HbH). (SELECT ONE)

38. A 27-year-old woman complains of constant back pain. She recently had an episode of severe chest and back pain that required narcotic medications, blood transfusions, and lots of fluids to treat. On examination, she is afebrile, with midthoracic tenderness on palpation. X-rays of the spine reveal periosteal reaction of the eighth thoracic vertebra She has a chronic blood disorder where bone infarction can occur that may be difficult to distinguish from osteomyelitis. (SELECT ONE)

Questions 39 through 41

(A) loss of Achillis tendon reflex
(B) increased perioperative morbidity
(C) renal concentration defect
(D) helmet cells and schistocytes are common
(E) occurs most commonly in the first trimester
(F) renal papillary necrosis
(G) cardiac arrhythmias
(H) increased HbH
(I) responds to folic acid
(J) paresthesias

For each patient with a hematologic disorder, select the most likely complications or associated conditions.

39. A 63-year-old woman with lymphoma has been treated with vincristine for many months.

She has now developed dose-limiting side effects from this drug. (SELECT TWO)

40. A 19-year-old woman is positive for sickle cell disease. (SELECT TWO)

41. A 24-year-old pregnant woman is found to be anemic. (SELECT ONE)

DIRECTIONS (Questions 42 through 59): Each of the numbered items in this section is followed by answers. Select the ONE lettered answer that is BEST in each case.

42. A 32-year-old woman has had a previous child with beta-thalassemia. She has just been confirmed as being 6 weeks pregnant. She is worried that the current pregnancy may also be affected. Which of the following methods is most likely to establish an accurate prenatal diagnosis?

(A) fetal ultrasound at 12 weeks
(B) cord blood electrophoresis
(C) chorionic villus sampling
(D) buccal mucosal cytology of both parents
(E) electrophoresis of amniotic fluid

43. A 27-year-old female presents with easy fatigue and light-headedness. She also has a dry cough and fever for the past few days. On examination, she is pale, her lungs are clear, and the rest is normal. A chest x-ray (CXR) shows patchy bilateral infiltrates; the hemoglobin is 8.4 g/dL, reticulocyte count of 6%, and many spherocytes on the peripheral blood film. Which of the following is the most likely significance of the spherocytosis on the blood film?

(A) multiple long bone fracture
(B) hereditary elliptocytosis
(C) Coombs'-positive hemolytic anemia
(D) glucose-6-phosphate dehydrogenase (G6PD) deficiency
(E) leukemia

44. A 25-year-old woman is pregnant for the first time. At prenatal assessment, she is found to have blood group A and Rh(D)-negative. Her husband is tested and he is Rh(D)-positive.

Which of the following is the most appropriate initial test to determine her risk for hemolytic disease of the newborn (erythroblastosis fetalis) due to Rh incompatibility?

(A) anti-Rh(D) antibody in maternal serum

(B) direct Coombs' test of maternal serum

(C) anti-Rh

(D) antibody in baby's serum

(D) ABO testing of the husband

(E) direct Coombs' test of neonate serum after birth

45. A 63-year-old man presents with fatigue, shortness of breath on exertion, and easy bruising. He has no prior history of bleeding disorders, and is not taking any medications. On examination, his conjunctivae are pale, he has palpable spleen, and there are multiple bruises and petechiae on his legs. A CBC reveals a hemoglobin of 8.3 g/dL, WBC of 2300/mL, and platelets of 30,000/mL. A blood film also shows multiple lymphocytes with prominent cytoplasmic projections. A bone marrow biopsy also shows similar cells in the marrow and marrow fibrosis. Which of the following is the most likely diagnosis? (See Fig. 5–5.)

(A) lymphoma

(B) myeloma

(C) myelofibrosis and myeloid metaplasia

(D) hairy cell leukemia

(E) chronic myelogenous leukemia

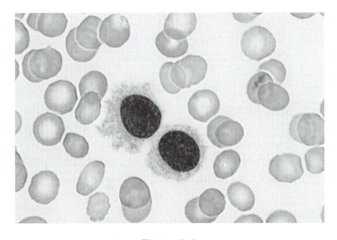

Figure 5–5.
(Reproduced, with permission, from Lichtman MA, et al. *Williams Hematology*, 7th ed. New York: McGraw-Hill, 2006:Plate XXI-7)

46. A 22-year-old long-distance runner is found to be mildly anemic. He is asymptomatic; his stool is negative for occult blood, and the ferritin level is 200 ng/mL. Which intervention is most likely to result in return of the hemoglobin to normal?

(A) using more supportive footwear

(B) iron replacement

(C) folate replacement

(D) altering his exercise program

(E) investigating and treating gastrointestinal (GI) pathology

47. A 49-year-old man presents with jaundice, nausea, and vomiting. He has a history of chronic alcoholism, and is currently drinking over one bottle of red wine a day. On physical examination, he is jaundiced and pale with a large tender liver. Laboratory data include hemoglobin of 9 g/dL, WBC of 4200/mL, and platelet count of 80,000/mL. His liver enzymes and bilirubin are also elevated. Ultrasound of the abdomen reveals liver enlargement with no bile duct obstruction, a normal size spleen, and no ascites. Which of the following is the most likely toxic effect of alcohol on the bone marrow?

(A) developing erythrocytes and myelocytes

(B) mature polymorphonuclear leukocytes

(C) mature red cells

(D) mature platelets

(E) eosinophils

48. A 22-year-old medical student donates his blood as part of a clinical study. He is discovered to have persistent HbF (fetal hemoglobin) levels. He feels well, and his clinical examination is normal. Which of the following features about this condition is most likely true?

(A) cause of sickling red cells

(B) disease of infants only

(C) variant of thalassemia major

(D) anemia exacerbated by fava beans

(E) benign genetic abnormality

49. A 19-year-old man had his spleen removed a year ago after a motorcycle accident. Which of the following findings on the blood film are most consistent with a previous history of splenectomy? (See Fig. 5–6.)

(A) increase in macrophages

(B) leukopenia

(C) polycythemia

(D) increased reticulocytes

(E) red cells with nuclear fragments

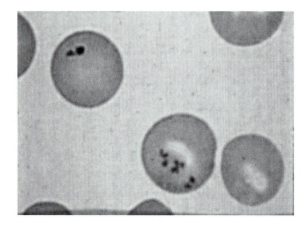

Figure 5–6.

50. A 49-year-old man is involved in a motor vehicle accident, resulting in large amounts of blood loss and hypotension. He is initially given normal saline at the accident site, and on arrival at the hospital, the trauma team orders an emergent blood transfusion with type O "universal donor" packed red cells. Which of the following is a possible complication of unmatched type O blood?

(A) type O donors have a higher incidence of hepatitis C virus

(B) type O donors have a shorter survival time when transfused than do other cell types

(C) at times type B blood may be mistyped as type O

(D) type O donors may have high titers of anti-A and anti-B in their plasma

(E) conversion of the recipient to type O blood

51. A 9-year-old boy presents with fever, feeling unwell, and easy bruising on his legs. On examination he is pale, blood pressure 100/60 mm Hg, pulse 100/min, and temperature 37.8°C. His lungs are clear, abdomen is soft with a palpable spleen, and there are petechiae and bruises on his legs. His CBC reveals a hemoglobin of 8.5 g/dL, WBC of 17,000/mL, and platelets of 30,000/mL. A blood film reveals neutropenia and leukemic lymphoblasts. Which of the following is the most appropriate initial diagnostic test to confirm the diagnosis?

(A) monospot test

(B) bone marrow aspirate and biopsy

(C) CT scan abdomen

(D) chest x-ray

(E) lumbar puncture and cerebrospinal fluid (CSF) fluid for cytology

52. A 50-year-old White woman presents with a 3-week history of tiredness and pallor. A family member has noted some yellowness of her eyes, but she denies darkening of the urine. Physical examination reveals only slight jaundice. Laboratory data include hemoglobin of 9 g/dL, reticulocyte count of 8%, a bilirubin in the serum of 2 mg/dL (indirect reacting), and some microspherocytes on peripheral smear. The direct antiglobulin test (Coombs') is positive. Which of the following is the most likely cause for her anemia?

(A) blood loss externally

(B) decreased red cell production

(C) ineffective erythropoiesis

(D) intravascular hemolysis

(E) extravascular hemolysis

53. A 24-year-old man is suspected of having mycoplasma pneumonia based on his symptoms of dry cough and chest x-ray findings. He is also anemic with hemoglobin of 10.5 g/dL, and hemolytic anemia from cold agglutinins is suspected. Which of the following is consistent with hemolytic anemia?

(A) increased haptoglobin level

(B) increased bilirubin in the urine

(C) increased reticulocyte count

(D) increased myoglobin in the blood

(E) increased hemopexin in the blood

54. A 57-year-old man, with a history of chronic alcohol ingestion, is admitted to the hospital with acute alcoholic intoxication and lobar pneumonia. Physical examination reveals pallor; a large, tender liver; and consolidation of the right lower lobe. Laboratory data include hemoglobin of 7 g/dL, WBC of 4000/mL, and platelet count of 85,000/mL.Which of the following is the most likely factor for the anemia?

(A) hemolysis

(B) hemobilia

(C) vitamin B_{12} deficiency

(D) toxic marrow suppression

(E) hemoglobinopathy

55. A 82-year-old woman is brought to the hospital because of functional decline at home and an inability to care for herself. She has a prior history of hypertension and dyslipidemia, and her medications include hydrochlorothiazide and atorvastatin. She looks disheveled, pale, and has muscle wasting; her heart and lungs are clear and there are no focal neurologic findings. Her hemoglobin is 9 g/dL, MCV 105 fL, WBC 4500/mL, and platelets 100,000/mL. The blood film shows macrocytic RBCs and hypersegmented neutrophils. Which of the following vitamin deficiencies is most likely responsible for her pancytopenia?

(A) B_{12} (cyanocobalamin)

(B) folate

(C) pyridoxine

(D) thiamine

(E) riboflavin

56. A 39-year-old man with chronic alcoholism is brought to the hospital after a fall, while intoxicated. He has completely recovered except for a bruise on his shoulder. His only abnormality is low hemoglobin of 9.6 g/dL, the platelets and WBC are normal. Additional tests including ferritin, vitamins B_{12}, and folate are normal. Which of the following findings is most likely to be seen on his peripheral blood film?

(A) macrocytosis

(B) basophilia

(C) red cell fragments

(D) increased platelet adhesiveness

(E) atypical lymphocytes

57. A 56-year-old woman presents with feeling light-headed when standing up and 3 days of passing dark black stools. She has past history of chronic viral hepatitis B, and has developed cirrhosis. On examination she is alert, blood pressure is 90/60 mm Hg supine and 76/60 mm Hg standing. Her abdomen is distended with signs of ascites, nontender, and there are multiple bruises on the legs. Her hemoglobin is 9.0 g/dL, platelets 90,000/mL, albumin 3 g/dL, bilirubin 1.3 mg/dL, and international normalized ratio (INR) 2.5 (prothrombin time [PT] 25 seconds). Which of the following coagulation factors are most likely deficient in this patient?

(A) V and VIII

(B) VIII, IX, XI, and XII

(C) XIII

(D) II, V, VII, IX, X, and XI

(E) II, VII, IX, and X

58. A 18-year-old man, of Italian extraction, is found to have a hypochromic microcytic anemia of 10 g/dL. In addition, there is a fair degree of anisocytosis, poikilocytosis, and targeting on the blood film. The WBC is 9500/mL, the platelet count is 240,000/mL, and the reticulocyte count is 7%. The spleen is palpated 5 cm below the left costal margin. Which of the following is the most likely diagnosis?

(A) sickle cell trait

(B) thalassemia minor

(C) HbS-C disease

(D) sideroblastic anemia

(E) hereditary spherocytosis

59. A 28-year-old man, originally from West Africa, is found on routine examination to have splenomegaly. His hemoglobin is 9.5 g/dL, and blood film examination reveals target cells. Which of the following is the most likely abnormal hemoglobin in this man?

   (A) HbM
   (B) HbS
   (C) Hb Zurich
   (D) HbC
   (E) Hb Barts

DIRECTIONS (Questions 60 through 73): Each set of matching questions in this section consists of a list of lettered options followed by several numbered items. For each numbered item, select the appropriate lettered option(s). Each lettered option may be selected once, more than once, or not at all. EACH ITEM WILL STATE THE NUMBER OF OPTIONS TO SELECT. CHOOSE EXACTLY THIS NUMBER.

Questions 60 through 64

   (A) iron deficiency anemia
   (B) beta-thalassemia trait
   (C) anemia of chronic disease
   (D) sideroblastic anemia

For each patient with a hypochromic microcytic anemia, select the most likely diagnosis.

60. A 42-year-old man is feeling chronically fatigued. His hemoglobin is 11.5 g/dL, and the blood film is hypochromic and microcytic. The serum iron is increased, total iron-binding capacity (TIBC) is normal, ferritin is increased, and HbA2 is decreased. (SELECT ONE)

61. An 18-year-old woman is feeling chronically fatigued. Her hemoglobin is 11.5 g/dL, RBC count 5,900,000/mL, and the blood film is hypochromic and microcytic. The serum iron is normal, TIBC is normal, ferritin is normal, and HbA2 is elevated. (SELECT ONE)

62. A 67-year-old man presents with fatigue due to a low hemoglobin value of 9.2 g/dL. The blood film shows hypochromic microcytic cells. His serum iron is decreased, TIBC is increased, ferritin is decreased, and HbA2 is normal. (SELECT ONE)

63. A 43-year-old man, in hospital for 2 weeks with pancreatitis, is anemic with hemoglobin of 9.7 g/dL and MCV 79 fL. The blood film shows slightly microcytic hypochromic red cells, and the reticulocyte count is 0.5 %. The serum is iron decreased, TIBC is decreased, serum ferritin is increased, and HbA2 normal. (SELECT ONE)

64. A 52-year-old man is complaining of fatigue. His physical examination is normal, but his hemoglobin is low at 8.9 mg/dL. The reticulocyte count is 0.5 %, serum iron and TIBC are normal, and ferritin is elevated. A bone marrow aspirate reveals erythroid precursors that have accumulated abnormal amounts of mitochondrial iron. (SELECT ONE)

Questions 65 through 69

   (A) spherocytes
   (B) schistocytes
   (C) sickle cells
   (D) burr cells
   (E) agglutinated cells
   (F) Heinz bodies

For each of the following conditions, select the most likely RBC morphology.

65. Found in severe liver disease. (SELECT ONE)

66. Represent precipitated Hb. (SELECT ONE)

67. Caused by loss of red cell membrane. (SELECT ONE)

68. Caused by polymerization of an abnormal Hb. (SELECT ONE)

69. Caused by trauma to red cell membranes. (SELECT ONE)

Questions 70 through 73

    (A) von Willebrand's disease

    (B) hemophilia A

    (C) hemophilia B

    (D) thrombotic thrombocytopenic purpura (TTP)

For each patient with a bleeding disorder, select the most likely diagnosis.

70. A 23-year-old man presents with prolonged nose bleeds. He has always noted easy bruising, and ongoing bleeding after minor cuts. There is no prior history of surgery or dental procedures. His hemoglobin is 14.5 g/dL, platelets 200,000/mL, and PT/PPT is normal. Further testing reveals that the bleeding time is elevated; the factor VIII level is reduced, as is the ristocetin cofactor assay. (SELECT ONE)

71. An 18-year-old man develops excessive bleeding 2 hours after wisdom tooth extraction. He has a history of easy bruising after playing sports, and of minor cuts that rebleed. His examination is normal, except for the tooth extraction site, which is still oozing blood. His hemoglobin is 14.8 g/dL, platelets 230,000 mL, PT is normal, and partial thromboplastin time (PTT) is elevated. A bleeding time is normal, factor VIII level is reduced, factor IX is normal, and ristocetin cofactor assay is normal. (SELECT ONE)

72. A 19-year-old man is brought to the hospital after injuring his knee playing football. The knee is swollen and painful to move. He has no prior history of bleeding disorders. Arthrocentesis of the knee reveals 20 cc of blood. Further investigations show that his platelets are 170,000/mL, PT is normal, PTT is elevated, bleeding time is normal, factor VIII is normal, factor IX is reduced, and the ristocetin cofactor assay is normal. (SELECT ONE)

73. A 27-year-old woman presents with nose bleeds, rash on her feet, and fevers. She looks unwell, pale, jaundiced, and there are multiple petechiae on her feet. The lungs are clear, heart sounds normal, and abdomen is soft with no palpable spleen or liver. Her bilirubin is 2 mg/dL (mostly indirect), aspartate amino transferase (AST), alanine amino transferase (ALT), alkaline phosphatase (ALP) are normal. The hemoglobin is 8.7 g/dL, platelets 24,000/mL, PT/PTT normal, and bleeding time is elevated. The blood film reveals anemia, thrombocytopenia, and red cell fragments. (SELECT ONE)

Answers and Explanations

1. **(D)** The symptoms are typical of cryoglobulinemia. Cryoglobulins are antibodies that precipitate under cold conditions and are associated with several diseases. There are three main types of cryoglobulin syndromes based on the immunoglobulin composition of the precipitating antibody. Most cryoglobulinemic vasculitis is Type II or mixed and seen secondary to hepatitis C virus infection. Cold agglutinin disease would present with hemolytic anemia. The other syndromes would not generally be temperature sensitive. *(Lichtman, pp. 1857–1858)*

2. **(E)** The syndrome is caused by cold-precipitable proteins (cryoglobulins) that are found in plasma or serum. These cryoproteins can be of three classes. Type 1 are single component (immunoglobulin G, M, or A [IgG, IgM, IgA]), Type 2 are called "mixed cryoglobulins" (usually IgG molecules complexed with IgM molecules having anti-IgG reactivity), and Type 3 are polyclonal immunoglobulins with anti-immunoglobulin activity. Cryoglobulinemia is small vessel vasculitis (not medium), and platelet aggregation is not an important mechanism for the vessel injury. *(Lichtman, pp. 1857–1858)*

3. **(D)** Auer bodies are slender, pink, staining rods containing lysozyme, and are exclusively seen in AML. Although similar to normal azurophilic granules in content and staining properties, they are distinguished by their gigantic size. Special stains can enhance the detection of Auer bodies. They are only seen in a minority of cases. The Philadelphia chromosome is a feature of choric myelogenous leukemia (CML), and a high leukocyte alkaline phosphatase level is seen in patients with a high WBC due to a leukemoid reaction. *(Lichtman, pp. 1186, 1192)*

4. **(B)** This is a case of chronic myelogenous leukemia. The reciprocal translocation involves the long arms of 22 and 9, and results in translocation of the ABL proto-oncogene from chromosome 9 adjacent to a portion of the BCR gene on chromosome 22. The resultant abnormal chromosome 22 is known as the Philadelphia (Ph1) chromosome. *(Lichtman, pp. 1244–1245)*

5. **(A)** An increased amount of HbF or HbA2 would be expected. As beta-chains are decreased in beta-thalassemia, the excess alpha-chains combine with gamma- and delta-chains to make HbF and HbA2, respectively. *(Lichtman, p. 652)*

6. **(A)** Graft-versus-host disease is a frequent complication of hematopoietic cell transplantation. It is caused by a reaction of immunologically competent donor derived T cells that react with recipient tissue antigens. It can be acute or chronic. Numerous treatment regimens involving methotrexate, glucocorticoids, cyclosporine, and other drugs are used in treatment. *(Lichtman, pp. 309–312)*

7. **(B)** In hemophilia A, there are decreased levels of functioning factor VIII. This can be due to reduced amounts of normal VIII, the presence of a functionally abnormal protein, or a combination of both. The activated partial thromboplastin time (APTT) is prolonged, and the prothrombin consumption test is abnormal. The prothrombin time, thrombin clotting time,

and bleeding time are usually normal. *(Lichtman, pp. 1870–1871)*

8. **(E)** Hypernephroma, cerebellar hemangiomas, hepatoma, and giant uterine myomas are the tumors associated with secondary polycythemia. Endocrine disorders, hypoxia, and high-affinity hemoglobins can also cause secondary polycythemia. *(Lichtman, pp. 781–786)*

9. **(C)** Heterophil antibodies react against sheep red cells and are not absorbed out by the guinea pig kidney. They are positive in patients with infectious mononucleosis. In 90% of cases, liver enzymes are elevated. Examination of the blood film reveals a lymphocytosis with atypical lymphocytes. *(Lichtman, p. 1137)*

10. **(A, D, I)** Hemoglobin C is abnormal hemoglobin where lysine has been substituted for glutamic acid at the sixth position of the beta-chain. Homozygous C red cells are often target-shaped with "extra" membrane to make them less osmotically fragile. However, cells containing principally HbC are more rigid than normal and their fragmentation in the circulation may result in microspherocytes. Intracellular crystals and oxygenated HbC can be seen. The spleen is invariably enlarged. Women can become pregnant and tolerate the pregnancy well. *(Lichtman, p. 684)*

11. **(B, F, J)** Bone lesions in myeloma are destructive, but the alkaline phosphatase is usually normal, indicating little blastic activity. Osteolysis, when combined with immobilization, can lead to hypercalcemia. It is usually mediated by an osteoclast-activating factor from neoplastic myeloma cells in the adjacent marrow. Bone pain can be severe. Bence Jones proteinuria and myeloma cells in the marrow are typical. If cryoglobulinemia occurs, it is type I. *(Lichtman, pp. 1505–1506)*

12. **(A, D, L)** Hemolytic anemias are not associated with erythroid hypoplasia of the marrow. Erythroid hyperplasia is present except during infections or insults that lead to regenerative

crises. As a result, there is usually an increased number of reticulocytes and elevated fecal and urinary urobilinogen. Decreased RBC survival is a hallmark of the disease. *(Lichtman, pp. 405–408)*

13. **(B, H, K)** Microcytic hypochromic anemias are caused by disorders of iron, globin, heme, or porphyrin metabolism and are not seen in thiamine deficiency. *(Lichtman, pp. 526–527)*

14. **(D, F, K)** Postsplenectomy thrombocytosis usually resolves within 2 months. Both acute blood loss and chronic iron deficiency can increase platelets. Hemolytic anemia is associated with both increased reticulocytes and thrombocytosis. Thromboembolic or hemorrhagic phenomena are more common in essential thrombocytosis rather than secondary causes. *(Lichtman, p. 1785)*

15. **(C)** Iron chelation with desferrioxamine will reduce the toxicity from iron overload if given regularly in high doses. The most lethal toxicity of iron load is iron infiltration of the myocardium, with resultant dysfunction and death. *(Lichtman, p. 657)*

16. **(C)** Bone marrow examination is most likely to show increased erythroid-to-myeloid ratio. Erythroid hyperplasia is common to all hemolytic anemias, and megaloblastic features may develop unless folate is supplied. *(Lichtman, p. 737)*

17. **(C)** The present treatment of choice for thalassemia minor is purely supportive. Care is taken to watch for anemia during intercurrent illness, due to a regenerative crisis. *(Lichtman, pp. 657–658)*

18. **(E)** Reactive thrombocytosis is usually transitory, without thromboembolism, hemorrhage, splenomegaly, or leukocytosis. Causes of secondary thrombocytosis include chronic inflammatory disorders (e.g., rheumatoid arthritis), acute inflammatory disease, acute or chronic blood loss, and malignancy. Recovery from thrombocytopenia ("rebound") can also result in very high platelets. A common cause is withdrawal from alcohol. *(Lichtman, pp. 1786–1787)*

19. **(E)** Steroids cause decreased numbers of eosinophils to circulate, so that eosinophilia may be seen in Addison's disease, for example. Beta-blockers may cause eosinophilia by blocking beta-adrenergic eosinopenia. Atopic and nonatopic chronic asthma are frequently associated with mild eosinophilia. Numerous allergic diseases, allergic rhinitis, atopic dermatitis, and urticaria can also cause eosinophilia. Parasites are the most common worldwide cause of eosinophilia, but other infections rarely cause it. *(Lichtman, pp. 869, 870)*

20. **(D)** Febrile reactions to leukocytes may be severe and cause hypotension, especially in repeatedly transfused patients. Antibodies to platelets can also develop. Usually, at least seven transfusions are required to induce sensitization. *(Lichtman, pp. 2166–2167)*

21. **(C)** The painful crisis seen in patients with sickle cell disease is due to vaso-occlusive disease where microvascular ischemic injury occurs to tissues. Acute illness, dehydration, and infections are common precipitants for this type of crisis. Because sickle cell anemia is a chronic hemolytic anemia, the reticulocyte is chronically elevated, except in aplastic crises, and erythrocyte life span is shortened. Infection is the most common precipitant of an aplastic crisis, particularly those caused by parvovirus B19. Sequestration crisis (hemoglobin level <6 mg/dL) is sudden massive pooling of red cells in the spleen resulting in hemodynamic instability. Hemolytic crisis is the sudden further reduction in red cell life span marked by falling hemoglobin, jaundice, and increased reticulocyte count. *(Lichtman, p. 675)*

22. **(E)** A serum ferritin determination would be most helpful. Iron stores in thalassemia are normal or increased. Some of the increase may be secondary to injudicious iron therapy. *(Lichtman, pp. 527–528)*

23. **(E)** The diagnosis of autoimmune hemolytic anemia requires demonstration of immunoglobulin and/or complement in the patient's RBC. The broad-spectrum Coombs' test is an excellent screen. *(Lichtman, p. 729)*

24. **(C)** Clopidogrel selectively inhibits platelet activation induced by ADP. It works as an ADP-receptor blocker. Other antiplatelet drugs such as ASA are COX-1 inhibitors, and dipyridamole modulates cAMP levels. *(Lichtman, pp. 291–293)*

25. **(B)** Heparin appears to act as catalyst in the inactivation of thrombin and factors XA, IXA, XIA, and by antithrombin III. However, not all patients with thrombosis and heparin resistance have antithrombin III deficiency. *(Lichtman, pp. 1988–1989)*

26. **(A)** Iron deficiency is the most common cause of anemia in infancy. Sixty percent of body iron concentration at birth is contained in circulating Hb. Milk is a poor source of iron, so the most common cause of iron deficiency in infancy is prolonged breast or bottle feeding. Cereals are high in iron content. *(Lichtman, pp. 520–521)*

27. **(C)** The 2,3-bisphosphoglycerate (2,3-BPG) binds to the central cavity of the heme molecule and changes the configuration in favor of oxygen release. The other common factors that affect oxygen affinity are temperature and pH. The oxygen affinity of Hb is easily characterized by P50; the oxygen tension at which Hb is half-saturated. *(Lichtman, p. 606)*

28. **(B)** Group AB has neither anti-A nor anti-B antibodies, as both A and B antigens are on the red cells. Persons with type AB blood are considered "universal recipients." It is a rare blood group (only 2–3% of population); if large amounts of blood are required in an AB individual, any type of blood (A, AB, B, O) can be used as long as the plasma is removed from the donor blood (in other words packed RBCs are used). *(Kasper, pp. 662–664)*

29. **(B)** There is lytic destruction of the 6th rib with a pathologic fracture and an extrapleural mass. The most common manifestation of multiple myeloma is multiple, "punched-out" lesions in the flat and tubular bones. Some may appear as discrete lytic lesions and remain as solitary lesions. *(Lichtman, p. 1510)*

30. **(A)** The diagnosis is AVN of the femoral head. Bone complications occur frequently in patients with sickle cell anemia. Infarcted areas of bone and bone marrow can become sites of infection (osteomyelitis) with *Staphylococcus aureus* or salmonella, but the lack of fever and clinical signs in this patient suggest AVN. Infarction of the femoral head nutrient artery leads to AVN and chronic joint pain. The humeral head is also at risk of AVN. Septic arthritis is a less common complication. *(Lichtman, p. 676)*

31. **(E)** Autoimmune hemolytic anemia is the most likely diagnosis. Spherocytosis is seen as well in burn victims, in microangiopathic hemolysis, and in congenital spherocytosis. *(Lichtman, p. 737)*

32. **(E)** Clopidogrel is an ADP-receptor blocker, and inhibits platelet activation induced by ADP. This results in a prolongation of bleeding time that is greater than that produced by acetylsalicylic acid (ASA). The effects last for 4–10 days after discontinuation. Clopidogrel is a prodrug that relies on an active metabolite for its effect, and is marginally more effective than ASA for certain conditions like stroke and acute coronary syndrome. The effect on bleeding time is additive to that of ASA. *(Lichtman, p. 292)*

33. **(F)** Fish oils cause a slight prolongation of the bleeding time. The mechanism is twofold: they reduce platelet arachidonic acid, and as well they compete with arachidonic acid for cyclooxygenase. Other foods that may affect platelet function include garlic, onions, and black tree fungus (found in Chinese cuisine). *(Lichtman, p. 1838)*

34. **(C)** A number of factors influence the rate and degree of HbS aggregation, including concentration of HbS in the cell, cellular dehydration, and the length of time in deoxyconformation. *(Lichtman, p. 672)*

35. **(D)** The patients with homozygous HbC disease have mild hemolysis, splenomegaly, target cells, and HbC crystals. Unlike sickle cell disease, the prognosis is favorable. *(Lichtman, pp. 684–685)*

36. **(A)** In beta-thalassemia, there is excess production of alpha-chains, which precipitate and destroy red cell precursors. *(Lichtman, p. 633)*

37. **(B)** HbH (four beta-chains) most commonly results from the compound heterozygous state for alpha-plus-thalassemia and either deletion or nondeletion alpha-plus-thalassemia. However, the phenotypic expression of the disease is quite variable. *(Lichtman, p. 651)*

38. **(C)** If the bone infarction occurs in proximity to a joint, an effusion can develop. The underlying pathology is a vaso-occlusive phenomenon. Bone infarction can appear like osteomyelitis (radiographically and clinically), which is problematic since patients with sickle cell disease are also at increased risk of osteomyelitis. *(Lichtman, p. 676)*

39. **(A, J)** Neurotoxicity is the dose-limiting side effect of vincristine. Neurologic toxicity is usually the result of a cumulative dose and usually begins when the total dose exceeds 6 mg/m^2. Paresthesia of fingers and feet and loss of deep tendon reflexes are the usual initial manifestation. Continual administration may lead to severe motor weakness, particularly in the elderly. Constipation can also occur as a result of autonomic neuropathy. Syndrome of inappropriate antidiuretic hormone (SIADH) with hyponatremia can occur. *(Lichtman, pp. 256–257)*

40. **(C, F)** The renal concentrating defect and positive sickle prep are constant, but occlusive phenomena in the kidney can result in hematuria from papillary necrosis. This occurs when the red cells are prone to sickle cell formation under hypoxic stress. *(Lichtman, pp. 676–677)*

41. **(I)** The megaloblastic anemia of pregnancy is the most common of all folate-deficient states. Dilutional anemia and iron deficiency also occur in pregnancy. In pregnancy, a low Hb concentration may simply be due to a disproportionate increase in plasma volume, rather than a true anemia. The exact hormonal mechanism is unknown. Folate levels fall during pregnancy; therefore, frank deficiency is most common in the third trimester. *(Lichtman, p. 489)*

42. **(C)** Chorionic villus sampling in the first trimester with deoxyribonucleic acid (DNA)-based diagnosis has a high degree of accuracy. Cord blood electrophoresis is suitable for screening high-risk infants at birth. *(Lichtman, p. 659)*

43. **(C)** Spherocytes are seen on the blood film in patients with moderate to severe hemolytic anemia. This patient has autoimmune hemolytic anemia due to cold agglutinins related the pneumonia. Spherocytosis is not associated with G6PD deficiency, trauma, or leukemia. The typical changes in G6PD deficiency include the presence of Heinz bodies. The cell morphology is not usually changed unless hemolysis is very severe. In hereditary spherocytosis, the Coombs' test is negative. *(Lichtman, p. 737)*

44. **(A)** Testing the mother for the presence of Rh(D) antibodies (alloimmunization) is done by indirect Coombs' test of the maternal serum with known Rh(D) positive cells. Prevention of Rh immunization by the administration of Rh antibody (via Rh immune globulin) has been an effective preventive measure for this disorder. This condition is usually associated with a positive Coombs' test using the baby's RBCs and a positive indirect Coombs' test using the mother's serum. ABO hemolytic disease of the newborn is clinically mild because the antigens are not fully expressed in utero. *(Lichtman, p. 751)*

45. **(D)** This patient has hairy cell leukemia, which is a rare form of adult of leukemia (2–3%). The disease is characterized by "hairy" cells in blood and bone marrow, splenomegaly, and pancytopenia. The lymphocytes have characteristic cytoplasmic projections, which give the disease its name. Treatment with the purine analogue, such as cladribine, produces complete remission in hairy cell leukemia. Recombinant alpha-interferon is not as effective. *(Lichtman, p. 1385)*

46. **(D)** Supportive footwear will decrease the likelihood of "march" hemolysis, but this rarely causes anemia. Similarly, although 20% of long-distance runners have GI blood loss, this is rarely of a magnitude to explain anemia. Most elite athletes have increases in both plasma volume and red cell mass, but the increase in plasma volume is greater, resulting in a dilutional-type anemia. This is physiologically beneficial (increased O_2 transport with increased blood fluidity), so there is no reason to cease exercising to correct the Hb. *(Lichtman, p. 415)*

47. **(A)** Alcohol is directly toxic to dividing and maturing cells, but may also affect neutrophil function. The hematologic effects of alcohol may be direct or indirect, via diet, infection, liver disease, and GI disease. The resulting hematologic abnormalities may be profound. *(Lichtman, pp. 557–558)*

48. **(E)** HbF is evenly distributed among red cells, unlike the increased F in other conditions. It is a heterogeneous condition, and can be classified into deletion and nondeletion forms. Clinically, it can have features similar to mild thalassemia. *(Lichtman, p. 655)*

49. **(E)** The spleen normally functions to pit nuclei and their fragments from red cells. These nuclear fragments are called Howell-Jolly bodies. The spleen has immune functions and filter functions. It also enhances iron reutilization, and acts as a reservoir and blood-volume regulator. In disease states, it can be a site of extramedullary hematopoiesis. *(Lichtman, p. 777)*

50. **(D)** Anti-A and anti-B in the donor plasma are usually absorbed in the recipient's tissues but have the capacity to harm recipient cells. *(Lichtman, p. 2165)*

51. **(B)** In acute lymphoblastic leukemia (ALL), a bone marrow analysis is the most important test in confirming the diagnosis. Once the diagnosis of ALL is established, CSF fluid (leukemic cells in the CSF can be identified in up to a third of *all* patients at diagnosis) and CXR are important tests in the workup of the patient. It is the most common malignancy in children under age 15 in the United States, accounting for 25% of all cancers in White children. It is less common in Black children. *(Lichtman, pp. 1324–1326)*

52. **(E)** This patient has autoimmune hemolysis and the red cell destruction is extravascular, usually occurring in the liver, spleen, or other reticuloendothelial sites. It liberates unconjugated bilirubin causing jaundice. Intrinsic causes of hemolytic anemia are usually inherited, and are a result of abnormalities of membranes, red cell enzymes, globins, or heme. Extrinsic hemolysis is a result of mechanical forces, chemicals or microorganisms, antibodies, or sequestration in the monocyte-macrophage system. *(Lichtman, pp. 406–407)*

53. **(C)** In hemolytic anemia the haptoglobin is decreased, reticulocyte count increased, and unconjugated bilirubin increased. There is no bilirubin in the urine because unconjugated bilirubin is not cleared by the kidney as it is tightly bound to plasma proteins. *(Lichtman, p. 737)*

54. **(D)** Anemia is usually multifactorial in alcoholics and includes marrow suppression, GI bleeding, hemorrhagic diathesis, and nutritional deficiency. *(Lichtman, pp. 557–558)*

55. **(B)** The macrocytosis and hypersegmented neutrophils suggests a megaloblastic anemia due to either folate or vitamin B_{12} deficiency. Folate deficiency results from decreased intake and malabsorption. Body folate stores are meager (only 3 months on average, compared to a few years for vitamin B_{12}), and therefore easily depleted when intake is poor. Alcohol itself can depress folate levels acutely, and also can cause pancytopenia directly. *(Lichtman, pp. 477, 488)*

56. **(A)** Macrocytosis is frequently seen in patients with chronic alcoholism for multiple reasons including vitamin B_{12} or folate deficiency, chronic liver disease, and also from the direct toxic effects of alcohol on red cells. Because both iron deficiency and folate deficiency are very common in alcoholics, a dimorphic blood film can also be seen (macrocytes, hypersegmented neutrophils, and hypochromic microcytes can be found) on the same slide. *(Lichtman, pp. 557–558)*

57. **(D)** Coagulation factors II, V, VII, IX, X, and XI would most likely be deficient. These are some of the factors that are synthesized in the liver. Factors II, VII, IX, and X are the vitamin K-dependent factors, which are also synthesized in the liver. *(Lichtman, p. 1953)*

58. **(B)** Thalassemia minor usually represents a heterozygous state and is often asymptomatic. Symptoms may develop during periods of stress such as pregnancy or severe infection. Hemoglobin values are usually in the 9–11 g/dL range. The red cells are small and poorly hemoglobinized. *(Lichtman, p. 651)*

59. **(D)** HbC characteristically produces targeting in the peripheral blood and also hemoglobin crystals in the cells. HbC is found in 17–28% of West Africans. Splenomegaly is a fairly constant feature, but most patients are quite asymptomatic. *(Lichtman, p. 684)*

60. **(D)** Sideroblastic anemia is associated with an increased serum iron and ferritin. TIBC is generally normal. HbA2 is usually decreased. *(Lichtman, pp. 823–825)*

61. **(B)** The beta-thalassemia trait is characterized by normal iron studies and an elevated HbA2. *(Lichtman, p. 652)*

62. **(A)** Iron deficiency is characterized by low serum iron and ferritin and an increase in TIBC. HbA2 is normal. *(Lichtman, pp. 524–526)*

63. **(C)** Anemia of chronic disease is characterized by decreased serum iron and TIBC, an elevated ferritin, and normal HbA2. *(Lichtman, pp. 567–568)*

64. **(D)** Erythroid precursors that have accumulated abnormal amounts of iron are called ringed sideroblasts. Sideroblastic anemia can be either inherited or acquired. Common acquired causes are ingestion of certain drugs, alcohol, or toxins such as lead or zinc. The beta-thalassemia trait is diagnosed by demonstrating an elevated HbA2, iron deficiency by iron studies and ferritin levels, and anemia of chronic disease by demonstrating

a chronic disease. Sideroblastic anemia generally requires a bone marrow aspiration revealing ringed sideroblasts for diagnosis. *(Lichtman, p. 823)*

65. **(D)** Burr cells and stomatocytes are found in severe liver disease and might result from abnormal membrane lipids. *(Lichtman, pp. 15–16)*

66. **(F)** Heinz bodies (precipitated Hb) are found in disorders with unstable Hb or after oxidant stress. *(Lichtman, pp. 15–16)*

67. **(A)** Spherocytes are caused by loss of membrane, as in hereditary spherocytosis or autoimmune hemolytic anemia. *(Lichtman, pp. 15–16)*

68. **(C)** Sickle cell disease results in polymerization of HbS and the characteristic sickle cells. *(Lichtman, pp. 15–16)*

69. **(B)** Schistocytes are caused by traumatic disruption of the red cell membrane (e.g., microangiopathic syndromes). *(Lichtman, pp. 15–16)*

70. **(A)** von Willebrand's disease is the most common inherited bleeding disorder. The abnormal plasma glycoprotein, von Willebrand factor (vWF), has two major functions: facilitating platelet adhesion and serving as a carrier for factor VIII. The disease is heterogeneous in its manifestations but can be very severe (type III disease). Evaluation reveals a prolonged bleeding time and decreased factor VIII activity. *(Lichtman, pp. 1935–1937)*

71. **(B)** Hemophilia A results from a deficiency or dysfunction of the factor VIII molecule. It is a sex-linked disease affecting 1 in 10,000 males. The PTT is prolonged, but the bleeding time is characteristically normal. *(Lichtman, pp. 1870–1874)*

72. **(C)** Hemophilia B is clinically indistinguishable from hemophilia A and is also inherited via the X chromosome. The bleeding time is usually normal, but the PTT is usually elevated. Differentiation from hemophilia A requires factor assay. *(Lichtman, pp. 1880–1881)*

73. **(D)** TTP is a fulminant disorder that can be fatal. It has been associated with malignancy, pregnancy, metastatic cancer, and high-dose chemotherapy. Most often, the classical tests of hemostasis and platelet function are normal. The classical symptoms include fever, thrombocytopenia, microangiopathic hemolytic anemia, renal failure, and fluctuating neurologic defects. *(Lichtman, p. 2034)*

CHAPTER 6

Oncology
Questions

DIRECTIONS (Questions 1 through 30): Each of the numbered items in this section is followed by answers. Select the ONE lettered answer that is BEST in each case.

1. A 19-year-old man presents with multiple lymph nodes in his neck. He reports no current infectious symptoms, and his monospot test is negative. On examination, he has blanching skin lesions on his face and conjunctivae, multiple large lymph nodes in his neck, and poor coordination when tested by tandem walking. He has past history of poor coordination and walking difficulty as well as recurrent sinopulmonary infections. A biopsy of the lymph node is positive for lymphoma. He is diagnosed with a hereditary disorder that is autosomal dominant, and is associated with defective deoxyribonucleic acid (DNA) repair mechanisms. Which of the following is the most likely diagnosis?

   (A) neurofibromatosis
   (B) tuberous sclerosis
   (C) ataxia-telangiectasia
   (D) von Hippel-Lindau syndrome
   (E) Peutz-Jeghers syndrome

2. A 33-year-old male immigrant from Taiwan presents with increasing right upper quadrant (RUQ) pain. The pain is dull, and it does not radiate or change with eating. On examination the abdomen is soft, there is a mass in the RUQ, and no ascites is clinically detected. He has a prior history of hepatitis B. His laboratory investigations reveal hepatitis B surface antigen (HBsAg) positive, hepatitis B surface antibody (HBsAb) negative, aspartate amino transferase (AST) 60 U/L, alanine amino transferase (ALT) 72 U/L, and an elevated alpha-fetoprotein level. Which of the following is the most likely diagnosis? (See Fig. 6–1.)

   (A) hepatoma
   (B) hepatocellular carcinoma (HCC)
   (C) metastatic cancer
   (D) hepatic hemangioma
   (E) liver cirrhosis

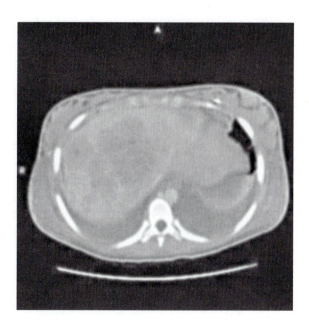

Figure 6–1.

3. A 42-year-old man received radiation exposure at a nuclear power plant in Eastern Europe. He is now concerned about his future cancer risk. Which of the following statements is correct?

(A) malignancies occur within 10 years of exposure

(B) leukemia has the shortest latency period of all malignancies

(C) large exposure is required to develop the most serious malignancies

(D) risk increases with advancing age at the time of exposure

(E) therapeutic radiation therapy given without chemotherapy does not increase the risk of a second malignancy

4. A 25-year-old woman has recently moved to a new city. She comes today for her first routine visit and annual physical assessment. She asks you about screening tests for cancer at her age. Which of the following cancer screening tests are recommended for her age group?

(A) mammography every 5 years

(B) Pap smear at least every 3 years

(C) stool for occult blood

(D) chest x-ray (CXR) every 3 years

(E) physical examination of the breast by a physician

5. A 25-year-old woman presents with intermittent double vision and fatigue. Her symptoms are worse at the end of the day. She reports no other focal muscle weakness or sensory symptoms. On examination her eye movements, motor strength, and reflexes in the upper and lower limbs are normal. Repetitive handgrip exercises cause loss of strength in the grip. A CXR reveals an anterior mediastinal mass. Which of the following is the most likely diagnosis of the anterior mediastinal mass?

(A) teratoma

(B) thyroid

(C) thymoma

(D) lymphoma

(E) mediastinal cyst

6. A 64-year-old man presents with symptoms of difficulty swallowing and weight loss of 10 lb. He has no prior history of heartburn, stomach ulcers, or difficulty swallowing. He smokes one pack a day for the past 45 years and drinks approximately 5 oz of alcohol a day. He is thin appearing, there are no oral lesions, and the remaining examination is normal. Esophago-scopy reveals a midesophageal narrowing with ragged ulcerating, and biopsies are taken. Which of the following is the most likely diagnosis?

(A) adenocarcinoma of esophagus

(B) esophageal web

(C) achalasia

(D) squamous cell carcinoma of esophagus

(E) esophageal leiomyoma

7. A 62-year-old man presents with dark tarry stools and light-headedness. Upper endoscopy finds an ulcerating lesion in his stomach and biopsies confirm gastric cancer. Which of the following is a risk factor for carcinoma of the stomach?

(A) *Helicobacter pylori* infection

(B) high socioeconomic status

(C) high protein diet

(D) high alcohol consumption

(E) high fat diet

8. A young man with leukemia is treated with methotrexate. Which of the following is the mechanism of action of this drug?

(A) preventing absorption of folic acid

(B) inhibiting dihydrofolate reductase

(C) preventing formation of messenger ribonucleic acid (mRNA)

(D) forming a cytotoxic metabolite

(E) preventing proper functioning of membrane adenosine triphosphatase (ATPase)

9. A 52-year-old man presents with abdominal pain and weight loss. He describes a dull "gnawing" pain located in the epigastric region radiating to the back. The abdominal examination is normal with no hepatosplenomegaly or masses palpated. A computerized tomography (CT) scan of the abdomen reveals a 3-cm mass in the pancreas. Which of the following statements regarding cancer of the pancreas is true?

(A) tumors of the pancreas are divided almost equally between those arising from the exocrine portion and those arising from the endocrine portion

(B) most endocrine tumors of the pancreas are malignant

(C) the body of the pancreas is the most common site of malignancy

(D) adenocarcinoma is the most common pancreatic cancer

(E) extension is through local invasion; metastases are a late manifestation

10. A 73-year-old man was born in Taiwan and came to the United States 3 years ago. He is known to be HBsAg positive. Which of the following findings suggests the development of HCC?

(A) hepatomegaly
(B) hepatic bruits
(C) ascites
(D) jaundice
(E) all of the above

11. A 47-year-old man presents with dark black stools and vague crampy abdominal pain. On examination he is pale, blood pressure 100/70 mm Hg, pulse 110/min, and the abdomen is soft and nontender. Rectal examination confirms melena, and the patient is transfused 2 units of packed red blood cells. Upper endoscopy does not identify the source of bleeding, so a small bowel barium study is ordered. It reveals a small bowel tumor. Which of the following statements concerning small bowel tumors is correct?

(A) carcinoid is a common cause of small bowel tumors

(B) malignant adenocarcinoma most frequently occurs in the duodenum

(C) malignant tumors bleed more frequently than benign tumors

(D) Peutz-Jeghers syndrome is characterized only by benign hamartoma

(E) most primary gastrointestinal (GI) lymphomas are located in the ileum

12. A 58-year-old man is newly diagnosed with colon cancer and undergoes surgical resection of the tumor. The pathology result reports no lymph node involvement, the lesion is 4 cm in size and involves the muscularis layer. His preoperative evaluation for distal metastases was negative. Which of the following factors is most important in predicting prognosis and survival in patients with colon cancer?

(A) age under 40
(B) male gender
(C) rectal bleeding
(D) small tumor size
(E) depth of tumor penetration

13. A 64-year-old woman presents with abnormal vaginal discharge and postmenopausal bleeding. Pelvic examination reveals a bulky uterus and no adnexal masses. She undergoes a dilation and curettage (D&C), and the pathology is positive for adenocarcinoma. Which of the following is correct about carcinoma of the uterine endometrium?

(A) not associated with diabetes mellitus and obesity

(B) most common in postmenopausal woman

(C) associated with multiparity

(D) common in Jews and Muslims

(E) associated with herpes simplex virus type 2 (HSV-2) infection

14. You are seeing a 62-year-old woman with a family history of breast cancer. She is worried about her future risk of breast cancer, since her mother died of breast cancer at the age of 63. Which of the following features is also a recognized risk factor for breast cancer?

   (A) early onset of menopause
   (B) early onset of menarche
   (C) late-life radiation exposure
   (D) multiparity
   (E) early full-term pregnancy

15. A 67-year-old man complains of shortness of breath on exertion and right-sided chest pain. The pain is constant in nature; he has no fever or chills and no sputum production. On examination, air entry to the left lower lobe is reduced and the area is dull on percussion. The CXR reveals left lower lobe pleural effusion, pleural thickening with calcification (plaques), and lower lobe fibrosis. Further history from the patient is significant in that he is a lifetime nonsmoker, and that he worked as a pipe fitter until retiring 2 years ago. Which of the following is the most likely diagnosis?

   (A) adenocarcinoma
   (B) squamous cell carcinoma
   (C) sarcoidosis
   (D) lymphoma
   (E) mesothelioma

16. A 23-year-old notices left leg pain after returning from a ski trip. The pain persists for 2 months, and he presents for medical evaluation after noticing a lump on his calf. On examination, there is a 2-cm nonmobile mass in his anterior shin. A magnetic resonance imaging (MRI) scan suggests the lesion is arising from the tibia, and a biopsy reveals bone sarcoma. Which of the following statements about bone sarcoma is correct?

   (A) distal bone sarcomas have a better prognosis
   (B) lung metastases are a late sign
   (C) local lymph node involvement is very common

   (D) articular cartilage is a common plane for tumor spread
   (E) skip metastases within the same bone are common and unrelated to prognosis

17. A 19-year-old woman notices axillary lymphadenopathy and presents for evaluation. She has noticed the lymph nodes for over a month. She has no fever, chills, weight loss, or night sweats. On examination, she has multiple mobile nontender lymph nodes in both axilla, and no cervical or inguinal lymph nodes. No spleen is palpable, and the rest of the examination is normal. A monospot test is negative, and a complete blood count (CBC) and biochemistry are normal. A biopsy of one lymph node reveals Hodgkin's disease (HD), nodular sclerosing variety. A bone marrow biopsy is arranged. Which of the following tests is also part of the routine staging evaluation for patients with HD?

   (A) positron emission tomography (PET) scan
   (B) gallium scan
   (C) CT of chest, abdomen, and pelvis
   (D) staging laparotomy
   (E) bone scan

18. A 23-year-old man is newly diagnosed with Hodgkin's lymphoma. Which of the following is the most likely presenting symptom of this type of lymphoma?

   (A) coincidentally detected mediastinal mass
   (B) fixed tender inguinal lymph node involvement
   (C) mobile nontender cervical lymph nodes
   (D) fixed nontender axillary nodes
   (E) mobile tender axillary nodes

19. A 68-year-old man presents with left axillary adenopathy that on biopsy reveals a low-grade lymphocytic lymphoma. Which of the following statements is correct?

   (A) staging in this type of disorder is not relevant
   (B) if disease is widespread, early aggressive chemotherapy will result in an improved prognosis for survival

(C) the disease is likely to be widespread at the time of diagnosis

(D) untreated, the prognosis is measured in months

(E) his age is not a relevant factor in treatment

20. A 63-year-old man presents with a new skin rash on his chest. The lesions are well-defined red-colored plaques. A skin biopsy of the lesion reveals lymphoma. Further diagnostic evaluation does not reveal any evidence of a visceral malignancy. Which of the following characteristics about this disease is correct?

(A) it is invariably a precursor to leukemia

(B) it is of T-cell origin

(C) it has no specific geographic distribution

(D) it has a high likelihood of cure

(E) it is related to sun exposure

21. A 65-year-old man, with a 45-pack-per-year history of smoking, presents with hematuria and flank pain. He reports no fever, chills, or dysuria, but he has lost 15 lb. On examination the abdomen is soft, no mass is felt, and there is no flank tenderness on percussion. His hemoglobin (Hb) is 18.5 g/dL, and his liver enzymes are normal. A CT scan of the abdomen reveals a mass in the left kidney with involvement of the renal vein. Which of the following is the most likely diagnosis?

(A) renal cyst

(B) renal cell carcinoma

(C) renal metastases

(D) renal abscess

(E) lymphoma

22. A 53-year-old woman presents with a 1-cm invasive carcinoma of the breast, detected on mammography. She feels well and has no other symptoms. On examination the lump is palpable, and there are no axillary lymph nodes. Which of the following is the most appropriate local therapy for her tumor?

(A) simple mastectomy with axillary dissection

(B) radiation therapy to breast and axilla

(C) local excision plus radiation therapy

(D) local excision and axillary dissection followed by radiation therapy

(E) local excision and axillary sampling

23. A 68-year-old woman presents to her attending physician feeling unwell and having lost 10 lb. Physical examination reveals left axillary lymphadenopathy. Biopsy reveals well-differentiated adenocarcinoma. Liver scan and bone scan suggest widespread metastases. Which statement concerning her further management is correct?

(A) the response rate for metastatic adenocarcinoma (well-differentiated) of unknown primary site is so poor that no investigation or treatment is indicated

(B) special stains might guide management

(C) extensive workup, including colonoscopy, abdominal CT scan, and mammography, will define subsets that benefit from treatment

(D) special studies of the excised lymph node are not useful in determining the site of origin

(E) metastatic breast cancer is the most common cause of adenocarcinoma of unknown primary site in women

24. A 47-year-old woman with cancer phobia comes to the office for counseling. Which of the following statements is true?

(A) cancer is the most common cause of death in the United States

(B) cancer is the most common cause of death in middle-aged women

(C) incidence rates for cancer are generally higher in women than men

(D) colon and rectum cancers have the highest mortality rate when considering both men and women

(E) about 25% of all cancers in the United States are due to environmental factors

25. A 63-year-old man, with chronic heartburn symptoms for many years, presents for reevaluation because of increased abdominal discomfort. He is taking a proton pump inhibitor for his symptoms but experiences little relief. He undergoes upper endoscopy that reveals no masses or tumors, but there is esophagitis. Biopsy of the lower esophagus reveals columnar cells. Which of the following statements is correct?

    (A) it is a major risk factor for squamous cell cancer of the esophagus

    (B) it can be found in up to 20% of patients undergoing esophagoscopy for esophagitis

    (C) the histologic changes include development of keratinized squamous cells

    (D) medical control of reflux will decrease the likelihood of malignant changes

    (E) only 10% of patients with Barrett's esophagus may develop malignancy

26. A 59-year-old man develops jaundice and pruritus. He has no abdominal pain, and on physical examination he is icteric, the liver span is 10 cm, and no masses are felt. Ultrasound reveals dilated intrahepatic bile ducts. He undergoes endoscopic retrograde cholangiopancreatography (ERCP), which suggests a cholangiocarcinoma. Which of the following is the most likely predisposing factor for cholangiocarcinoma?

    (A) smoking

    (B) excess alcohol intake

    (C) chronic hepatitis B virus (HBV) infection

    (D) history of ulcerative colitis or sclerosing cholangitis

    (E) gallstones

27. A 53-year-old woman notices a lump in her left breast. She reports no symptoms of breast discharge or previous breast disease. She is postmenopausal, menarche was at age 13, and her family history is negative for breast cancer. Examination reveals a 2-cm palpable lump, which is mobile and nontender, and there are no axillary lymph nodes. Biopsy of the lump is positive for breast cancer, and she undergoes a lumpectomy and lymph node dissection. Which of the following factors is important in deciding about adjuvant therapy for breast cancer?

    (A) menopausal status

    (B) tumor size

    (C) endocrine receptor status

    (D) lymph node status

    (E) all of the above

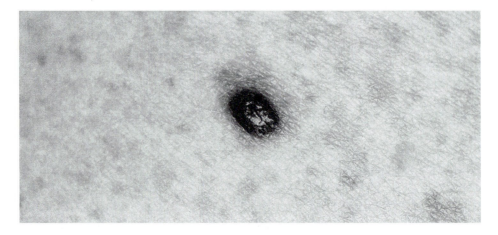

Figure 6–2.
(Reproduced, with permission, from Wolff K and Johnson RA, *Fitzpatrick's Color Atlas & Synopsis of Clinical Dermatology*, 5th ed. New York: McGraw-Hill, 2005:175.)

28. A 45-year-old man is worried about a dark pigmented skin lesion on his arm. The "mole" is 3 mm wide, symmetric with a regular border and even pigmentation. He reports no change in size or other symptoms. Which of the following is the most appropriate next step in management? (See Fig. 6–2.)

 (A) observation only

 (B) excisional biopsy

 (C) punch biopsy

 (D) chemotherapy, then surgical excision

 (E) surgical excision and regional node dissection

29. A 73-year-old man presents with fatigue and multiple lymph nodes in his neck. He has multiple large nontender lymph nodes in his neck and axilla. The spleen is not palpable, and the remaining examination is normal. A biopsy of the lymph node reveals lymphocytic lymphoma. Which of the following factors predicts poor prognosis?

 (A) no extranodal involvement

 (B) poor performance status

 (C) age <60

 (D) low serum lactate dehydrogenase (LDH) levels

 (E) fever and weight loss

30. An asymptomatic 74-year-old man has a high erythrocyte sedimentation rate (ESR) noted on routine blood work done in a yearly physical examination. A follow-up protein electrophoresis reveals a monoclonal immunoglobulin G (IgG) spike. Which of the statements would suggest a plasma cell myeloma, rather than a monoclonal gammopathy of unknown significance?

 (A) Bence Jones protein 2 g/day

 (B) normal hemoglobin

 (C) M component level of 2 g/dL

 (D) bone marrow plasma cells of 5%

 (E) normal serum calcium level

DIRECTIONS (Questions 31 through 63): Each set of matching questions in this section consists of a list of lettered options followed by several numbered items. For each numbered item, select the appropriate lettered option(s). Each lettered option may be selected once, more than once, or not at all. EACH ITEM WILL STATE THE NUMBER OF OPTIONS TO SELECT. CHOOSE EXACTLY THIS NUMBER.

Questions 31 through 37

 (A) Hispanic Americans

 (B) White Americans

 (C) Black Americans

 (D) Native Americans

 (E) Chinese Americans

 (F) Japanese Americans

 (G) Filipino Americans

For each type of cancer, select the most likely ethnic group.

31. Have the lowest cancer rates for both sexes. (SELECT ONE)

32. Have very high rates of melanoma. (SELECT ONE)

33. Have the highest rates for breast, corpus uteri, and ovarian cancers. (SELECT ONE)

34. Have especially high rates for cervical cancer. (SELECT ONE)

35. Have elevated rates for nasopharynx and liver cancers. (SELECT ONE)

36. Have high rates for stomach cancer. (SELECT ONE)

37. Have high cancer rates, at least partially, due to socioeconomic factors. (SELECT ONE)

Questions 38 through 42

    (A) alcoholic beverages

    (B) alkylating agents

    (C) arsenic

    (D) asbestos

    (E) benzene

    (F) ultraviolet radiation

    (G) Epstein-Barr virus

    (H) hepatitis B virus (HBV)

    (I) human papillomavirus (HPV)

    (J) vinyl chloride

For each patient with cancer, select the most likely etiologic agent.

38. A 56-year-old man notices an ulcer on his tongue. The lesion persists for a month and becomes more painful and larger in size. There is a 5-mm pale lesion on the lateral border of his tongue, and the remaining examination is normal. A biopsy of the site is positive for squamous cell cancer. (SELECT ONE)

39. A 68-year-old man develops shortness of breath on exertion and right-sided chest pain. Air entry is reduced to the right lower lobe and the area is dull on percussion. A CXR reveals a right pleural effusion. A CT scan of the chest reveals a pleural-based tumor in the right lower lobe, and areas of calcification on the pleura. A biopsy of the lesion is positive for mesothelioma. (SELECT ONE)

40. A 64-year-old woman notices a nodule on her face that persists for more than a month. It appears as a raised lesion with small vessels on it. Excisional biopsy of the lesion confirms a diagnosis of basal cell carcinoma. (SELECT ONE)

41. A 54-year-old woman has postmenopausal vaginal bleeding. There is no associated pain or systemic symptoms, and speculum examination reveals an irregular appearance to the cervix, which bleeds easily when samples are taken for a Pap smear. The diagnosis is cervical cancer. (SELECT ONE)

42. A 58-year-old woman presents with RUQ abdominal discomfort. She has no history of gallstones, and on examination, there is a firm mass in the RUQ. Ultrasound of the liver reveals a 6-cm solitary lesion in the liver, and her alpha-fetoprotein level is elevated. (SELECT ONE)

Questions 43 through 47

    (A) cancer metastatic to the lung

    (B) squamous cell cancer of the lung

    (C) adenocarcinoma of the lung

    (D) small cell cancer of the lung

    (E) large cell cancer of the lung

For each of the following findings, select the most likely type of lung cancer.

43. The most common type of lung cancer in the United States. (SELECT ONE)

44. Has the best prognosis of all malignant lung cancers. (SELECT ONE)

45. Most likely to cause nonmetastatic hypercalcemia. (SELECT ONE)

46. Associated with syndrome of inappropriate antidiuretic hormone (SIADH). (SELECT ONE)

47. Associated with myasthenic syndrome (Eaton-Lambert syndrome). (SELECT ONE)

Questions 48 through 52

    (A) methotrexate

    (B) cytarabine

    (C) 5-fluorouracil (5-FU)

    (D) bleomycin

    (E) doxorubicin

    (F) pamidronate

    (G) cisplatin

    (H) busulfan

    (I) cyclophosphamide

    (J) vincristine

For each patient with an adverse reaction, select the most likely chemotherapeutic agent

48. A 23-year-old man notices numbness in his hands and feet. On examination, there is distal loss of sensation to touch, and vibration in all four limbs. He recently finished chemotherapy for testicular cancer. (SELECT ONE)

49. A 56-year-old woman is receiving chemotherapy for lymphoma for the past year. Her liver enzymes have been persistently elevated for the last 2 months. She has no prior history of chronic liver disease, and screening tests for viral hepatitis are negative. A liver biopsy indicates early hepatic fibrosis. (SELECT ONE)

50. A 64-year-old man is receiving chemotherapy for squamous cell cancer of the lung. He has now developed erythema, induration, thickening, and eventual peeling of the skin on the fingers, palms, and soles of his feet. (SELECT ONE)

51. A 54-year-old woman received adjuvant chemotherapy for breast cancer 1 year ago. She now presents with symptoms and signs of congestive heart failure. An echocardiogram confirms decreased left ventricular function. (SELECT ONE)

52. A 34-year-old man is undergoing preconditioning high-dose chemotherapy for a bone marrow transplant. On the third day of treatment, he develops hematuria. (SELECT ONE)

Questions 53 through 55

(A) anaplastic thyroid cancer
(B) follicular cancer of the thyroid
(C) lymphoma of the thyroid
(D) papillary cancer of the thyroid
(E) medullary thyroid cancer

For each of the following statements, select the most likely type of thyroid cancer.

53. Has the best prognosis of all thyroid malignancies (SELECT ONE)

54. Is proportionately more common in Blacks than Whites (SELECT ONE)

55. Is associated with a specific marker (SELECT ONE)

Questions 56 through 59

(A) lymphocyte-predominant Hodgkin's disease (HD)
(B) nodular-sclerosing HD
(C) mixed-cellularity HD
(D) lymphocyte-depleted HD, reticular type
(E) lymphocyte-depleted HD, diffuse fibrosis type
(F) all variants of HD

For each of the following statements, select the most likely type of Hodgkin's disease (HD).

56. The only form of HD more common in women (SELECT ONE)

57. Reed-Sternberg cells can be difficult to locate in this variant (SELECT ONE)

58. This variant has a particularly good outcome (SELECT ONE)

59. Can be accompanied by a nonnecrotizing epithelioid granulomatous reaction (SELECT ONE)

Questions 60 through 63

(A) nonsteroidal anti-inflammatory drugs (NSAIDs)
(B) opioids
(C) amphetamines
(D) anticonvulsants
(E) phenothiazines
(F) butyrophenones
(G) steroids

For each patient with metastatic cancer pain, select the most likely treatment choice.

60. A 52-year-old woman has metastatic breast cancer with boney metastases. She is taking hydromorphone for the pain but is still experiencing back pain. She is reluctant to take more of the hydromorphone since she become very drowsy with higher doses. This group of medications is particularly useful for pain from bony metastases. (SELECT ONE)

61. A 74-year-old man with metastatic prostate cancer develops shooting pains in his left leg and constant back pain. Further evaluation reveals a pathologic compression fracture of the lumbar spine and involvement of the nerve roots in his lower spine causing the pain. He is started on a medication to help reduce the symptoms, but a limitation of the drug is leukopenia and thrombocytopenia. (SELECT ONE)

62. A 68-year-old woman was treated for melanoma 3 years ago. She now presents with constant headaches, nausea, vomiting, and left-sided weakness. A CT scan reveals two masses in the right parietal lobe consistent with metastatic melanoma. She is started on medication to help reduce her symptoms of headaches and nausea. (SELECT ONE)

63. A 65-year-old man has metastatic lung cancer and severe bone and chest pain. He is started on morphine and ibuprofen to control the pain but is still not comfortable. Further gradual increases in the morphine dose achieve good pain control but he becomes drowsy on the appropriate dose and is unable to do much. He is started on a medication that can be useful in controlling opioid-induced sedation. (SELECT ONE)

Answers and Explanations

1. **(C)** Ataxia-telangiectasia is inherited in an autosomal recessive manner. It is associated with non-Hodgkin's lymphoma, acute lymphocytic leukemia, and stomach cancer. Associated immunoglobulin A (IgA) (± immunoglobulin E [IgE]) deficiency predisposes to infection as well. All the other conditions listed are inherited in an autosomal dominant manner, and a positive family history is much more likely. *(Kasper, p. 2423)*

2. **(B)** Only the chronic carrier state increases HCC risk, not previous infection. The majority, but not all, of HCC associated with HBV occurs in the setting of cirrhosis (60–90%). Because the latency period of HBV infection is 35 years, before HCC supervenes, early-life infection is strongly correlated with HCC. The chronic carrier state of HBsAg in endemic areas, such as Taiwan, is associated with a relative risk of over 100 for the development of HCC. Over half the chronic carriers of HBsAg in such a population will die of cirrhosis or HCC. In Taiwan, where childhood vaccination was introduced in 1984, the death rate from childhood HCC has already declined. *(Devita, pp. 533–534)*

3. **(B)** Radiation-induced malignancies tend to occur at the age where that particular malignancy would normally occur. Therefore, the latency period can be 40 years or more. The latency period tends to be shortest (5–7 years) for leukemia. The risk for most malignancies is greatest with early-life radiation, and evidence suggests that therapeutic radiation confers excess risk as well. The amount of exposure determines the likelihood of developing malignancy, not its severity. *(Devita, pp. 197–198)*

4. **(B)** There is universal agreement on the need for regular Pap smears in young women. There is no need to screen for colon cancer (fecal occult blood) or lung tumors (CXR), particularly at this age. Mammography, if indicated for screening, would be only for older women. Many authorities recommend breast self-examination as well as physical examination by a physician. *(Kasper, pp. 444–446)*

5. **(C)** All of the given responses are potential anterior mediastinal masses, but when an anterior mediastinal mass presents with myasthenia gravis the diagnosis of thymoma is essentially established. Myasthenia gravis occurs as a paraneoplastic process of the thymoma. The ocular and muscle fatigue symptoms are characteristic of myasthenia. About 5–10% of patients with thymoma will also have hypogammaglobulinemia. About 5% of patients with thymoma will have autoimmune pure red cell aplasia. *(Kasper, pp. 2518–2523)*

6. **(D)** The history of weight loss and dysphagia suggests carcinoma of the esophagus, and squamous cell carcinoma is a disease that occurs in older men who drink and smoke heavily. Smoking and or excessive drinking are considered etiologic factors in the development of squamous cell carcinoma. Adenocarcinomas arise within dysplastic columnar epithelium in the distal esophagus, usually in the presence of chronic gastric reflux. *(Kasper, pp. 523–524)*

7. **(A)** Low dietary vitamin C, and high salt and nitrate consumption predispose to gastric cancer, as does ingestion of smoked foods. Smoking is a risk factor, but alcohol is not.

H. pylori is another important risk factor, since it causes gastritis that eventually leads to chronic atrophic gastritis, metaplasia, dysplasia, and then carcinoma. *(Kasper, pp. 524–525)*

8. **(B)** The most likely mode of action of methotrexate is by tightly binding dihydrofolate reductase (DHFR), which maintains the intracellular folate pool in its fully reduced form as tetrahydrofolates. These compounds are required in the de novo synthesis of pyrimidines and purines. *(Kasper, p. 476)*

9. **(D)** Adenocarcinoma is the most common cancer of the pancreas. The proximal pancreas is the most common site, with only 20% occurring in the body and 5–10% in the tail. About 95% of the tumors arise from the exocrine portion of the gland, and these are usually malignant. Most of the endocrine tumors are benign. Early development of metastases is characteristic of pancreatic adenocarcinoma. *(Kasper, pp. 537–538)*

10. **(E)** For most patients, the development of HCC is the first manifestation of their underlying liver disease. The most common presentation is with RUQ pain, mass, and weight loss, but hepatic decompensation with jaundice and ascites is also common. About 25% of patients have hepatic bruits. *(Kasper, pp. 533–534)*

11. **(B)** Adenocarcinoma, the most common malignancy of the small bowel, is most common proximally, particularly in the duodenum. Small bowel lymphomas are most common in the ileum, but the stomach is the most common site of GI lymphoma. Carcinoids usually present with local symptoms. Carcinoid syndrome is present only with hepatic metastases. Benign tumors bleed more frequently than malignant ones. Malignant adenocarcinomas can occur in Peutz-Jeghers syndrome. *(Kasper, pp. 531–533)*

12. **(E)** Depth of tumor penetration (Dukes stage) is the most important prognostic factor in the 5-year survival in patients with colon cancer. Rectal bleeding is a good prognostic sign, perhaps because surface erosion manifests early. Young age, male gender, and location in the rectum all indicate a poorer prognosis. Unlike

most tumors, no correlation with tumor size and prognosis has been established for colon cancer. *(Kasper, pp. 527–531)*

13. **(B)** Carcinoma of the cervix is common in young women. For endometrial cancer, the peak is from age 55 to 60. Endometrial cancer is associated with nulliparity, diabetes mellitus, and obesity. Cervical cancer is associated with human papilloma virus (HPV) infection. There is tremendous variation in incidence of cervical cancer based on geography, ethnicity, and sexual history. *(Kasper, pp. 556–557)*

14. **(B)** Breast cancer risk is reduced by 20% for each year that menarche is delayed. Early menopause, natural or surgical, also decreases risk. Early (age 18 or 19) full-term pregnancy and multiparity decrease the risk. Radiation exposure is a risk factor primarily in adolescence and is marginal after the age of 40. In summary, there are three important dates in the assessing the risk of breast cancer: age of menarche, age of first full-term pregnancy, and age of menopause. *(Kasper, p. 517)*

15. **(E)** The history of being a pipe fitter suggests asbestos exposure, and the CXR finding of pleural plaques and lower lobe fibrosis confirms prior asbestos exposure. The classic associated cancer is mesothelioma. However, in 30–50% of cases, no history of asbestos exposure is apparent. The average age on presentation is 60, and this is typically many years after the exposure. The most common presenting symptoms are dyspnea and nonpleuritic chest pain. Smoking injury in patients with asbestos exposure increases the risk of other lung cancers such as adenocarcinoma or squamous cell carcinoma. *(Kasper, pp. 1522–1523)*

16. **(A)** Overwhelmingly, the major prognostic factor in osteosarcoma is location of the tumor. Pelvic and axial lesions do worse than those in the extremities, and survival is better in tibial tumors than femoral tumors. Lung metastases are very common. *(Kasper, pp. 558–561)*

17. **(C)** CT imaging of the chest, abdomen, and pelvis is part of the staging workup for patients

with HD. Other components of staging include CBC, lytes, LDH, CXR, and bone marrow biopsy. PET and gallium scanning are not always done, and are usually helpful at the completion of treatment to document remission. The purpose of staging laparotomy is to determine whether radiation alone will be used for treatment. As chemotherapy usage increases, the necessity for staging laparotomy decreases. *(Kasper, pp. 654–655)*

18. **(C)** The most characteristic presentation of Hodgkin's disease is that of enlarged, superficial cervical or supraclavicular lymph nodes in a young person. The nodes are usually freely moveable, nontender, and not painful. Occult presentation with intrathoracic or intra-abdominal disease is unusual. *(Kasper, pp. 654–655)*

19. **(C)** About 85% of low-grade lymphocytic lymphomas are widespread at the time of diagnosis. However, staging is still important as radiation therapy can be curative for localized (stage I, II) disease. Because the prognosis for this malignancy is measured in years, it has been difficult to demonstrate a survival benefit for aggressive chemotherapy. The poor prognosis for lymphoma in older patients might be a result of less-aggressive therapy. *(Kasper, pp. 648–649)*

20. **(B)** Cutaneous lymphomas are of T-cell origin and are more common in other parts of the world, such as Japan. Patients with adult T-cell lymphoma-leukemia (ATLL) have acute fulminant courses characterized by skin invasion and leukemic cells. This syndrome is clearly related to human T-cell lymphotropic virus-I (HTLV-I), and there is a possibility that HTLV-I, or another retrovirus, might be the agent for mycosis fungoides and Sézary syndrome. ATLL responds poorly to treatment and therapy for the low-grade malignancies controls symptoms but does not result in cure. *(Kasper, p. 653)*

21. **(B)** Age, history of smoking, and polycythemia in a patient with hematuria strongly suggests a renal cell carcinoma. The elevated hemoglobin represents increased erythropoietin production and is not related to prognosis. Involvement along the renal vein and metastases to the lung is also characteristic of renal cell carcinoma. Elevated liver enzymes and weight loss can represent nonmetastatic effects of malignancy and can reverse with resection. Almost half of patients will have a palpable abdominal mass on presentation. The CT of the thorax is a useful test because three-quarters of those with metastatic disease will have lung metastases. *(Kasper, pp. 541–542)*

22. **(D)** Breast-conserving surgery is now recommended for small tumors. Radiation therapy will decrease local recurrence rates. For tumors <1 cm, adjuvant therapy is indicated only if axillary nodes are positive. Therefore, in this case, an axillary dissection will provide important therapeutic information. However, this is an area of rapidly changing knowledge and practice. *(Kasper, pp. 519–520)*

23. **(B)** Patients with adenocarcinoma of unknown origin are typically elderly and have metastatic tumors at many sites. Generally, the prognosis is poor, but some subsets, in which effective treatment is available, can be identified by clinical criteria with only moderate investigations. These include peritoneal carcinomatosis in women (responds to treatment for ovarian cancer), predominant skeletal metastases in men (can reflect prostatic cancer), and women with axillary lymphadenopathy (can reflect breast cancer). In the latter scenario, studies for estrogen and progesterone receptors are very useful in guiding therapy. *(Kasper, pp. 562–563)*

24. **(B)** When men and women of all ages are considered, cardiovascular diseases are the most common cause of death. However, among women age 35–74 years, cancer is the leading cause of death. Lung cancer is the number one cause of death from cancer, when both men and women are considered. Men generally have higher incidence rates for cancer: breast, gallbladder, and thyroid cancers are the exceptions. It is felt that 75–80% of all cancers in the United States are due to environmental factors. The environmental contribution is estimated by comparing age-adjusted U.S. rates of specific cancers to the rates for the country with the lowest risk. *(Devita, pp. 228–250)*

25. **(B)** Barrett's esophagus, characterized by a columnar cell-lined esophageal mucosa, is a major risk factor for adenocarcinoma of the esophagus. Although acid reflux may be a predisposing factor, there is no evidence that either medical or surgical antireflux measures alter the outcome. It is found in about 20% of patients undergoing endoscopy for esophagitis, and up to 50% may develop a malignancy. *(Kasper, p. 222)*

26. **(D)** Worldwide, the presence of liver flukes (e.g., *Clonorchis sinensis*) is the most likely predisposing factor for cholangiocarcinoma. Part of this increased risk is caused by the development of hepatolithiasis. The highest rate of cholangiocarcinoma is found in Southeast Asia. It is thought that liver flukes and a diet high in nitrosamine are the prime reasons for this. In North America, primary sclerosing cholangitis and chronic ulcerative colitis are the most common predisposing factors. Cholelithiasis, alcohol, smoking, and chronic hepatitis B are not known to be risk factors. *(Kasper, p. 536)*

27. **(E)** The size of the tumor is a prognostic factor, as is knowing menopausal status, endocrine receptor status, and lymph node involvement. These four factors are used to decide who will benefit from adjuvant chemotherapy, radiotherapy, or tamoxifen treatment. *(Kasper, pp. 520–522)*

28. **(A)** Observation alone is adequate for this lesion. The "ABCD" rules are helpful in distinguishing benign skin lesions from malignant melanoma. (A) asymmetry, benign lesions are symmetric; (B) border irregular, most nevi have clear-cut borders; (C) color variation, benign lesions have uniform color; (D) diameter, >6 mm is more likely to be malignant. In addition, recent rapid change in size is also helpful in distinguish benign from malignant lesions. Thickness of the tumor is the most important prognostic factor in the majority of cases, and ulceration indicates a more aggressive cancer with a poorer prognosis. Although cumulative sun exposure is a major factor in melanoma (e.g., more frequent near the equator), it cannot explain such things as the more common occurrence of some types in relatively young people. It is possible that brief, intense exposure to sunlight may contribute to, or initiate, carcinogenic events. *(Kasper, pp. 500–502)*

29. **(B)** Prognosis of patients with non-Hodgkin's lymphoma is best assessed with the International Prognostic Index. It is an index with five clinical risk factors that helps to predict the 5-year survival. Poor prognostic factors are age >60 years, high serum LDH level, poor performance status (either Eastern Cooperative Oncology Group [ECOG] >2, or Karnofsky <70), Ann Arbor stage III or IV, or >1 extranodal involvement. *(Kasper, p. 647)*

30. **(A)** IgG spikes >3.5 g/dL or IgA >2 g/dL strongly suggest myeloma rather than monoclonal gammopathies of undetermined significance (MGUS). MGUS is suggested when the spike is <3.5 g/dL, the marrow has fewer than 10% plasma cells, and the Bence Jones proteinuria is <1.0 g/day. Depressed hemoglobin levels, elevated calcium levels, progressive bone lesions, and impaired renal function suggest more advanced stages of multiple myeloma. *(Kasper, pp. 658–660)*

31. **(D)** Native Americans of both sexes have low cancer rates, but cancer rates (for women) for stomach, biliary tract, cervix, and kidney are surprisingly high. *(Devita, pp. 228–240)*

32. **(B)** Whites have high rates for melanoma, lymphoma, leukemia, and lip cancer. *(Devita, pp. 228–240)*

33. **(B)** Whites have high rates for breast, corpus uteri, testis, bladder, brain, colon, and rectum cancer. *(Devita, pp. 228–240)*

34. **(A)** Although Hispanic Americans have relatively low cancer rates (66% of that for White Americans and 54% of that for Black Americans), they do have high rates for cancer of the cervix. *(Devita, pp. 228–240)*

35. **(E)** Chinese Americans have a rate of nasopharyngeal cancer 23 times greater than White Americans and liver cancer rates 7 times greater than White Americans. *(Devita, pp. 228–240)*

36. **(F)** Japanese Americans have a threefold increase in stomach cancer rate compared to White Americans, but this is lower than rates in Japan. *(Devita, pp. 228–240)*

37. **(C)** The excess risk of cancers of the stomach, esophagus, lung, and cervix among Black Americans is diminished when socioeconomic variations are factored in. *(Devita, pp. 228–240)*

38. **(A)** Alcoholic beverages combine with tobacco smoking to increase cancer of the mouth and, by causing cirrhosis, can lead to liver cancer. *(Devita, pp. 241–250)*

39. **(D)** Asbestos exposure causes more deaths from lung cancer (two-fold increase) than from mesothelioma (hundredfold increase) because the latter tumor is so rare. *(Devita, pp. 241–250)*

40. **(F)** Sun exposure severe enough to cause sunburn is associated with increased risk of melanoma, whereas other skin cancers are more related to cumulative exposure. *(Devita, pp. 241–250)*

41. **(I)** Although causation is not definite, a high proportion of cervical cancers reveal HPV-16 and HPV-18 on biopsy. HPV has also been isolated from vulvar, penile, and anal cancers. *(Devita, pp. 241–250)*

42. **(H)** Cirrhosis, related to chronic HBV infection, is a leading cause of HCC. *(Devita, pp. 241–250)*

43. **(C)** Adenocarcinoma is now the most common form of lung cancer, accounting for 40% of the total cases. *(Devita, p. 928)*

44. **(B)** Because of its tendency for early exfoliation and obstruction, squamous cell cancer is often detected at an earlier stage. Even correcting for this, there is some suggestion that its prognosis is still better, perhaps because of its slow growth rate. *(Devita, p. 928)*

45. **(B)** Nonmetastatic hypercalcemia occurs in up to 15% of all squamous cell cancers due to the production of parathyroid hormone related peptide (PTH-rP). This is a paraneoplastic phenomenon. *(Devita, p. 933)*

46. **(D)** SIADH occurs in up to 10% of all small cell cancers of the lung. SIADH, Cushing's syndrome, and neurologic paraneoplastic syndromes usually occur with small cell lung cancer, not nonsmall cell lung cancer. *(Devita, p. 985)*

47. **(D)** Eaton-Lambert syndrome is unusual, but small cell lung cancer causes the majority of cases that are paraneoplastic. *(Devita, pp. 985, 2530)*

48. **(G)** Cisplatin is used for the treatment of many different cancers including testicular cancer. Its major toxicities are renal, ototoxicity, myelosuppression, and peripheral neuropathy. The neuropathy is dose- and duration-dependent. *(Kasper, p. 475)*

49. **(A)** Liver toxicity is most common when methotrexate is used on a daily basis, such as for psoriasis. Myelosuppression and GI mucositis are the most common side effects in cancer therapy. *(Devita, p. 392)*

50. **(D)** Although lung injury is the most serious complication of bleomycin, this unusual skin reaction is more frequent, occurring in almost 50% of patients. *(Devita, pp. 453–454)*

51. **(E)** Doxorubicin can cause a cumulative, dose-dependent cardiomyopathy that can result in congestive heart failure. However, an acute, non-dose-related myocarditis-pericarditis can also occur. It can cause arrhythmias, heart failure, or pericardial effusions. *(Devita, pp. 425–427)*

52. **(I)** Cyclophosphamide causes hemorrhagic cystitis in up to 10% of patients because active metabolites are excreted. Adequate hydration and frequent urination can decrease the frequency of this complication. *(Devita, pp. 363–365)*

53. **(D)** Papillary cancer has the best prognosis of all thyroid cancers. Although it is seven times more common than follicular cancer, fewer people die from it. Even with follicular cancer, most patients will die of other diseases. In common

with other thyroid cancers, age seems to be an independent risk factor for poor prognosis. *(Devita, pp. 1746–1750)*

54. **(B)** Although well-differentiated thyroid cancer is twice as common in Whites than in Blacks, the proportion that is follicular is more than twice as high in Blacks. *(Devita, pp. 1746–1750)*

55. **(E)** Serum calcitonin elevation is specific for medullary thyroid cancer and is the most specific tumor marker now available. When combined with provocative agents (e.g., calcium, pentagastrin), it is also very sensitive. In the familial syndrome, provocative tests have been superseded by genetic studies. *(Devita, p. 1757)*

56. **(B)** Nodular sclerosing Hodgkin's disease is more common in women, and is particularly common in younger age groups but can occur at any age. *(Devita, p. 2347)*

57. **(A)** In lymphocyte-predominant Hodgkin's disease, multiple sections often have to be examined to find Reed-Sternberg cells. Some authorities question whether such cells are necessary for diagnosis of this form. Variants, often called lymphocytic and histiocytic (L&H) or popcorn cells, are often frequently found. *(Devita, p. 2345)*

58. **(A)** Most patients with lymphocyte-predominant Hodgkin's disease have clinically localized disease and are asymptomatic; the prognosis is usually favorable. However, it accounts for only 4–5% of cases. *(Devita, p. 2346)*

59. **(F)** This is a frequent accompaniment of Hodgkin's disease and can be found in involved lymph nodes, and may be extensive enough to obscure the presence of Hodgkin's disease. Rather than evidence of occult involvement, the presence of granulomas implies stage for stage, a better prognosis than those without this reaction. *(Devita, pp. 2344–2352)*

60. **(A)** Prostaglandins play a role in bone resorption in metastatic disease, perhaps explaining the effectiveness of NSAIDs for this type of pain. Aspirin has been shown to have an anti-tumor effect in an animal bone tumor model. *(Devita, p. 2992)*

61. **(D)** Carbamazepine is an anticonvulsant used widely as an adjuvant analgesic for neuralgic pain caused by either tumor infiltration or surgical nerve injury. Because cancer patients commonly have compromised hematologic reserve, leukopenia and thrombocytopenia caused by carbamazepine may limit its use. *(Devita, pp. 2993, 2999)*

62. **(G)** Steroids are useful for controlling pain in patients with leptomeningeal metastases or headache from increased intracranial pressure. *(Devita, p. 3000)*

63. **(C)** Usually, sedation can be controlled by altering opioid dosage, or switching to a drug with a shorter half-life, as well as stopping other sedating medications. If this fails, amphetamine, methylphenidate, and caffeine can be used to counteract the sedative effect. *(Devita, p. 3001)*

Diseases of the Nervous System
Questions

1. A 69-year-old woman presents to the clinic with memory difficulty. The patient's daughter is concerned because she is having difficulty doing her finances, such as paying bills. Memory impairment testing reveals the poor ability to generate lists of words or copy diagrams (intersecting pentagons). Her remaining physical examination is normal. Which of the following anatomic findings is most likely with her condition?

   (A) atrophy of the medial temporal lobes
   (B) atrophy of the entire frontal and temporal lobes
   (C) cranial nerve involvement
   (D) transient episodes of hemiplegia
   (E) atrophy of the caudate

2. A 38-year-old man presents with involuntary facial grimacing, shrugging of the shoulders, and jerking movements of the limb. His father was similarly affected. There is also a history of mood changes for the past 3 months. On examination, he appears restless with intermittent slow movements of his hands and face. He has difficulty performing rapid finger movements, and tone is decreased in the upper and lower limbs. Which of the following is most likely to represent the progression of his illness?

   (A) a normal life span
   (B) a 50% chance of only male children being similarly affected
   (C) mental deterioration
   (D) eventual development of rigidity
   (E) development of hemiparesis

3. An 18-year-old woman has periodic episodes that begin with severely decreased vision, followed by ataxia, dysarthria, and tinnitus. The symptoms last for 30 minutes and are then followed by a throbbing occipital headache. Which of the following is the most likely diagnosis?

   (A) vertebral-basilar insufficiency
   (B) chronic basilar artery dissection
   (C) classic migraine
   (D) ophthalmoplegic migraine
   (E) basilar migraine

4. A 6-month-old child presents with recurrent seizures and poor development. The evaluation reveals a baby with hydrocephalus, impaired movement of the extremities, hypotonia, and retinal abnormalities. A computerized tomography (CT) scan demonstrates large ventricles and calcified lesions. Which of the following is the most likely diagnosis?

   (A) Tay-Sachs disease
   (B) congenital hydrocephalus
   (C) kernicterus
   (D) toxoplasmosis
   (E) congenital neurosyphilis

5. A 74-year-old woman develops acute neurologic symptoms and presents to the emergency room. An urgent magnetic resonance imaging (MRI) scan demonstrates acute occlusion in the right posterior cerebral artery. Which of the following clinical symptoms is she most likely to have?

   (A) homonymous hemianopia
   (B) total blindness
   (C) expressive aphasia
   (D) ataxia and dysarthria
   (E) a right-sided hemiplegia

6. A 53-year-old man complains of clumsiness with both hands, like having difficulty doing up buttons or using his keys. Physical examination reveals fasciculations of his thigh and forearm muscles; diffuse muscle weakness, loss of muscle bulk, and increased tone in the upper and lower limbs. There is generalized hyper-reflexia, and positive Babinski signs bilaterally. Which of the following is the most likely natural progression of this condition?

   (A) a long history of remissions and exacerbations
   (B) sensory loss in the distribution of peripheral nerves
   (C) focal seizures
   (D) a progressively downhill course
   (E) cogwheel rigidity

7. A 38-year-old man presents with involuntary facial grimacing, shrugging of the shoulders, and jerking movements of the limb. His father was similarly affected. There is also a history of mood changes for the past 3 months. On examination, he appears restless with intermittent slow movements of his hands and face. He has difficulty performing rapid finger movements, and tone is decreased in the upper and lower limbs. Which of the following treatments is helpful in suppressing the movements?

   (A) gamma-aminobutyric acid (GABA)-mimetic agents
   (B) inhibitors of GABA metabolism
   (C) cholinergic agents
   (D) dopamine receptor blockers
   (E) centrally acting cholinesterase inhibitors

8. A 22-year-old woman presents with acute vision loss and pain in the left eye, but no other symptoms. On examination she appears well, visual acuity is not possible, and she can only perceive movement and bright light. The direct papillary reflex is absent but the indirect (consensual) response is normal. The optic disc is edematous. Which of the following symptoms is also most likely present in patients with this condition?

   (A) limb weakness
   (B) hemiplegia
   (C) cervical myelopathy
   (D) sphincter impairment
   (E) seizures

9. A 63-year-old man developed a transient episode of vertigo, slurred speech, diplopia, and paresthesias. He is symptom-free now, and clinical examination is entirely normal. His past medical history is significant for hypertension and dyslipidemia. Which of the following is the most likely cause for symptoms?

   (A) posterior circulation transient ischemic attack (TIA)
   (B) anterior communicating artery aneurysm
   (C) hypertensive encephalopathy
   (D) pseudobulbar palsy
   (E) occlusion of the middle cerebral artery

10. A 75-year-old woman presents with symptoms of visual change and facial weakness. On examination, the pupils are equal and reactive to light, the fundi appear normal, and there is a right homonymous visual field defect. Which of the following is the most likely cause of the right homonymous hemianopia?

   (A) right optic nerve
   (B) chiasm
   (C) right optic radiations
   (D) right occipital lobe
   (E) left optic radiations

11. A 10-year-old boy has multiple tan-colored patches on his skin, and freckle-like skin changes in his armpit area. The rest of clinical examination is normal. Which of the following conditions is also found in patients with this disorder as they get older?

(A) bilateral eighth nerve tumors

(B) irregular small pupils

(C) multiple cutaneous and subcutaneous tumors

(D) cataracts

(E) hip involvement

12. A 44-year-old man presents with involuntary movements of his face, shoulders, and arms. His father had a similar condition. There is also a history of mood changes for the past 6 months. On examination, he appears restless with intermittent slow movements of his hands and face. He has difficulty performing rapid finger movements, and tone is decreased in the upper and lower limbs. Which of the following is the most likely diagnosis?

(A) Parkinson's disease

(B) Huntington's chorea

(C) amyotrophic lateral sclerosis (ALS)

(D) spinal muscular atrophy

(E) Sydenham's chorea

13. A 56-year-old man is brought to the emergency department by his wife because of memory loss and difficulty walking. She has noticed personality changes, truancy from work, and lack of personal care over the past 1 year. On examination he appears unkempt, smells of urine, and is uncooperative. He cannot recall the date or season, and gets angry when asked questions. His answers are often fabricated when checked with his wife. The blood pressure is 150/90 mm Hg, pulse 100/min, and he is diaphoretic and tremulous. His gait is wide based, and motor strength and reflexes are normal. His ocular movements are normal but there is nystagmus on lateral gaze. In the past he has had multiple admissions for alcohol withdrawal. Which of the following is the most appropriate next step in management?

(A) prophylactic phenytoin administration

(B) prophylactic diazepam administration

(C) prophylactic carbamazepine administration

(D) calcium administration

(E) steroid administration

14. A 60-year-old man with diabetes acutely develops double vision and discomfort in his left eye. On examination, there is ptosis of the left eyelid, the eye is rotated down and out, and the pupil is 3 mm and reactive to light. The right eye is normal. Which of the following is the most likely diagnosis?

(A) fourth nerve palsy

(B) diabetic autonomic neuropathy

(C) third nerve palsy

(D) sixth nerve palsy

(E) seventh nerve palsy

15. A 48-year-old man complains of recurrent episodes of sudden-onset dizziness. He notices an abrupt onset of a spinning sensation when sitting up or lying down in bed. The symptoms last for 30 seconds and then resolve completely. He has no hearing change or other neurologic symptoms, and his physical examination is completely normal. A Dix-Hallpike maneuver reproduces his symptoms. Which of the following is the most likely mechanism for his vertigo symptoms?

(A) basilar migraine

(B) brain stem ischemic events

(C) benign cerebellar tumors

(D) calcium debris (calcium carbonate crystals) in the semicircular canals

(E) Meniere's disease

16. A 40-year-old man is injured in a car accident and fractures his left elbow. He now complains of numbness of his fourth and fifth fingers, and weakness in his hand grip. Neurologic findings confirm weakness of handgrip with weakness of finger abduction and adduction, and decreased sensation over the fifth finger and lateral aspect of fourth finger. Which of the following is the most likely diagnosis?

    (A) ulnar nerve injury
    (B) radial nerve injury
    (C) median nerve injury
    (D) carpal tunnel syndrome
    (E) axillary nerve injury

17. A 31-year-old woman complains of excessive sleepiness during the daytime for years despite adequate nighttime sleep. She has episodes of intense drowsiness three to four times a day, even when at work or while eating meals. She has sought medical attention in the past, after falling asleep while driving. She is slender and otherwise healthy and on no medications. Which of the following treatments is most likely indicated for her condition?

    (A) a device providing continuous positive airway pressure (CPAP) at night
    (B) oral surgery
    (C) tracheostomy
    (D) amphetamines
    (E) benzodiazepines at bedtime

18. A 43-year-old man is referred from the emergency department with memory loss and difficulty walking. He was brought in by his wife who has noticed personality changes, truancy from work, and lack of personal care over the past 2 years. On examination he appears unkempt, smells of urine, and is uncooperative. He cannot recall the date or season, and gets angry when asked questions. His answers are often fabricated when checked with his wife. His gait is wide-based, and there is loss of sensation in his feet up to the shins. His motor strength and reflexes are normal. His ocular movements are normal and there is no nystagmus. In the past he has had multiple admissions for alcohol withdrawal. Which of the following is the most likely diagnosis?

    (A) Wernicke's encephalopathy
    (B) Wernicke-Korsakoff syndrome
    (C) Alzheimer's dementia
    (D) Charcot-Marie-Tooth disease
    (E) vascular dementia

19. A 59-year-old woman has numbness and tingling in her feet. On examination, there are signs of involvement of the peripheral nerves in the form of decreased sensation, motor weakness, and distal reflex loss. The findings are symmetric. Which of the following medical conditions is most likely to explain her peripheral nerve findings?

    (A) heart disease
    (B) dermatomyositis
    (C) hypothyroidism
    (D) diabetes mellitus
    (E) adrenal insufficiency

20. A 94-year-old man presents with progressive headaches, light-headedness, drowsiness, and unsteady gait over 6 weeks. On examination, his blood pressure is 160/90 mm Hg, pulse 70/min, lungs clear, and he has no focal weakness. His gait is unsteady but sensation in the feet is normal. A CT scan reveals a hyperintense clot over the left cerebral cortex. Which of the following is the most likely cause for this clot?

    (A) is venous in origin
    (B) is arterial in origin
    (C) is from injury to the middle meningeal artery
    (D) is from a subarachnoid hemorrhage
    (E) is from injury to the middle cerebral artery

21. A 68-year-old man has many months history of progressive hearing loss, unsteady gait, tinnitus, and facial pain. An MRI scan reveals a tumor at the cerebellopontine angle. Which of the following cranial nerves is this tumor most likely to affect?

(A) fourth cranial nerve

(B) sixth cranial nerve

(C) eighth cranial nerve

(D) tenth cranial nerve

(E) eleventh cranial nerve

22. A 27-year-old woman presents with acute vision loss and pain in the left eye, but no other symptoms. On examination, she appears well, visual acuity is not possible, and she can only perceive movement and bright light. The direct pupillary reflex is absent but the indirect (consensual) response is normal. The optic disc is edematous. An example of the pathologic changes seen in her optic nerve are shown in Fig. 7–1 a. It shows a plaque of demyelination in the optic nerve as compared to a normal sample in Fig. 7–1 b. Which of the following is the most likely diagnosis?

(A) diabetic microvascular disease

(B) arteriosclerosis

(C) trauma

(D) multiple sclerosis

(E) Creutzfeldt-Jakob disease

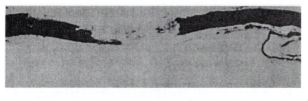

Figure 7–1a.

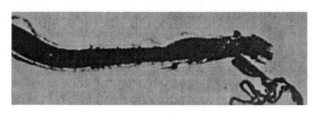

Figure 7–1b.

23. A 25-year-old man complains of excessive sleepiness during the daytime for years despite adequate nighttime sleep. He has sought medical attention after falling asleep while driving. He is slender and otherwise healthy and on no medications. Which of the following symptoms might he also complain about?

(A) excessive snoring (wife's report)

(B) automatic behavior (wife's report)

(C) restless sleep (wife's report)

(D) paresthesias

(E) morning headache

24. A 17-year-old woman presents with symptoms of a fine tremor of her hands. The tremor is best seen when her hands are stretched out. She is not on any medications and reports no alcohol use. Which of the following is the most likely diagnosis?

(A) hypopituitarism

(B) marijuana use

(C) hyperthyroidism

(D) myxedema

(E) iron overdose

25. A 19-year-old man has had progressive ataxia of gait and great difficulty in running. In the past year, he has developed hand clumsiness. Physical examination reveals pes cavus, kyphoscoliosis, and both cerebellar and sensory changes in the legs. There is a positive family history of Friedreich's ataxia. Where are the pathologic changes seen in this condition most likely to be found?

(A) spinal cord tracts

(B) basal ganglia

(C) cerebral cortex

(D) peripheral autonomic nerves

(E) peripheral motor nerves

26. A 24-year-old man presents with mild jaundice, tremor, and personality changes. Examination reveals slowness of finger movement, rigidity, and coarse tremor of the outstretched hands. As well there is abnormal slow movement of the tongue and pharynx resulting in a change in speech and occasional difficulty swallowing. He is icteric, the liver span is 10 cm, and no spleen is palpable. Which of the following findings is most likely seen in this condition?

    (A) a reduction of copper excretion in the urine
    (B) an increase of the serum ceruloplasmin content
    (C) no renal involvement
    (D) retention of normal neurologic movements
    (E) a peculiar greenish-brown pigmentation of the cornea

27. A 52-year-old man complains of episodes of severe unilateral, stabbing facial pain that is intermittent for several hours, and then disappears for several days. The pain is describes as "electric shock-like" and only lasts a few seconds. Physical examination of the face and mouth is entirely normal. Which of the following treatments is most effective for this condition?

    (A) morphine
    (B) indomethacin
    (C) cimetidine
    (D) carbamazepine
    (E) lidocaine (Xylocaine) gel

28. A 63-year-old woman develops symptoms of nausea, vomiting, and dizziness, which she describes as a to-and-fro movement of the room like as if she is on a boat. Which of the following findings suggests the vertigo is central in origin?

    (A) deafness
    (B) symptoms are more protracted but less severe
    (C) unidirectional nystagmus
    (D) visual fixation inhibits vertigo and nystagmus
    (E) spinning sensation is toward the fast phase of nystagmus

29. A 30-year-old woman complains of double vision, and easy fatigue with exercise. The fatigue improves with resting, but it is interfering with her work. Examination reveals ptosis and impaired eye movements with normal pupillary response. The double vision is brought out by asking her to look at the ceiling, and after a sustained interval, the eyes slowly drift down. Which of the following is the most likely diagnosis?

    (A) optic atrophy
    (B) ophthalmic zoster
    (C) paralysis agitans
    (D) Horner syndrome
    (E) myasthenia gravis

30. A 47-year-old woman presents with increasing headaches and visual changes. On examination, her pupils are normal and reactive to light, the extraocular movements are normal, and there are visual field defects of the outer half in both eyes (bitemporal hemianopsia). Which of the following is the most likely diagnosis?

    (A) pituitary adenoma
    (B) falx meningioma
    (C) craniopharyngioma
    (D) aneurysm of the internal carotid artery
    (E) glioblastoma

31. A 45-year-old man presents with weakness and fasciculations in his arms and legs. His cranial nerves are normal, but there is weakness of his left handgrip and right leg quadriceps with loss of muscle bulk. There are obvious fasciculations over the left forearm and right thigh. Tone is increased in the arms and legs and the reflexes are brisk. Which of the following is the most likely diagnosis?

    (A) amyotrophic lateral sclerosis (ALS)
    (B) myotonic muscular dystrophy
    (C) amyotonia congenita
    (D) tabes dorsalis
    (E) migraine

32. Which of the following is the most likely finding in a 79-year-old woman with Parkinson's disease?

    (A) constant fine tremor
    (B) muscle atrophy
    (C) akinesia
    (D) pupillary constriction
    (E) spontaneous remission

33. A 47-year-old man presents to the emergency room with symptoms of dizziness and difficulty walking. He describes his dizziness as a spinning sensation of the room with associated nausea and vomiting. Which of the following findings suggests the vertigo is peripheral in origin?

    (A) optic neuritis
    (B) tinnitus
    (C) bidirectional nystagmus
    (D) vertical nystagmus
    (E) visual fixation does not affect vertigo or nystagmus

DIRECTIONS (Questions 34 through 42): Each set of matching questions in this section consists of a list of lettered options followed by several numbered items. For each numbered item, select the appropriate lettered option(s). Each lettered option may be selected once, more than once, or not at all. EACH ITEM WILL STATE THE NUMBER OF OPTIONS TO SELECT. CHOOSE EXACTLY THIS NUMBER.

Questions 34 and 35

    (A) aqueductal stenosis
    (B) infectious process
    (C) enlarged foramina of Luschka
    (D) nutritional deficiency
    (E) agenesis of the corpus callosum
    (F) postvaccination
    (G) acoustic neuroma

For each patient with neurologic symptoms, select the most likely structural pathology.

34. A 77-year-old woman presents with headaches and difficulty walking. She has an unbalanced gait and falls easily, especially when trying to walk upstairs. The tone is normal and there are no cerebellar findings. A CT scan reveals enlarged ventricles. (SELECT ONE)

35. A 23-year-old woman presents with arm weakness, decreasing vision in her right eye, and difficulty with her balance. An MRI of the brain reveals multiple demyelinating lesions. (SELECT THREE)

Questions 36 through 39

    (A) basal ganglia hemorrhage
    (B) cerebellar hemorrhage
    (C) pontine hemorrhage
    (D) lobar intracerebral hemorrhage
    (E) cocaine-related hemorrhage
    (F) subarachnoid hemorrhage
    (G) arteriovenous malformation (AVM)
    (H) hypertensive encephalopathy
    (I) primary intraventricular hemorrhage

For each patient with altered level of consciousness, select the most likely diagnosis.

36. A 67-year-old man develops coma over a few minutes. He is unresponsive on arrival to the hospital. He has ataxic respirations and pinpoint, reactive pupils. Oculocephalic reflexes are absent. There is no motor response with noxious stimulation. (SELECT ONE)

37. A 74-year-old woman develops occipital headache, vomiting, and dizziness. She looks unwell, blood pressure 180/100 mm Hg, pulse 70/min, and respirations 30/min. She is unable to sit or walk because of unsteadiness. Over the next few hours, she develops a decline in her level of consciousness. (SELECT ONE)

38. A 52-year-old man, with poorly controlled hypertension in the past, presents with increasing headache, confusion, and vomiting. His blood pressure is 230/125 mm Hg, pulse 60/min, respirations 24/min, and there is papilledema. He has no focal deficits. (SELECT ONE)

39. A 24-year-old man has a history of recurrent throbbing headaches. He suddenly develops mild right-sided weakness. His blood pressure in the past has been normal but is now slightly elevated. (SELECT ONE)

Questions 40 through 42

   (A) hyperkalemia

   (B) facial nevi

   (C) weakness and atrophy of the hands

   (D) hypokalemia

   (E) mental retardation

   (F) fasciculations

   (G) hypercalcemia

   (H) convulsions

For each patient with a neurologic condition, select the most likely associated findings.

40. A 20-year-old man develops fatigue and severe muscle weakness of his limbs usually after eating a large meal. He is diagnosed with familial periodic paralysis. (SELECT ONE)

41. An 11-year-old girl with a diagnosis of tuberous sclerosis (SELECT THREE)

42. A 23-year-old woman with impaired pain and temperature sensation in her arms but normal light touch. A CT scan reveals dilatation of the central part of the spinal cord in the cervical region (syringomyelia). (SELECT TWO)

DIRECTIONS (Questions 43 through 58): Each of the numbered items in this section is followed by answers. Select the ONE lettered answer that is BEST in each case.

43. A 27-year-old woman complains of double vision and fatigue at the end of the day. Further history reveals difficulty in chewing food, and some weakness in climbing stairs. She has stopped running because of easy leg fatigue and leg weakness. The symptoms improve with resting. On examination, there is weakness of the eyelids, masticatory muscles, and thigh flexors. Her handgrip decreases with repetitive action. There is no sensory abnormality, and reflexes are normal. Which of the following is the most likely diagnosis?

   (A) hypercalcemia

   (B) myasthenia gravis

   (C) multiple sclerosis

   (D) thyroid storm

   (E) meningeal lymphoma

44. A 20-year-old man suffered a significant closed head injury after a diving accident. He is left with minor memory impairment but makes a full recovery. A few months later, he has a witnessed loss of consciousness with some arm and leg twitching. After the event, he is disoriented for 2 hours and then gradually returns to baseline. There was no incontinence or tongue biting, and his examination is normal. Which of the following is the most likely diagnosis?

   (A) syncope

   (B) generalized seizure

   (C) focal seizure

   (D) cardiac arrhythmia

   (E) drop attack

45. A 22-year-old woman presents with fever, headache, and confusion. She has not been herself for the past 2 days, including not going to work and forgetting events. On examination, she is moving all her limbs, but not oriented to place or time. The remaining examination is normal. A CT scan shows bilateral, small, low-density temporal lobe lesions. Cerebrospinal fluid (CSF) shows mononuclear cell pleocytosis, increased protein, and normal glucose. The electroencephalogram (EEG) shows bilateral periodic discharges from the temporal leads and slow-wave complexes at regular intervals of 2–3/sec. Which of the following is the most appropriate treatment for her condition?

(A) penicillin

(B) chloramphenicol

(C) acyclovir

(D) erythromycin

(E) steroids

46. A 67-year-old woman with hypertension presents with sudden onset of headache, vomiting, and left-sided weakness. On examination, she has weakness of the left face, hand, and leg (graded three out of five), blood pressure of 180/100 mm Hg, and respiration of 20/min. Which of the following is the most appropriate initial diagnostic test?

(A) CT scan with contrast

(B) MR scan with gadolinium

(C) CT scan without contrast

(D) MR cerebral angiogram

(E) conventional cerebral angiogram

47. A 77-year-old woman develops acute hoarseness, difficulty swallowing, dizziness, and falling to the right side. On examination, there is decreased sensation to pain on the right side of her face and left side of her body. The palate and pharynx move very little on the right side, and there is loss of coordination of the right arm and leg. Motor power in the arms and legs is normal. While attempting to walk, she falls to the right side, and complains of vertigo. An MRI scan confirms the diagnosis of the ischemic stroke. Which of the following is the most likely location of the stroke?

(A) right medial medulla

(B) right lateral medulla

(C) right internal capsule

(D) right parietal cortex

(E) right cerebellum

48. A 27-year-old woman, a recent immigrant from the Caribbean basin, has had progressive leg weakness. Physical examination reveals increased tone of both legs with weakness, clonus, extensor plantar responses, and brisk reflexes. There is also loss of vibration and position senses in the feet. The upper extremities are normal. A clinical diagnosis of tropical spastic paraparesis (TSP) is made. Which of the following is the most likely cause of this condition?

(A) human immunodeficiency virus (HIV) infection

(B) cytomegalovirus (CMV) infection

(C) human T-cell lymphotropic virus (HTLV)-1 infection

(D) thiamine deficiency

(E) central nervous system (CNS) tuberculosis infection

49. A 40-year-old woman complains of episodes of severe unilateral, stabbing facial pain that is intermittent for several hours, and then disappears for several days. Physical examination is entirely normal. Which of the following is the most likely diagnosis?

(A) trigeminal neuralgia

(B) herpes zoster

(C) acoustic neuroma

(D) Bell's palsy

(E) diabetic neuropathy

50. A 63-year-old man suddenly becomes acutely ill with headache and fever of 38.9°C. There is pain in the eye, and the orbits are painful to pressure. There is edema and chemosis of the conjunctivae and eyelids, and the eye bulbs are proptosed. Diplopia and ptosis are present, and the pupils are slow in reacting. Which of the following is the most likely diagnosis?

(A) cavernous sinus thrombosis

(B) chorioretinitis

(C) subarachnoid hemorrhage

(D) brain abscess

(E) none of the above

51. A 20-year-old woman presents with a history of rapid loss of vision in one eye. Examination reveals pain on movement of the eyeball. The appearance of the fundi is normal, but the afferent pupillary response is diminished. Perimetry shows a large central scotoma. Which of the following is the most likely diagnosis?

    (A) optic atrophy
    (B) papilledema
    (C) retrobulbar neuritis
    (D) amblyopia ex anopsia
    (E) hysteria

52. A 67-year-old man has two episodes of numbness on the left side of his body, which last 5 minutes. He now experiences transient loss of vision in his right eye lasting 2 minutes. On examination, his blood pressure is 155/90 mm Hg, pulse 80/min regular, and visual fields, extraocular movements, and pupils are all normal. The remaining motor and sensory examination is also normal. Which of the following is the most likely diagnosis?

    (A) posterior cerebral artery insufficiency
    (B) parietal lobe neoplasm
    (C) parasagittal meningioma
    (D) AVM
    (E) right internal carotid artery atherosclerosis

53. An 18-year-old man develops fever, headache, confusion, and generalized seizures. On examination, he is moving all his limbs, but incoherent. A CT scan shows bilateral, small, low-density temporal lobe lesions. CSF shows mononuclear cell pleocytosis, increased protein, and normal glucose. The EEG shows bilateral periodic discharges from the temporal leads and slow-wave complexes at regular intervals of 2–3/sec. Which of the following is the most appropriate next step in management?

    (A) angiography
    (B) observing response to therapy

    (C) cerebral biopsy
    (D) acute viral titers
    (E) CSF culture

54. A 24-year-old woman presents with foot and leg weakness that is progressively getting worse over the past 1 week. Initially, she developed tingling in her feet and noticed that they would drag, but now she has difficulty standing and walking due to the leg weakness. Three weeks ago she had a "chest cold," which resolved on its own. On examination, muscle bulk is normal, motor strength is two out of five in the quadriceps, and one out of five in the feet. Reflexes at the ankle and knee are absent, and sensation testing is normal. The upper limb examination is normal. The CSF protein is very high, glucose is normal, and cell count is slightly elevated. Which of the following is the most likely diagnosis?

    (A) diabetic neuropathy
    (B) alcoholic neuropathy
    (C) Guillain-Barré syndrome
    (D) cyanide poisoning
    (E) poliomyelitis

55. A 37-year-old woman complains of drooping eyelids, double vision, and fatigue at the end of the day. Further history reveals difficulty in chewing food, and some weakness in climbing stairs. The symptoms improve with resting. On examination, there is weakness of the eyelids, masticatory muscles, and thigh flexors. Her handgrip decreases with repetitive action. There is no sensory abnormality, and reflexes are normal. Her chest x-ray (CXR) is shown in Fig. 7–2 a and b. Which of the following is the most likely diagnosis?

    (A) bronchogenic carcinoma
    (B) Hodgkin's disease
    (C) teratoma
    (D) thyroid tumor with retrosternal extension
    (E) thymoma

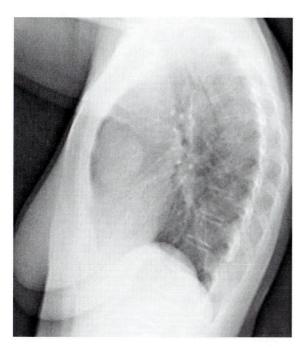

Figure 7–2a.

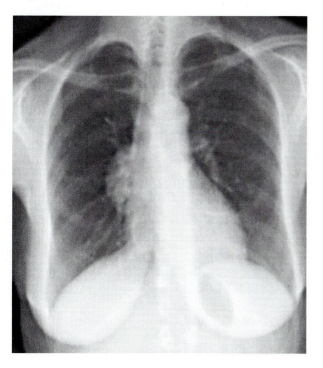

Figure 7–2b.

56. A 79-year-old woman is seen in the office for "dizziness." Which of the following findings would suggest true vertigo?

(A) the patient is taking multiple antihypertensives

(B) the symptoms are worse on standing

(C) she has had two falls

(D) the room is spinning around her

(E) a prior Holter monitor was negative during episodes of dizziness

57. A 65-year-old woman complains of recurrent episodes of sudden-onset dizziness and nausea. She notices an abrupt onset of a spinning sensation when rolling over or sitting up in bed. The symptoms last for 30 seconds and then completely resolve. She has no hearing change or other neurologic symptoms, and her physical examination is completely normal. A Dix-Hallpike maneuver reproduces her symptoms. Which of the following findings on vestibular testing favors the diagnosis of benign paroxysmal positional vertigo (BPPV) over central positional vertigo?

(A) no latency period

(B) no fatigability

(C) habituation occurs

(D) mild vertigo

(E) symptoms consistently the same from one set of tests to the next

58. A 23-year-old man complains of intermittent double vision and fatigue at the end of the day. Further history reveals difficulty in chewing food, and some weakness in climbing stairs. He has stopped working as a courier because of easy leg fatigue and weakness. The symptoms improve with resting. On examination, there is weakness of the eyelids, masticatory muscles, and thigh flexors. Having him look up at the ceiling for a long period brings on his double vision. His handgrip decreases with repetitive action. There is no sensory abnormality, and reflexes are normal. Which of the following treatments is contraindicated in this patient?

(A) anticholinergic drugs

(B) surgery

(C) plasmapheresis

(D) cyclophosphamide

(E) high-dose prednisone

DIRECTIONS (Questions 59 through 78): Each set of matching questions in this section consists of a list of lettered options followed by several numbered items. For each numbered item, select the appropriate lettered option(s). Each lettered option may be selected once, more than once, or not at all. EACH ITEM WILL STATE THE NUMBER OF OPTIONS TO SELECT. CHOOSE EXACTLY THIS NUMBER.

Questions 59 through 63

(A) simple partial seizure

(B) complex partial seizures

(C) tonic-clonic (grand mal) seizures

(D) absence (petit mal) seizures

(E) myoclonic seizures

(F) status epilepticus

For each patient with clinical symptoms and signs, select the most likely seizure type.

59. A 55-year-old man presents with increasing shortness of breath, decreased urine output, malaise, nausea, and vomiting. He has a history of hypertension, chronic renal failure, and coronary artery disease. His laboratory data reveal very high urea and creatinine, consistent with acute on chronic renal failure. He also notes having intermittent "twitching" in his arms and legs that started recently. (SELECT ONE)

60. A 24-year-old woman complains of having intermittent bouts of smelling burning rubber followed by lip smacking and chewing movements as observed by others. During these spells, she does not respond to questions. There has never been any complete loss of consciousness during these episodes either. An MRI of the brain reveals temporal lobe sclerosis. (SELECT ONE)

61. A teenager has a long history of "daydreaming" in school. EEG reveals evidence of a generalized seizure disorder, but there has never been a history of convulsive muscular activity. (SELECT ONE)

62. A 23-year-old woman has a history of repetitive involuntary movements of her right hand associated with abnormal facial movements. At times, the movements spread to involve the entire arm. (SELECT ONE)

63. This form of epilepsy almost always starts in childhood. (SELECT ONE)

Questions 64 through 68

(A) phenytoin

(B) carbamazepine

(C) phenobarbital

(D) primidone

(E) sodium valproate (valproic acid)

(F) ethosuximide

(G) lorazepam

(H) trimethadione

For each type of seizure, select the most appropriate therapy.

64. Is the drug of choice for absence attacks (SELECT ONE)

65. Is the drug of choice for myoclonic seizures (SELECT ONE)

66. Is the drug of choice for tonic-clonic (grand mal) seizures (SELECT THREE)

67. Is the drug of choice for partial seizures (SELECT TWO)

68. Is the drug of choice for status epilepticus (SELECT ONE)

Questions 69 through 73

(A) essential anisocoria

(B) Horner syndrome

(C) tonic pupils (Holmes-Adie syndrome)

(D) Argyll Robertson pupils

(E) midbrain pupils

(F) atropinized pupils

(G) oculomotor palsy

For each patient with a pupillary abnormality, select the most likely diagnosis.

69. A 63-year-old man is noticed to have asymmetric pupils. He is completely well and has no symptoms. On examination, the left pupil is small, round, and has a brisk response to light and near stimuli (accommodation). There is also ptosis of the left eyelid, but no other ocular movement abnormality or symptoms of double vision. (SELECT ONE)

70. A 23-year-old woman is noticed to have irregular pupils on routine examination. She has one large pupil, which has minimal response to light stimulation, but it does respond to accommodation. The eye movements are normal and she experiences no double vision. (SELECT ONE)

71. A 57-year-old woman presents for evaluation of memory loss. She is noticed to have small, irregular pupils that respond poorly to light but pupillary response to accommodation is normal. (SELECT ONE)

72. A 24-year-old man notices different size pupils. The left pupil is 1 mm larger than the right. Both pupils respond normally to light and accommodation. The discrepancy in the pupils is still there in low, medium, and bright light conditions. He reports no other visual symptoms. (SELECT ONE)

73. A 64-year-old woman is having double vision and severe headaches. On examination, the left pupil is dilated compared to the right, and the light response is diminished. (SELECT ONE)

Questions 74 through 78

(A) anterior horn cell
(B) peripheral nerve
(C) neuromuscular junction
(D) muscle

For each patient with muscle weakness, select the most likely anatomic site for the disorder.

74. A 48-year-old man complains of muscle weakness in his right hand (dominant hand). On examination, the hand muscles are smaller than on the left, and the reflexes are decreased out of proportion to weakness. (SELECT ONE)

75. A 26-year-old woman complains of early fatigue and weakness in doing strenuous activity. Her symptoms are worse near the end of the day. She appears well, muscle bulk, tone, and reflexes are normal. Handgrip strength decreases with repetitive testing. (SELECT ONE)

76. A 63-year-old woman has noticed weakness in her right hand such that she is having difficulty writing and doing up buttons. On examination, there is marked atrophy of the forearm and hand muscles with fasciculations. Tone is increased and reflexes are brisk. Sensory testing in the hand is normal. There are also fasciculations on her thighs, which she has never noticed before. (SELECT ONE)

77. A 49-year-old man notices weakness and numbness in his left hand. He had recently slipped on a wet floor and injured his elbow. Examination of the hand reveals predominantly weakness to abduction and adduction and sensory loss over the fourth and fifth fingers. (SELECT ONE)

78. A 67-year-old man with lung cancer notices symptoms of weakness in his arms and legs. He describes difficulty in rising out of chair or going upstairs, but no pain or discomfort. On examination, proximal muscle strength is four out of five in the upper and lower limbs, but the reflexes, tone, and sensation are normal. He has a colored rash on his eyelids, and raised papules on his knuckles. (SELECT ONE)

Answers and Explanations

1. **(B)** Alzheimer's disease can be quite diffuse, but there is particular involvement of the medial temporal lobes and cortical association areas. The atrophy of the hippocampus is particularly marked. Microscopic examination reveals neurofibrillary tangles and amyloid plaques. *(Ropper, p. 901)*

2. **(C)** This is a case of Huntington's chorea. It is an autosomal dominant gene (found on the short arm of chromosome 4), and male and female children are equally affected. Movement disorder, mental deterioration, and personality change are the hallmarks of the disease, but can be very subtle initially. The disease starts typically between ages 35 and 40 (although the variation is wide) and runs its course in about 15 years. The akinetic rigid variety (Westphal variant) of Huntington's typically has a child-hood onset. *(Ropper, p. 910)*

3. **(E)** Basilar migraine can be very dramatic, and can resemble ischemia in the territory of the basilar posterior cerebral arteries. The visual symptoms of basilar migraine typically affect the whole of both visual fields, and can even cause temporary cortical blindness. There can also be an alarming period of coma or quadri-plegia. *(Ropper, p. 151)*

4. **(D)** Toxoplasmosis is the most likely diagnosis. The infection has a predilection for the CNS and the eye, and produces encephalitis in utero. Symptoms can be evident in the first few days of life. Infants born with active disease may have fever, rash, seizures, and hepatosplenomegaly at birth. *(Ropper, p. 882)*

5. **(A)** Occlusion of the right posterior cerebral artery is most likely to cause homonymous hemianopia. This artery conveys blood to the inferior and medial portion of the posterior temporal and occipital lobes and to the optic thalamus. *(Ropper, p. 677)*

6. **(D)** This man has amyotrophic lateral sclerosis (ALS). The disease causes neuronal loss in the anterior horns of the spinal cord and motor nuclei of the lower brain stem. The disease is one of constant progression, rather than remis-sions and exacerbations, and death usually occurs within 5 years. There is no sensory loss and no seizure diathesis, because only the motor system is involved. There can be signs of hyperreflexia and spasticity, depending on the balance of upper and lower motor neuron damage, but not cogwheel rigidity. *(Ropper, p. 939)*

7. **(D)** There are disturbances of norepinephrine, glutamic acid decarboxylase, choline acetyl-transferase, GABA, acetylcholine, and somato-statin, but their significance is poorly understood. Dopamine blocking agents (e.g., haloperidol) can be used to treat psychosis and ameliorate chorea but do not alter the course of disease. Presynaptic dopamine depletors such as clozapine, reserpine, or tetrabenazine can be used for chorea as well, but have significant side effects. Antidepressants are helpful for symptomatic treatment. Most patients eventually end up in an institution. *(Ropper, p. 913)*

8. **(A)** This patient has multiple sclerosis (MS). Weakness or numbness in one or more limbs is the initial manifestation of disease in about half

the patients. Other common initial presentations include optic neuritis (25%) and acute myelitis. Hemiplegia, seizures, and cervical myelopathy (in older patients) occur occasionally as the initial manifestation. Sphincter impairment usually occurs later in the disease. *(Ropper, p. 777)*

9. **(A)** Posterior circulation TIA is suggested by the transient episodes. The basilar artery is formed by the two vertebral arteries and supplies the pons, the midbrain, and the cerebellum. With vertebrobasilar TIAs, tinnitus, vertigo, diplopia, ataxia, hemiparesis, and bilateral visual impairment are common findings. *(Ropper, p. 692)*

10. **(E)** The hemianopia is due to a lesion of the left optic radiations. The posterior cerebral artery arises from the basilar artery but is sometimes a branch of the internal carotid. With posterior cerebral artery lesions affecting the occipital cortex, it is possible for the hemianopia to be an isolated finding. *(Ropper, p. 218)*

11. **(C)** The two common forms of neurofibromatosis (NF-1 and NF-2) are genetically distinct. NF-1 is the type with multiple café au lait spots and is associated with axillary or inguinal freckling, iris hamartomas (Lisch nodules), peripheral neurofibromas, and bony abnormalities (including kyphoscoliosis). NF-2 is associated with CNS tumors, particularly bilateral eighth nerve tumors. Skin lesions are spare or absent, and early lens opacities can occur. *(Ropper, p. 869)*

12. **(B)** Huntington's chorea is the most likely diagnosis given the hereditary nature of this patient's illness (autosomal dominants). It differs from Sydenham's chorea by its gradual onset and slow choreic movements versus brusque jerks seen in Sydenham's. The caudate nucleus and putamen are both severely involved in Huntington's chorea, and degeneration of the caudate nucleus results in enlarged lateral ventricles (with a "butterfly" appearance on CT). Atrophy is very widespread in the brain and includes the cerebral cortex. A decrease in glucose metabolism as revealed on positron emission tomography (PET) scan *precedes* the evidence of tissue loss. *(Ropper, p. 911)*

13. **(B)** Prophylactic administration of diazepam in a withdrawing alcoholic can prevent or reduce severe syndromes such as delirium tremens (DTs). Prophylactic phenytoin, however, is not helpful. A calm, quiet environment with close observation and frequent reassurance is very important. Vitamin administration (especially thiamine) is important, but frequently, severe magnesium depletion slows improvement. *(Ropper, pp. 1010–1011)*

14. **(C)** Third nerve palsy can result in ptosis of the eyelid. There is also loss of the ability to open the eye, and the eyeball is deviated outward and slightly downward. With complete lesions, the pupil is dilated, does not react to light, and loses the power of accommodation. In diabetes, the pupil is often spared. The sixth cranial nerve can also be affected by diabetes, but this is much less common. *(Ropper, p. 1135)*

15. **(D)** This person has benign paroxysmal positional vertigo (BPPV), which is characterized by sudden-onset brief episodes of vertigo lasting less than a minute. The symptoms are usually brought on by head movement. The cause is commonly attributed to calcium debris in the semicircular canals, known as canalithiasis. The debris is loose otoconia (calcium carbonate) within the utricular sac. Although BPPV can occur after head trauma, there is usually no obvious precipitating factor. It generally abates spontaneously and can be treated with vestibular rehabilitation. *(Ropper, p. 261)*

16. **(A)** Injury to the ulnar nerve results in impaired adduction and abduction of the fingers. The nerve is commonly injured in elbow dislocations and fractures. The fibers arise from the eighth cervical and the first thoracic segments. The ulnar is a mixed nerve with sensory supply to the medial hand. *(Ropper, p. 1168)*

17. **(D)** This woman does not have risk factors for sleep apnea (older age, snoring, obesity) and likely has narcolepsy. Adrenergic stimulant drugs such as methylphenidate or amphetamines help the sleepiness, and tricyclic compounds can help the cataplexy. Strategically planned naps can also be helpful. *(Ropper, p. 348)*

18. **(B)** The combination of symptoms is typical of chronic alcohol abuse. The mental symptoms are suggestive of Wernicke-Korsakoff syndrome. A distal limb sensory-motor neuropathy is also typical of alcoholism. Confusion, tremulousness, and disorientation are typical for acute alcohol intoxication. Wernicke's encephalopathy is a symptom complex of ophthalmoplegia, ataxia, nystagmus, and acute confusional state. *(Ropper, p. 984)*

19. **(D)** These signs and symptoms develop in a fairly large percentage of patients with diabetes mellitus. Loss of proprioceptive sensation together with absent reflexes superficially resembles tabes dorsalis. If sensory loss is severe, Charcot's joints can develop. *(Ropper, pp. 1134–1135)*

20. **(A)** A subdural hematoma is almost always of venous origin and secondary to a minor or severe injury to the head, but may occur in blood dyscrasias or cachexia in the absence of trauma. Acute subdural hematomas commonly present with a fluctuating level of consciousness and significant cerebral damage. Chronic subdurals may also present with seizures or papilledema. *(Ropper, pp. 758–759)*

21. **(C)** An acoustic neuroma is most likely to lead to a palsy of the eighth cranial nerve. Deafness, headache, ataxia, tinnitus, and diplopia are seen, as well as facial paresthesias. Acoustic neuromas represent 5–10% of all intracranial tumors. They develop from Schwann cells and generally grow very slowly. They may be very large before symptoms develop. *(Ropper, p. 572)*

22. **(D)** Visual loss in multiple sclerosis varies from slight blurring to no light perception. Other eye symptoms include diplopia and pain. The classic syndrome of optic or retrobulbar neuritis occurs commonly at some point in the disease, and it is the presenting symptom in 25% of cases. *(Ropper, p. 777)*

23. **(B)** The early age of onset and otherwise good health suggest a diagnosis of narcolepsy, which is usually accompanied by other symptomatology. Hypnagogic hallucinations are almost always visual. They occur most frequently at the onset of sleep, either during the day or at night. They are generally very vivid. Cataplexy is a brief loss of muscle power without loss of consciousness. The patient is fully aware of what is going on. The paralysis may be complete or partial. Automatic behavior with amnesia is a common manifestation of the narcolepsy-cataplexy syndromes, occurring in 50% of cases. Automatic behavior can be confused with complex partial seizures. Paresthesias are not part of narcolepsy syndrome. Snoring, restless sleep, and morning headache suggest sleep apnea. *(Ropper, p. 510)*

24. **(C)** In hyperthyroidism, neurologic symptoms include tremors of the hands, exophthalmos, lid lag, stare, and muscle weakness. Muscle weakness of hyperthyroidism affects the pelvic girdle and, to a lesser extent, the shoulder girdle. Reflexes are normal or increased, and sensation is normal. It must be differentiated from myasthenia gravis, which may also accompany thyrotoxicosis. *(Ropper, p. 80)*

25. **(A)** This young man has Friedreich's ataxia, associated with a gene defect on chromosome 9. The pathologic changes are found in the spinal cord tracts. Degeneration is seen in the posterior columns, the lateral corticospinal tract, and the spinocerebellar tracts. Ataxia, sensory loss, nystagmus, reflex changes, clubfeet, and kyphoscoliosis are the characteristic findings. The heart is frequently involved, and cardiac disease is a common cause of death. *(Ropper, pp. 931–934)*

26. **(E)** In Wilson's disease, there is usually a reduction of the serum ceruloplasmin content. Signs and symptoms of injury to the basal ganglia are accompanied by cirrhosis of the liver. Renal involvement is characterized by persistent aminoaciduria. The most common neurologic finding is tremor. The corneal pigmentation (Kayser-Fleischer ring) is the most important diagnostic finding on physical examination. If it is absent, any neurologic findings cannot be ascribed to Wilson's disease. *(Ropper, pp. 830–831)*

27. **(D)** This patient has trigeminal neuralgia. Carbamazepine (an anticonvulsant drug) is given in doses varying from 600 to 1200 mg/day. Phenytoin has also been used. The two drugs can also be used in combination. Operative procedures include alcohol injection of the nerve or ganglion, partial section of the nerve in the middle or posterior fossa, decompression of the root, and medullary tractotomy. Radiofrequency surgery can destroy pain fibers but spare motor fibers. *(Ropper, pp. 161–163)*

28. **(B)** In central vertigo, the vertigo can be mild and chronic. In peripheral disease, the symptoms are generally more severe, but finite (although often recurrent). *(Ropper, p. 265)*

29. **(E)** In myasthenia gravis, weakness of the facial and levator palpebrae muscles produces a characteristic expressionless face, with drooping of the eyelids. Weakness of the ocular muscles may cause paralysis or weakness of individual muscles, paralysis of conjugate gaze, ophthalmoplegia, or a pattern similar to internuclear ophthalmoplegia. The presence of normal pupillary responses to light and accommodation with weakness of extraocular muscles, levators, and orbicularis oculi is almost completely diagnostic of myasthenia. *(Ropper, pp. 1250–1251)*

30. **(A)** Adenomas of the pituitary gland constitute approximately 7% of intracranial tumors, with the chromophobic type being the most common. With macroadenomas, some degree of pituitary insufficiency is common, and half the patients have headaches. With microadenomas, the other pituitary functions may be completely normal. *(Ropper, p. 575)*

31. **(A)** The most common initial symptom of ALS is weakness and wasting of the extremities. The fasciculations can be a very prominent part of the disease. This is rare in other neurologic disorders. *(Ropper, p. 939)*

32. **(C)** The characteristic triad in Parkinson's disease (Tremor, Rigidity, Akinesia) has been expanded to include Postural instability. This forms the mnemonic **TRAP**. Autonomic instability is also common. Findings on examination also include masklike facies, dysarthria, stooped posture, and abnormal gait. *(Ropper, pp. 916–917)*

33. **(B)** Tinnitus and deafness may be found in peripheral vertigo, but not central. The nystagmus is usually unidirectional and is never vertical. Visual fixation inhibits vertigo and nystagmus during testing in peripheral vertigo. *(Ropper, p. 260)*

34. **(A)** Adults may develop hydrocephalus as a result of occlusion of CSF pathways by tumors in the third ventricle, brain stem, or posterior fossa. In adults, the symptoms of obstructive hydrocephalus include headache, lethargy, malaise, incoordination, and weakness. Seizures do not usually occur. Dementia, altered consciousness, ocular nerve palsies, papilledema, ataxia, or corticospinal tract signs may be present. *(Ropper, p. 535)*

35. **(B, D, F)** Myelin is a complex protein lipid carbohydrate structure, which forms part of the cell membrane of the oligodendroglia. Vascular lesions cause demyelination because of ischemia. Papovaviruses can cause progressive multifocal leukoencephalopathy in patients with HIV infection, or less commonly, malignancy. Acute disseminated encephalomyelitis has been described after smallpox or rabies vaccination. Nutritional deficiencies can also cause demyelination (e.g., pernicious anemia with vitamin B_{12} deficiency). *(Ropper, p. 771)*

36. **(C)** Pontine hemorrhage is associated with impaired oculocephalic reflexes and small, reactive pupils. It generally evolves over a few minutes, usually with coma and quadriplegia. The prognosis is poor, and death often occurs within hours. *(Ropper, p. 714)*

37. **(B)** Cerebellar hemorrhage, when mild, may present with only headache, vomiting, and ataxia of gait. Patients may complain of dizziness or vertigo. The eyes may be deviated to the side opposite the hemorrhage. Nystagmus is not common, but an ipsilateral sixth nerve palsy can occur. This is the only type of intracerebral hemorrhage that commonly benefits from surgical intervention. *(Ropper, p. 741)*

38. **(H)** Hypertensive encephalopathy is an unusual complication of chronic hypertension and, nowadays, is almost never the initial presentation of hypertension. Intracerebral hemorrhage into the cerebellum, pons, and thalamus are usually due to spontaneous rupture of small, penetrating arteries and are also associated with hypertension. The lack of physical findings argues against one of these hemorrhagic processes. Cocaine-related hemorrhage is caused by acute hypertension. Subarachnoid hemorrhage is more likely caused by an aneurysm, and lobar intracerebral hemorrhage is frequently caused by nonhypertensive factors such as amyloid angiopathy, AVMs, and aneurysms. *(Ropper, p. 728)*

39. **(G)** AVMs are more frequently seen in men and, although present from birth, do not usually become symptomatic until later in life. The peak incidence of symptoms is between ages 10 and 30. The headaches can be similar to migraine, or it can be more diffuse. It can also present with seizure or rupture. Hemorrhage can be massive or minimal when rupture does occur. *(Ropper, p. 723)*

40. **(D)** The most common familial periodic paralysis syndrome is usually associated with low potassium, but there are less common forms characterized by high or normal potassium. It is characterized by recurrent attacks of weakness or paralysis of the somatic musculature, with loss of the deep tendon reflexes. Preventive therapy includes potassium supplementation and possibly a low carbohydrate, low salt, high potassium diet. Imipramine and acetazolamide are said to be useful in acute attacks. *(Ropper, p. 1270)*

41. **(B, E, H)** Tuberous sclerosis is an autosomal dominant disease with a wide variety of clinical phenotypes. Lesions occur in the nervous system, skin, bones, retina, kidney, and elsewhere. The skin lesions include facial nevi (fibroma molluscum) and patches of skin fibrosis. Hard nodules are found throughout the brain. Seizures and mental retardation can occur. *(Ropper, pp. 866–867)*

42. **(C, F)** Syringomyelia is characterized by a dissociated sensory loss. Atrophy of the muscles can result in a clawhand deformity. Fasciculations are commonly found. *(Ropper, pp. 1084–1085)*

43. **(B)** The most common presenting symptoms relate to weakness of eye muscles, causing ptosis or diplopia. Difficulty in chewing, dysarthria, and dysphagia are also common. The differential diagnosis includes all diseases that cause weakness of oropharyngeal or limb muscles. These include the muscular dystrophies, ALS, and progressive bulbar palsies, among others. Most other conditions do not improve after injection of edrophonium or neostigmine. *(Ropper, pp. 1250–1251)*

44. **(B)** This man had a generalized posttraumatic seizure. The prolonged confusion after the event suggests seizure rather than syncope. In the majority of cases, seizures do not develop until several months after the injury, 6–18 months being the most common interval. The more severe the injury, the greater the likelihood of seizures. For severe injuries, some authorities recommend prophylactic anticonvulsants for 1–2 years. There is no firm evidence for this, however. *(Ropper, p. 291)*

45. **(C)** This patient has herpes simplex virus encephalitis. Acyclovir selectively inhibits viral deoxyribonucleic acid (DNA) polymerase. Acyclovir is currently the treatment of choice because of better efficacy and less toxicity than previous drugs. Because it is so nontoxic, therapy can be started even if the diagnosis is only presumptive. *(Ropper, p. 639)*

46. **(C)** CT scan is still superior to MRI in certain circumstances, particularly in the emergency setting, for diagnosing acute subarachnoid hemorrhage, intracerebral bleeding, fractures of the face, temporal bone, and base of the skull. A CT is useful in evaluating patients with osseous spinal stenosis and spondylosis, but an MRI is preferred if there are neurologic defects. *(Ropper, p. 16)*

47. **(B)** The lateral medullary syndrome (also known as Wallenberg syndrome) causes ipsilateral numbness but also contralateral involvement of pain and thermal sense by affecting the

spinothalamic tract. It can be caused by occlusion of the vertebral arteries; posterior-inferior cerebellar arteries; and superior, middle, or inferior medullary arteries. Ipsilateral ataxia and falling to the side of the lesion are common. Ipsilateral paralysis of the tongue is characteristic of medial medullary syndrome, which also causes contralateral paralysis of arm and leg. Paralysis of the body is not characteristic of lateral medullary syndrome, but ipsilateral paralysis of palate and vocal cord does occur. Ipsilateral Horner syndrome, nystagmus, diplopia, vertigo, nausea, and vomiting are characteristic. *(Ropper, pp. 678–679)*

48. **(C)** TSP is frequently associated with a retroviral (HTLV-1) infection that can be spread through blood transfusion, sexual contact, intravenous drug use, and vertical transmission from mother to child. It is slowly progressive, and bladder involvement is characteristic. Sensory symptoms are usually mild, and a true sensory level is almost never found. On occasion, cranial nerve findings, frontal release signs, and cerebellar signs (tremor, dysmetria) are present. *(Ropper, pp. 647–648, 1059)*

49. **(A)** The cause of trigeminal neuralgia (tic douloureux) is unknown, although some cases may be caused by compression of the trigeminal nerve by arteries or veins of the posterior fossa. The pain occurs in paroxysms and is strictly limited to one or more branches of the fifth cranial nerve. Paroxysms may be brief or last up to 15 minutes. There is no objective sensory loss, but the patient may complain of hyperesthesia of the face. Watering of the eye on the involved side may occur during an attack. *(Ropper, pp. 161–163)*

50. **(A)** Cavernous sinus thrombosis is usually secondary to traumatic, neoplastic, or suppurative processes in the orbit, the nasal sinuses, or the upper half of the face. The optic discs are swollen, and there may be numerous surrounding small or large hemorrhages if the orbital veins are occluded. Visual acuity is normal or moderately impaired. Involvement of the cranial nerves in the cavernous sinus (third, fourth, sixth, and V1 and V2 divisions of the fifth) causes diplopia, ptosis, and sensory loss on the face. *(Ropper, p. 735)*

51. **(C)** In the vast majority of cases, retrobulbar neuritis occurs as an episode in a demyelinating disease such as multiple sclerosis. It is the first manifestation of multiple sclerosis in 15% of cases and occurs at some point in 50% of all patients with the disease. The course of the retrobulbar neuritis is that of gradual spontaneous improvement. *(Ropper, p. 213)*

52. **(E)** Internal carotid artery insufficiency is the most likely diagnosis. Abnormalities are found in the extracranial arteries in more than one-half of the patients with symptomatic cerebral infarction. Current treatment is carotid endarterectomy for severe stenosis and aspirin therapy for lesser degrees of stenosis. *(Ropper, pp. 686–692)*

53. **(B)** The patient's findings strongly suggest herpes simplex encephalitis. This is generally caused by herpes simplex virus type 1 (HSVI). When the disease is suspected, appropriate antiviral therapy (acyclovir) should be started immediately. CT scan is not helpful in diagnosis because it becomes positive only late in the disease, but MRI scans may be helpful. Brain biopsy, once the diagnostic test of choice, is the most definitive test but is rarely performed. *(Ropper, pp. 638–639)*

54. **(C)** Guillain-Barré syndrome often appears days to weeks after a viral upper respiratory or gastrointestinal (GI) infection. The initial symptoms are due to symmetric limb weakness. Paresthesias may be present. Unlike most other neuropathies, proximal muscles may be affected more than distal muscles early in the disease. Tendon reflexes are usually lost within a few days. Protein content of the CSF is usually high within a few days of onset. *(Ropper, pp. 1121–1122)*

55. **(E)** This patient has myasthenia gravis and the thymus tissue is often abnormal, with encapsulated tumors occurring in about 15% of cases. Almost all thymomas occur in patients over age 30. Even without thymoma, thymectomy can result in remission in patients with generalized myasthenia. Its benefit is delayed for months or more, so it is not an emergency treatment for myasthenia. *(Ropper, p. 1252)*

56. (D) Vertigo is defined as an illusory or hallucinatory feeling of movement of the body or environment, usually spinning. Dizziness can be caused by multiple factors in the elderly, including orthostatic hypotension, hypoglycemia, and depression. *(Ropper, p. 257)*

57. (C) Patients with BPPV, in contrast to those with central positional vertigo, have a latent period from the time of onset of the offending position to development of symptoms. With maintenance of the position, patients with BPPV become less symptomatic (fatigability), and repeated positioning also lessens the symptoms (habituation). As well, in BPPV, although the symptoms are usually severe, they can be quite variable from one testing period to the next. *(Ropper, p. 261)*

58. (A) Anticholinergic drugs exacerbate the underlying defects. Cholinergic drugs are largely inhibitors of cholinesterase. Prednisone may improve as many as 80% of patients. Thymectomy helps patients with no thymoma, but thymoma patients do not do as well. Plasmapheresis benefits most patients but needs to be repeated at intervals. *(Ropper, pp. 1256–1258)*

59. (E) Myoclonic seizures are sudden, brief, single, or repetitive muscle contractions involving one body part or the entire body. Loss of consciousness does not occur unless other types of seizures coexist. These seizures can be idiopathic or associated with Creutzfeldt-Jakob disease, uremia, hepatic failure, subacute leukoencephalopathies, and some hereditary disorders. Recent evidence has linked a variant form of Creutzfeldt-Jakob disease with bovine spongiform encephalopathy (BSE), a prion disease of cattle. This variant form usually presents with ataxia and behavior changes prior to myoclonus and dementia. *(Ropper, pp. 87–89)*

60. (B) Complex partial seizures were once classified as temporal lobe epilepsy. Although the temporal lobe (especially the hippocampus or amygdala) is the most common site of origin,

some seizures have been shown to originate from mesial parasagittal or orbital frontal regions. *(Ropper, p. 277)*

61. (D) Pure absence seizures consist of the sudden cessation of ongoing conscious activity without convulsive muscular activity or loss of postural control. They can be so brief as to be inapparent but can last several minutes. There is usually no period of postictal confusion. *(Ropper, p. 274)*

62. (A) Simple partial seizures can occur with motor, sensory, autonomic, or psychic symptoms. When a partial motor seizure spreads to adjacent neurons, a "Jacksonian march" can occur (e.g., right thumb to right hand and right arm to right side of face). Face and hand movements are frequently linked because their cortical controlling regions are adjacent. *(Ropper, pp. 275–276)*

63. (D) Absence seizures almost always begin in young children (age 6–14). They may first present as learning difficulties in school. The EEG is diagnostic, revealing brief 3-Hz spike and wave discharges occurring synchronously throughout all the leads. *(Ropper, p. 274)*

64. (E) Valproic acid can be used for typical and atypical seizures, myoclonic seizures, and tonic-clonic seizures. It causes little sedation and does not impair cognition. However, the blood count and liver tests must be monitored for a time after initiation of therapy to ensure the safety of the patient. *(Ropper, p. 293)*

65. (E) Valproic acid is the drug of choice for atypical absence seizures and myoclonic seizures. *(Ropper, p. 293)*

66. (A, B, E) Phenytoin is the first choice for tonic-clonic seizures; it can cause gum hyperplasia and hirsutism, which are particularly unpleasant side effects in young women. Lymphadenopathy, ataxia, incoordination, confusion, and cerebellar toxicity can also occur. Carbamazepine and valproic acid are also options for the initial treatment of tonic-clonic seizures. *(Ropper, p. 293)*

67. **(A, B)** Carbamazepine is the initial choice for partial seizures. Phenytoin is also an option. *(Ropper, p. 292)*

68. **(G)** Lorazepam or diazepam is the treatment of choice for status epilepticus. Diazepam intravenously (IV) at 2 mg/min up to 20 mg, or lorazepam IV (0.1 mg/kg) at no faster than 2 mg/min, is initially given followed by phenytoin loading (15–18 mg/kg) no faster than 50 mg/min. *(Ropper, p. 297)*

69. **(B)** Horner syndrome results in a small, round pupil on one side. Light and near reaction is brisk, and response to mydriatics and miotics is normal. The affected pupil will not dilate in the dark, so darkness accentuates the anisocoria. The syndrome is often idiopathic but can be caused by neoplasm, brain stem stroke, or carotid dissection. *(Ropper, pp. 464–465)*

70. **(C)** The tonic pupil (Holmes-Adie syndrome) is caused by a parasympathetic lesion at or distal to the ciliary ganglion. The pupil is large and usually unilateral, with absent response to light. A bright room, by causing constriction of the normal pupil, accentuates the anisocoria. The tonic pupil can be associated with Shy-Drager syndrome, amyloidosis, or diabetes. However, it is most commonly seen in otherwise healthy young women. *(Ropper, p. 243)*

71. **(D)** Argyll Robertson pupils are small, irregular, and often bilateral. The response to light is impaired, but the response to near vision is preserved. Argyll Robertson pupils can be a manifestation of syphilis, a treponemal infection. It can also be associated with lesions of the dorsal midbrain (obstructive hydrocephalus, pineal region tumors) and after aberrant regeneration. *(Ropper, p. 242)*

72. **(A)** This patient has physiologic or essential anisocoria, which can be seen in up to 20% of the population at some time. Its hallmarks are a normal response to light and accommodation and the asymmetry is maintained in different lighting conditions. It can also be variable from day to day. *(Ropper, p. 243)*

73. **(G)** Compression of the oculomotor nerve (third cranial nerve) results in paresis of the oculomotor muscles supplied by the nerve and symptoms of double vision. The parasympathetic fibers running along the outside of the nerve are also affected resulting in dilation of the pupil. Increased intracranial pressure from any mass lesion (blood, abscess, or tumor) leading to uncal herniation and compression of the nerve is the usual cause. *(Ropper, p. 230)*

74. **(B)** Peripheral nerve lesions result in reflex loss greater than the degree of weakness. Reflex loss is variable in anterior horn cell disease and decreased proportionately in muscle disease. In neuromuscular junction disorders, reflexes are characteristically normal. *(Ropper, pp. 1113–1114)*

75. **(C)** Diurnal fluctuations and pathologic fatigue are common in disorders of neuromuscular transmission (e.g., myasthenia gravis). *(Ropper, pp. 1250–1251)*

76. **(A)** In diseases of the anterior horn cell (such as ALS), atrophy is marked and early. Muscle disease can result in marked atrophy, but much later in the course of the disease. Atrophy is generally moderate in peripheral nerve disease and absent in disorders of the neuromuscular junction. *(Ropper, p. 939)*

77. **(B)** Peripheral nerve disease is the most likely to cause distal weakness and is the only one of the four to also cause sensory symptoms. *(Ropper, p. 1168)*

78. **(D)** Dermatomyositis is one of the inflammatory myopathies that has a characteristic rash on the eyelids (heliotrope) and knuckles (Gottron's papules). It is associated with certain cancers as a paraneoplastic syndrome. The muscle enzyme creatine kinase (CK) is elevated is most cases, but the condition is painless. Symptoms are those of proximal muscle weakness, with normal reflexes and tone on examination. *(Ropper, pp. 1204–1205)*

CHAPTER 8

Kidneys
Questions

DIRECTIONS (Questions 1 through 37): Each of the numbered items in this section is followed by answers. Select the ONE lettered answer that is BEST in each case.

1. A 25-year-old woman presents with nausea and vomiting of 2 days duration. She is not on any medications and was previously well until now. Her physical examination is normal except for a postural drop in her blood pressure from 110/80 mm Hg supine to 90/80 mm Hg standing. Her serum electrolytes are sodium 130 mEq/L, potassium 3 mEq/L, chloride 90 mEq/L, bicarbonate 30 mEq/L, urea 50 mg/dL, and creatinine 0.8 mg/dL. Which of the following electrolytes is most likely to be filtered through the glomerulus but unaffected by tubular secretion?

   (A) potassium
   (B) sodium
   (C) bicarbonate
   (D) urea
   (E) creatinine

2. Ten days after a kidney transplant, a 32-year-old man develops allograft enlargement, fever, oliguria, and hypertension. Which of the following is the most likely diagnosis?

   (A) steroid hyperglycemia
   (B) erythrocytosis
   (C) hyperacute rejection
   (D) acute rejection
   (E) renal artery stenosis

3. A 19-year-old man presents with malaise, nausea, and decreased urine output. He was previously well, and his physical examination is normal except for an elevated jugular venous pressure (JVP) and a pericardial rub. His electrolytes reveal acute renal failure (ARF). Which of the following findings on the urinalysis is most likely in keeping with acute glomerulonephritis (GN)?

   (A) proteinuria
   (B) white blood cell casts
   (C) granular casts
   (D) erythrocyte casts
   (E) hyaline casts

4. A 24-year-old woman presents with nausea, vomiting, anorexia, and gross hematuria. She had a sore throat 2 weeks ago that resolved on its own. On examination, her blood pressure is 160/90 mm Hg, pulse 90/min, JVP is 7 cm, heart sounds are normal, there is 1+ pedal edema, and the lungs are clear. She has a renal biopsy. Which of the following electron microscopy findings on the renal biopsy is most likely in keeping with poststreptococcal GN?

   (A) diffuse mesangial deposits
   (B) no deposits
   (C) electron-dense endothelial deposits
   (D) closed capillary lumen
   (E) subepithelial humps

5. A 74-year-old man is brought to hospital because of urinary retention. He has a Foley catheter inserted to relieve the obstruction, and 1500 cc of urine is emptied from his bladder. Over the next few hours, he has 200cc/h of urine output. Which of the following urine electrolyte values is most likely in keeping with his diagnosis?

(A) high sodium
(B) low potassium
(C) high specific gravity
(D) low pH
(E) osmolality >500 mOsm/kg

6. A 68-year-old woman has used large amounts of analgesic for years to relieve severe headaches and arthritis. She now has an elevated urea and creatinine consistent with chronic renal failure. Which of the following changes in the kidney is most likely seen with her diagnosis?

(A) glomerulosclerosis
(B) papillary necrosis and tubulointerstitial inflammation
(C) cortical necrosis
(D) tubular necrosis
(E) nephrolithiasis

7. A 64-year-old woman develops severe diarrhea 2 weeks after finishing antibiotics for pneumonia. She has also noticed decreased urine output despite drinking lots of fluids. On examination, she has a postural drop in her blood pressure, the JVP is low, and the abdomen is soft but diffusely tender. Despite giving 4 L of normal saline, her urine output remains low. The urinalysis is positive for heme-granular casts and the urine sodium is 42 mEq/L. Which of the following medications should be held during the recovery phase of this woman's ARF?

(A) acetaminophen
(B) digoxin
(C) lorazepam
(D) enalapril
(E) simvastatin

8. A 64-year-old woman has metabolic alkalosis and the bicarbonate level is 34 mEq/L. Which of the following is the most likely cause?

(A) diuretic use
(B) hyperkalemia
(C) mineralocorticoid deficiency
(D) diarrhea
(E) angiotensin-converting enzyme (ACE)-inhibitor use

9. A 32-year-old man with sickle cell anemia is seen for routine follow-up. He feels well at the present time, but in the past he has had many sickle cell crises, which have resulted in kidney injury. Which of the following renal abnormalities is most likely to be seen in him?

(A) inability to acidify the urine
(B) granular casts
(C) inability to concentrate the urine
(D) pyuria
(E) salt-losing state

10. A 63-year-old man with an 8-year history of recurrent severe arthritis in his large toes has an elevated creatinine level. Which of the following mechanisms is the most likely explanation for his renal impairment?

(A) GN
(B) vascular injury
(C) uric acid kidney stones
(D) distal tubular atrophy
(E) renal parenchymal uric acid crystals

11. A 67-year-old man presents with symptoms of renal colic. Plain x-rays of the abdomen reveal no obvious stone. An intravenous pyelogram (IVP) is ordered to confirm the clinical diagnosis. Which of the following coexisting medical conditions increases the risk of contrast-induced nephropathy?

(A) hyperparathyroidism
(B) pyelonephritis
(C) nephrolithiasis
(D) hypernephroma
(E) multiple myeloma

12. A 64-year-old man presents with weight gain, shortness of breath, easy bruising, and leg swelling. On examination, his blood pressure is 140/80 mm Hg, pulse 100/min, JVP 4 cm, heart sounds normal, and lungs are clear. There is a 3+ pedal and some periorbital edema. Investigations include a normal chest x-ray (CXR), electrocardiogram (ECG) with low voltages, anemia, high urea and creatinine, and 4 g/day of protein in the urine. A renal biopsy, which shows nodular deposits that have an apple-green birefringence under polarized light when stained with Congo red. Which of the following is the most likely diagnosis?

    (A) amyloidosis
    (B) multiple myeloma
    (C) diabetic nephropathy
    (D) minimal change disease
    (E) immunoglobulin A (IgA) nephropathy

13. A 74-year-old man presents with fatigue, shortness of breath on exertion, and back and rib pain, which is made worse with movement. Investigations reveal he is anemic, calcium, urea, and creatinine are elevated. X-rays reveal multiple lytic lesions in the long bones and ribs, and protein electrophoresis is positive for an immunoglobulin G (IgG) paraprotein. Which of the following is the most likely mechanism for the renal injury?

    (A) plasma cell infiltrates
    (B) tubular damage by light chains
    (C) glomerular injury
    (D) vascular injury by light chains
    (E) uric acid crystals

14. A 77-year-old man with a mass in the lung develops asymptomatic hyponatremia. His JVP is 4 cm, heart sounds are normal, and the lungs are clear. The urine sodium is 64 mEq/L and osmolality 550 mOsm/kg. Which of the following is the most likely diagnosis?

    (A) nephrotic syndrome
    (B) syndrome of inappropriate antidiuretic hormone (SIADH) production

    (C) renal metastases from lung cancer
    (D) lung metastases from hypernephroma
    (E) renal tubular acidosis (RTA)

15. A 69-year-old man has lost a friend to prostate cancer, and would like to be evaluated for the disease. He has no urinary symptoms. Which of the following tests is most likely indicated to screen him for prostate cancer?

    (A) prostate ultrasound
    (B) digital rectal examination (DRE)
    (C) DRE and prostate specific antigen (PSA)
    (D) PSA
    (E) none of the above

16. A 63-year-old woman has Type II diabetes mellitus, which is well-controlled. Her physical examination is positive for peripheral neuropathy in the feet and nonproliferative retinopathy. A urinalysis is positive for proteinuria. Which of the following treatments is most likely to attenuate the course of renal disease?

    (A) calcium channel blockers
    (B) ACE inhibitors
    (C) hepatic hydroxymethylglutaryl-coenzyme A (HMG-CoA) inhibitors
    (D) dietary carbohydrate restriction
    (E) weight reduction

17. A 32-year-old man has trace proteinuria on dipstick urinalysis. A 24-hour urine collection reveals 380 mg/day of protein excretion in the urine. Which of the following statements concerning this degree of proteinuria is correct?

    (A) rarely requires any investigation
    (B) in systemic diseases, it has no prognostic values
    (C) can be caused by fever
    (D) is rarely reversible
    (E) always caused by tubular defects

18. A 56-year-old man is involved in a severe motor vehicle accident. He develops ARF after admission to hospital. One of the possibilities for his ARF is posttraumatic renal vein thrombosis. Which of the following findings is most likely to suggest renal vein thrombosis?

   (A) white cell casts on urinalysis
   (B) heme-granular casts
   (C) heavy proteinuria
   (D) urine supernatant pink and tests positive for heme
   (E) specific gravity >1.020

19. A 69-year-old woman presents with left flank pain and hematuria. Physical examination suggests a left-sided abdominal mass. Computerized tomography (CT) scan of the abdomen reveals a 5-cm mass in the left kidney. Which of the following laboratory abnormalities might also be present? (See Fig. 8–1.)

   (A) polycythemia
   (B) thrombocytopenia
   (C) hypocalcemia
   (D) leukocytosis
   (E) high renin hypertension

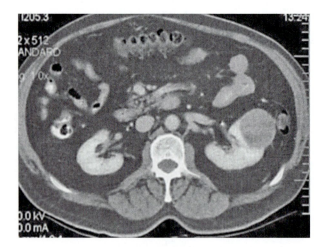

Figure 8–1.

20. A 60-year-old woman with heart failure and normal renal function is started on furosemide (Lasix) 80 mg/day. She notices a good diuretic response every time she takes the medication. A few weeks later, she is feeling unwell because of fatigue and muscle weakness, but her heart failure symptoms are better. Which of the following is the most likely explanation for her muscle weakness?

   (A) hyponatremia
   (B) hypernatremia
   (C) hypokalemia
   (D) hyperkalemia
   (E) anemia

21. A 57-year-old man, otherwise fine, is found to have low serum sodium on routine laboratory testing. His serum osmolality is low, but his urine osmolality is >150 mOsm/kg. Which of the following is most likely to be found on further evaluation?

   (A) massive edema
   (B) hyperkalemia
   (C) dehydration
   (D) elevated urea nitrogen
   (E) an intrathoracic lesion

22. A 78-year-old man is brought to the hospital because of nausea and vomiting. On examination he appears dry, his abdomen is soft, and the JVP is not visible. His laboratory tests reveal hypernatremia and his calculated free water deficit is approximately 3 L. In what part of the normal kidney is most of the water reabsorbed from?

   (A collecting ducts
   (B) proximal tubule
   (C) distal tubule
   (D) ascending loop of Henle
   (E) descending loop of Henle

23. A 64-year-old man is admitted for hematuria after slipping on an icy pavement. His physical examination is normal. A selective angiogram of the left kidney is shown in Fig. 8–2. Which of the following is the most likely diagnosis?

   (A) renal cell carcinoma
   (B) kidney contusion and laceration
   (C) transitional cell carcinoma

(D) renal hamartoma

(E) renal hemangioma

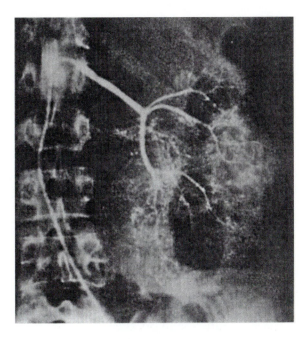

Figure 8–2.

24. A 64-year-old man presents with symptoms of malaise, shortness of breath, edema, and no urine output for 24 hours. His past medical history is not significant, and his only medication is daily aspirin. On examination his JVP is 4 cm, heart sounds are normal, lungs are clear, and the abdomen is soft. A Foley catheter is inserted into his bladder for 200 cc of urine, which is sent for urinalysis. His urine output still remains low. Which of the following is the most appropriate initial diagnostic test?

(A) renal ultrasound

(B) blood cultures

(C) urine cultures

(D) inferior vena cavagram with selective renal venogram

(E) blood urea nitrogen (BUN)/creatinine ratio

25. A 68-year-old woman develops new symptoms of burning when voiding. She has no fever, chills, or back discomfort. Her urinalysis reveals numerous white cells and bacteria. Which of the following medical comorbidities is most likely to coexist in this patient?

(A) anemia

(B) exercise

(C) diabetes mellitus

(D) influenza

(E) analgesic drug use

26. A 28-year-old woman presents with a recent episode of coughing up some blood, frequent nosebleeds, and now decreased urine output. A nasal mucosa ulcer was seen on inspection. Her urinalysis is positive for protein and red cells consistent with a GN. The CXR shows two cavitary lesions and her serology is positive for antineutrophil cytoplasmic antibodies (ANCA). Which of the following is the most likely diagnosis?

(A) Wegener's granulomatosis

(B) bacterial endocarditis

(C) Goodpasture's syndrome

(D) lupus erythematosus

(E) poststreptococcal disease

27. A 42-year-old man notices leg and facial swelling but no other symptoms. His examination is pertinent for 3+ pedal edema including periorbital edema. A 24-hour urine collection reveals 5 g of proteinuria. Which of the following is the most likely diagnosis?

(A) sickle cell disease

(B) medullary sponge kidney

(C) radiation nephritis

(D) staphylococcal infection

(E) amyloid disease

28. A 74-year-old woman develops acute sepsis from pneumonia and is admitted to the intensive care unit because of hypotension. She is started on antibiotics, and her blood pressure is supported with intravenous normal saline. Despite this she remains oliguric and develops ARF. Her urinalysis has heme-granular casts and the urine sodium is 56 mEq/L. Which of the following is the most likely cause of her ARF?

(A) nephrotoxic antibiotics
(B) acute infectious GN
(C) acute tubular necrosis (ATN)
(D) contrast nephropathy
(E) cholesterol emboli

29. A pregnant woman develops hypertension, edema, and proteinuria, at 34 weeks of gestation. Which of the following is not a risk factor for the development of this complication?

(A) first pregnancy
(B) diabetes mellitus
(C) twin pregnancy
(D) extreme of reproductive age
(E) human immunodeficiency virus (HIV) infection

30. A 30-year-old man presents with hematuria. His examination is normal except for an elevated blood pressure of 164/94 mm Hg. An ultrasound of the kidneys reveals multiple renal cysts in both kidneys. His father had a similar condition. Which of the following is not associated with this syndrome?

(A) liver cysts
(B) intracranial aneurysms
(C) autosomal dominant inheritance
(D) rheumatoid arthritis (RA)
(E) progression to end-stage renal failure

31. A 15-year-old boy develops renal colic. The stone is not recovered, but urinalysis reveals hexagonal crystals, and a cyanide-nitroprusside test on the urine is positive. Which of the following is the most likely diagnosis?

(A) cystinuria
(B) thalassemia
(C) hereditary glycinuria
(D) primary hyperoxaluria
(E) sarcoidosis

32. A 29-year-old man is stable 1 year post-kidney transplant. Which of the following complications of transplantation is the most likely cause of death?

(A) atherosclerotic disease
(B) opportunistic infection
(C) metabolic bone disease
(D) lung cancer
(E) lymphoma

33. A 37-year-old immunosuppressed patient with renal failure develops sepsis. Which of the following antibiotics, if used, would require a major reduction in dosage?

(A) erythromycin
(B) doxycycline
(C) tobramycin
(D) isoniazid (INH)
(E) amphotericin B

34. A 63-year-old woman presents for routine evaluation. She has had diabetes for the past 12 years with complications of neuropathy and retinopathy. You decide to screen her for renal complications of diabetes. Which of the following findings is not compatible with diabetic nephropathy?

(A) nephrotic range proteinuria
(B) microalbuminuria
(C) hypertension
(D) red blood cell (RBC) casts in urine
(E) renal tubular acidosis (RTA) type IV

35. A 24-year-old woman is dipstick positive for blood in her urine. This is repeated twice between menstrual periods and remains positive. Microscopic evaluation reveals RBCs, some of which are deformed and some in the form of casts. Which of the following is the most likely cause of the hematuria?

(A) urinary tract stones

(B) GN

(C) trauma

(D) benign renal tumor

36. A 63-year-old man becomes oliguric 2 days following an open cholecystectomy. Which of the following findings would suggest that prerenal ARF is a major factor in the etiology?

(A) postural hypotension

(B) fractional excretion of sodium is 3%

(C) specific gravity is 1.012

(D) the urine sodium is 30 mEq/L

(E) heme-granular casts on urine microscopy

37. A 46-year-old woman with nausea and vomiting presents to hospital because of light-headedness when standing and decreased urine output. She looks unwell; the blood pressure supine is 90/60 mm Hg and 80/60 mm Hg when standing. Her abdominal, heart, and lung examinations are normal. Which of the following laboratory values suggests prerenal azotemia in this patient?

(A) markedly elevated urea, unchanged creatinine

(B) unchanged urea, elevated creatinine

(C) little change in either creatinine or urea for several days after oliguria develops

(D) urea/creatinine ratio of 10

(E) urea/creatinine ratio of 25

DIRECTIONS (Questions 38 through 79): Each set of matching questions in this section consists of a list of lettered options followed by several numbered items. For each numbered item, select the appropriate lettered option(s). Each lettered option may be selected once, more than once, or not at all. EACH ITEM WILL STATE THE NUMBER OF OPTIONS TO SELECT. CHOOSE EXACTLY THIS NUMBER.

Questions 38 through 41

(A) central diabetes insipidus (DI)

(B) nephrogenic DI

(C) primary polydipsia

(D) osmotic diuresis

(E) hypercalcemia

For each patient with polyuria and polydipsia, select the most likely diagnosis.

38. A 21-year-old woman develops polydipsia and polyuria during pregnancy. (SELECT TWO)

39. A 19-year-old man develops polyuria and polydipsia after a head injury. (SELECT ONE)

40. A 19-year-old man and one of his two brothers has had polyuria and polydipsia since birth. Neither his sisters nor his parents are affected. (SELECT ONE)

41. A 27-year-old woman with well-controlled bipolar affective disorder, treated with lithium, develops polyuria and polydipsia. (SELECT ONE)

Questions 42 through 46

(A) metabolic acidosis

(B) metabolic alkalosis

(C) respiratory acidosis

(D) respiratory alkalosis

For each patient with new symptoms, select the most likely acid base disorder.

42. A 19-year-old girl develops sudden-onset non-bloody diarrhea. She was previously well and is not taking any medications or traveled anywhere recently. Her abdomen is soft and non-tender on examination, and the anion gap is normal. (SELECT ONE)

43. A 75-year-old man develops acute confusion and drowsiness after a dental procedure. He has a history of severe chronic lung disease due to smoking. Earlier in the day, he had a tooth extraction and afterwards was given acetaminophen with codeine (Tylenol # 3) for pain relief. (SELECT ONE)

44. A 74-year-old woman has symptoms of shortness of breath on exertion and waking up at night. Her physical examination reveals a JVP at 8 cm, extra third heart sound, lung crackles, and pedal edema. She is started on furosemide 80 mg/day for heart failure, while further investigations are performed. (SELECT ONE)

45. A 53-year-old woman is being treated for tuberculosis with INH and rifampin. (SELECT ONE)

46. A 69-year-old woman is taking large amounts of aspirin for osteoarthritis, and now complains of ringing in her ears and nausea. (SELECT ONE)

Questions 47 through 52

   (A) nephrogenic DI
   (B) central DI
   (C) primary polydipsia
   (D) solute diuresis
   (E) natriuretic syndrome

For each patient with increased urine output, select the correct diagnosis.

47. A 42-year-old man presents to hospital with dark black-colored stools and passing out while getting up. On examination he is diaphoretic, blood pressure 80/50 mm Hg supine, pulse 120/min, and the DRE is positive for melena. He is resuscitated in the emergency room. He has low urine output and develops renal failure from ATN. A few days later, his urine output increases to 200 cc/h. (SELECT ONE)

48. A 27-year-old woman presents because she is feeling unwell. Her examination is normal, but her serum sodium is 115 mEq/L. Her urine lytes: sodium 55 mEq/L, osmolality 100 mOsm/L. This condition causes the greatest amount of medullary washout. (SELECT ONE)

49. A 64-year-old man develops severe diarrhea after returning from a foreign holiday. He is hypovolemic clinically and is given normal saline. His serum sodium is 125 mEq/L and potassium is 2.5 mEq/L. He develops increased urine output with urine sodium of 10 mEq/L and osmolality of 200 mOsm/L. His polyuria can be caused by hypokalemia. (SELECT ONE)

50. A 34-year-old man is brought for evaluation because of bizarre behavior. He comments that he is voiding all the time of clear water-like urine. He has a past history of schizophrenia for which he is taking a major tranquilizer. (SELECT ONE)

51. A 38-year-old man is admitted to hospital for investigation of polyuria and a low serum sodium concentration. After a fluid deprivation test, there was no change in his urine osmolality. He was then given vasopressin (DDAVP) with no change in urine volume or urine osmolality after 2 hours. (SELECT ONE)

52. A 67-year-old man is admitted to hospital after a stroke. He has swallowing difficulties, and a nasogastric feeding tube is inserted to provide high protein content nutrition. After starting the tube feeds, he develops large amounts of urine output. His serum sodium is normal, and the urine values are sodium 60 mEq/L and osmolality 420 mOsm/L. (SELECT ONE)

Questions 53 through 58

   (A) congestive heart failure (CHF)
   (B) extrarenal sodium and fluid losses
   (C) SIADH
   (D) polydipsia
   (E) essential hyponatremia
   (F) renal failure
   (G) endocrine cause of hyponatremia
   (H) renal sodium and fluid losses
   (I) artifactual
   (J) osmotic
   (K) impaired diuresis

For each patient with hyponatremia, select the most likely diagnosis.

53. A 74-year-old man from a nursing home is not feeling well and is confused. He is not able to give any reliable history. His serum sodium is 120 mEq/L and osmolality is 265 mOsm/kg.

On examination, his blood pressure is 100/50 mm Hg, pulse 100/min, and neck veins are not visible. His urine sodium is 40 mEq/L and urine osmolality is 330 mOsm/kg. (SELECT ONE)

54. A 65-year-old woman is admitted to the hospital after a stroke resulting in left hemiparesis. She has no trouble swallowing and is on a full diet. One week later, on routine biochemistry, her sodium is 128 mEq/L and osmolality is 270 mOsm/kg. She has no symptoms and is euvolemic on clinical examination. Urine sodium is 40 mEq/L and urine osmolality is 450 mOsm/kg. (SELECT ONE)

55. A 42-year-old man is on amitriptyline for depression. Recently he has been feeling more lethargic and unwell. His clinical examination is normal. Serum sodium is 125 mEq/L and osmolality is 260 mOsm/kg, and urine sodium is 40 mEq/L and osmolality is 450 mOsm/kg. (SELECT ONE)

56. A 32-year-old man is feeling unwell and brought to the hospital. His serum sodium is 125 mEq/L. On examination, his blood pressure is 110/70 mm Hg, pulse 110/min supine, and sitting up causes him to feel light-headed with a drop in his blood pressure. His urine sodium is 5 mEq/L and urine osmolality is 800 mOsm/kg. (SELECT ONE)

57. A 57-year-old man is referred for assessment of his low serum sodium of 125 mEq/L. On examination, he has pitting edema and elevated neck veins. His urine sodium is 10 mEq/L and urine osmolality 350 mOsm/kg. (SELECT ONE)

58. A 63-year-old man is feeling unwell with symptoms of increased thirst and voiding. He is not taking any medications and there is no past medical history. Physical examination is normal, but his serum sodium is 130 mEq/L and serum osmolality is 310 mOsm/kg. (SELECT ONE)

Questions 59 through 63
(A) lower gastrointestinal (GI) losses
(B) prior use of diuretics

(C) RTA
(D) current use of diuretics
(E) malignant hypertension
(F) primary hyperaldosteronism
(G) glucocorticoid excess

For each patient with hypokalemia, select the most likely diagnosis.

59. A 30-year-old woman is having symptoms of muscle weakness and fatigue. On examination, her blood pressure is 120/80 mm Hg, pulse 80/min, JVP 4 cm, heart sounds normal, and lungs clear. Her serum potassium level is 2.5 mEq/L, and bicarbonate 30 mEq/L. The urine potassium is 10 mEq/L. (SELECT ONE)

60. A 55-year-old man is having symptoms of muscle weakness and fatigue. He has poorly controlled asthma and recently had an exacerbation. On examination, his blood pressure is 160/90 mm Hg, pulse 80/min, JVP 4 cm, heart sounds normal, and lungs clear. His serum potassium level is 2.5 mEq/L and bicarbonate 30 mEq/L. The urine potassium is 40 mEq/L. Plasma renin and aldosterone levels are low. (SELECT ONE)

61. A 44-year-old woman is having symptoms of muscle weakness and fatigue. On examination, her blood pressure is 120/80 mm Hg, pulse 80/min, JVP 4 cm, heart sounds normal, and lungs clear. Her serum potassium level is 2.5 mEq/L, bicarbonate 18 mEq/L, and anion gap is normal. The urine potassium is 40 mEq/L. (SELECT ONE)

62. A 30-year-old man is having symtoms of muscle weakness, fatigue, and headaches. On examination, his blood pressure is 180/100 mm Hg, pulse 80/min, JVP 4 cm, heart sounds normal, and lungs clear. His serum potassium level is 2.5 mEq/L and bicarbonate 30 mEq/L. The urine potassium is 40 mEq/L. Plasma renin is low and aldosterone is high. (SELECT ONE)

63. A 60-year-old woman is having symptoms of muscle weakness and fatigue. On examination, her blood pressure is 110/80 mm Hg, pulse 100/min, JVP 1 cm, heart sounds normal, and lungs clear. Her serum potassium level is 2.5 mEq/L, bicarbonate 15 mEq/L, and anion gap is normal. The urine potassium is 10 mEq/L. (SELECT ONE)

Questions 64 through 68

    (A) metabolic acidosis and respiratory acidosis

    (B) metabolic acidosis and respiratory alkalosis

    (C) metabolic alkalosis and respiratory acidosis

    (D) metabolic alkalosis and respiratory alkalosis

    (E) metabolic alkalosis and metabolic acidosis

For each of the following medical conditions, select the associated acid base disturbances.

64. Salicylate overdose (SELECT ONE)

65. Sepsis (SELECT ONE)

66. Chronic pulmonary disease on steroids (SELECT ONE)

67. Renal failure with vomiting (SELECT ONE)

68. Hepatic cirrhosis complicated by ARF (SELECT ONE)

Questions 69 through 73

    (A) diffuse proliferative GN

    (B) crescentic GN

    (C) focal proliferative GN

    (D) membranoproliferative GN

    (E) minimal change GN

    (F) focal segmental GN

    (G) membranous GN

    (H) deposition diseases

    (I) nonimmune basement membrane abnormalities

For each patient with GN, select the most likely diagnosis on renal biopsy.

69. A 14-year-old girl develops a rash, abdominal pain, and arthralgias. She is also experiencing some nausea, vomiting, and crampy abdominal pain. On examination, she has a palpable purpuric rash on her buttocks and lower legs, a tender abdomen, and no active joint inflammation. Her stools test positive for blood, and urinalysis reveals RBCs and RBC casts. Her renal function deteriorates rapidly over several days. A renal biopsy is performed. (SELECT ONE)

70. A 28-year-old woman has noticed increasing lower limb swelling and shortness of breath. She has a 2-year history of facial rash, hair loss, arthralgias, and thrombocytopenia. On examination, her blood pressure is 150/90 mm Hg, pulse 80/min, there is a maculo-papular rash on her face, JVP is 4 cm, heart sounds normal, lungs clear, and there is pedal and periorbital edema. Her creatinine is very high, and a renal biopsy is performed. (SELECT FOUR)

71. A 47-year-old woman with RA is being treated with nonsteroidal anti-inflammatory drugs (NSAIDs) and gold. She develops acute shortness of breath with hypoxemia and is admitted to the hospital. Admission urinalysis reveals 4+ proteinuria but no active sediment. A renal biopsy is performed. (SELECT ONE)

72. A 19-year-old man, who is otherwise healthy, is found to have RBCs in his urine. There is no proteinuria. Evaluation of his family reveals that his mother also has hematuria. She has minimal renal impairment and, other than being hard of hearing, is in good health. A renal biopsy might show. (SELECT ONE)

73. A 33-year-old man from Southeast Asia, without HIV infection, is diagnosed as having pulmonary tuberculosis. He is started on multiple medications, including INH and rifampin. Three months later, he has developed edema. Liver tests are normal, and serum creatinine is increased by 30% over baseline. Urinalysis reveals 4+ proteinuria. A renal biopsy is performed. (SELECT ONE)

Questions 74 through 77

    (A) polycystic kidney disease

    (B) medullary sponge kidney

    (C) medullary cystic disease

    (D) Liddle syndrome

    (E) Bartter syndrome

    (F) congenital nephrogenic DI

    (G) RTA type I

    (H) RTA type II

    (I) X-linked hypophosphatemia

    (J) cystinuria

    (K) Fanconi syndrome

For each patient with a medical problem, select the most likely diagnosis or renal impairment.

74. A 14-year-old boy is short in height and has had several fractures with minimal trauma. Physical examination reveals prominent costochondral junctions and bowed legs. This syndrome could be secondary to (SELECT FOUR)

75. A 43-year-old man had a subarachnoid hemorrhage from an intracranial aneurysm 8 years ago. He has also had progressive renal impairment associated with hematuria. The most likely diagnosis is (SELECT ONE)

76. An 18-year-old man is found to have metabolic alkalosis and hypokalemia. This could be secondary to (SELECT TWO)

77. A 28-year-old man presents with a kidney stone. He is married to his first cousin, and 6 months earlier, his 8-year-old son had a kidney stone as well. The most likely diagnosis is (SELECT ONE)

Questions 78 and 79

    (A) urinary osmolality >500

    (B) urinary sodium >40

    (C) urinary sodium <20

    (D) fractional sodium excretion >1%

    (E) RBCs in urine

    (F) granular casts in urine

For each patient with ARF, select the characteristic urine electrolyte and microscopy findings.

78. A 21-year-old woman presents with a 2-day history of abdominal pain, nausea, and vomiting. On examination, her blood pressure is 100/70 mm Hg, pulse 100/min, JVP is below sternal angle, and abdomen is diffusely tender. Her urine output is low and electrolytes reveal elevated urea and normal creatinine. (SELECT TWO)

79. A 63-year-old woman presents with left arm swelling, redness, fever, and symptoms of light-headedness. She has a prior history of hypertension and high cholesterol. On examination, her blood pressure is 80/50 mm Hg, pulse 120/min, there is a large area of cellulites on her left arm, and she appears flushed. She is admitted to the intensive care unit for management of sepsis and hypotension. On the second hospital day, she still has a low urine output, despite a normal blood pressure and heart rate. Her urea and creatinine have doubled since admission. (SELECT THREE)

Answers and Explanations

1. **(D)** Urea is filtered at the glomerulus, and thereafter, any movement in or out of tubules is a passive process depending on gradients, not secretion. Reabsorption of urea in the distal tubule and collecting duct, when urine flow is reduced, results in the disproportionate elevation of urea nitrogen over creatinine in prerenal azotemia. *(Kasper, p. 246)*

2. **(D)** Renal scans initially show a reduction in excretion with cortical retention. This is the most common type of rejection. Most acute rejections will respond to immunosuppressive agents if diagnosed early. In contrast, immediate nonfunction of a graft can be caused by damage to the kidney during procurement and storage. Such problems are becoming less frequent. Obstruction, vascular compression, and ureteral compression are other causes of primary nonfunction of a renal graft. *(Kasper, p. 1672)*

3. **(D)** Both granular and erythrocyte casts are present, but the latter indicate bleeding from the glomerulus and are most characteristically seen. Red cells reach the urine probably via capillary wall "gaps" and form casts as they become embedded in concentrated tubular fluid with high protein content. Proteinuria is invariably present but is not as specific. *(Kasper, pp. 250–251)*

4. **(E)** These humps are discrete, electron-dense nodules that persist for about 8 weeks and are highly characteristic of the disease. Light microscopy reveals diffuse proliferation, and immunofluorescence reveals granular immunoglobulin G (IgG) and C3. Most patients will recover spontaneously. *(Kasper, pp. 1680–1681)*

5. **(A)** The urine contains large amounts of potassium, magnesium, and sodium. The large volume is often appropriate for preexisting volume expansion, but careful attention to fluid and electrolytes is important to prevent hypokalemia, hypomagnesemia, hyponatremia or hypernatremia, and volume depletion. *(Kasper, p. 1724)*

6. **(B)** She has analgesic nephropathy, and chronic analgesic ingestion may lead to papillary necrosis and tubulointerstitial inflammation. Complete understanding of the pathogenesis is lacking, and may vary with different analgesics. Depletion of reducing equivalents such as glutathione may also play a role. *(Kasper, p. 1703)*

7. **(D)** Although all drugs should be reassessed at this time, and if appropriate, the dosage adjusted, drugs with known nephrotoxicity, such as ACE inhibitors and NSAIDs, should be stopped. *(Kasper, p. 1644)*

8. **(A)** Diuretics are a common cause for metabolic alkalosis since many patients take these medications for hypertension or CHF. Diarrhea causes a nonanion gap metabolic acidosis, and mineralocorticoid excess leads to metabolic alkalosis, primarily because of renal bicarbonate generation. Other major mechanisms for metabolic alkalosis include extracellular fluid (ECF) volume contraction, potassium depletion, and increased distal salt delivery. Less common causes are Liddle syndrome, bicarbonate loading (posthypercapnic alkalosis), and delayed conversion of administered organic acids. *(Kasper, pp. 265, 267–268)*

9. **(C)** In sickle cell anemia, the kidney is characterized by an inability to concentrate the urine because of functional tubule defects that occur as a result of ischemic injury. Papillary necrosis may also occur in patients with homozygous sickle cell disease or sickle cell trait during a sickle crisis. Some patients can develop glomerular injury (focal and segmental glomerular sclerosis) after many years from the anemia-induced hyperfiltration that occurs. *(Kasper, pp. 1709–1710)*

10. **(E)** The typical renal lesions in gout are urate crystals in the medulla or pyramids, with surrounding mononuclear and giant cell reaction. The degree of renal impairment, however, does not correlate with hyperuricemia, and the decline in renal function correlates with aging, hypertension, renal calculi, or unrelated nephropathy. *(Kasper, p. 1704)*

11. **(E)** The danger of ARF after IVP has led to caution, especially in patients with multiple myeloma. The patient should not be dehydrated if IVP is necessary. The risk is also increased in patients with diabetes mellitus or chronic renal failure. *(Kasper, pp. 1646–1647)*

12. **(A)** Renal amyloidosis can be primary (AL) or secondary amyloidosis (AA). The hallmark finding, nephrotic syndrome, is present in 25% of patients at presentation and probably develops ultimately in over 50%. The apple-green birefringence deposits under polarized light are diagnostic of amyloidosis, and not seen in any other renal disease. *(Kasper, p. 1689)*

13. **(B)** In multiple myeloma, tubular damage by light chains is almost always present. The injury is a direct toxic effect of the light chains or indirectly from the inflammatory response. Infiltration by plasma cells and glomerular injury is rare. Hypercalcemia may produce transient or irreversible renal damage as do amyloid and myeloma cell infiltrates. *(Kasper, p. 658)*

14. **(B)** The urine osmolality in patients with SIADH need not be hypertonic to plasma, but only inappropriately high compared with serum. The major characteristics of SIADH include hyponatremia, volume expansion without edema, natriuresis, hypouricemia, and normal or reduced serum creatinine level, with normal thyroid and adrenal function. *(Kasper, pp. 2102–2103)*

15. **(C)** Although an elevated PSA (>4) has the best positive predictive value, combining it with DRE is probably the most effective screening process. *(Kasper, p. 545)*

16. **(B)** It is very likely that control of hypertension and excellent glucose control will slow the development and course of renal disease in Type II diabetes mellitus. ACE inhibitors seem to decrease proteinuria and slow progression of renal disease. As renal function deteriorates, limiting dietary protein intake can also be beneficial. Calcium channel blockers have no extra effect beyond their antihypertensive effect. *(Kasper, pp. 2164–2165)*

17. **(C)** Persistent proteinuria should always be investigated and, if no cause can be found, yearly follow-up instituted. Mild proteinuria has significant prognostic value in diabetes. Mild proteinuria can be caused by glomerular or tubular causes. Functional causes of proteinuria such as fever, orthostasis, exercise, and heart failure are usually reversible. *(Kasper, p. 250)*

18. **(C)** Renal vein thrombosis is associated with heavy proteinuria and hematuria. Flank pain and pulmonary embolism can also occur. *(Kasper, p. 1707)*

19. **(A)** This patient likely has hypernephroma (renal cell carcinoma). Polycythemia is caused by the production of erythropoietin-like factors. There is no relationship to hypertension. The tumor frequently presents as metastatic disease. *(Kasper, pp. 541–542)*

20. **(C)** Hypokalemia can result in paralytic ileus, rhabdomyolysis, weakness, and cardiac repolarization abnormalities. It is a common complication along with hyponatremia of starting patients on diuretics. *(Kasper, p. 260)*

21. **(E)** Intrathoracic lesions may be benign or malignant, and the latter may secrete a substance similar to vasopressin. Bronchogenic carcinoma is the most common intrathoracic lesion causing SIADH. *(Kasper, pp. 2102–2103)*

22. **(B)** The largest volume of water is reabsorbed in the nephron at the proximal convolution. Maximally concentrated urine depends on ADH, which allows distal convoluted tubes and collecting ducts to become permeable to water. *(Kasper, pp. 1640–1641)*

23. **(A)** The diagnosis is renal cell carcinoma. There is marked hypervascularity of the left kidney. The arteries are irregular and tortuous, following a random distribution. There are small vessels within the renal vein that indicate the blood supply of the neoplastic thrombosis involving the renal vein. The kidney is enlarged and abnormally bulbous in the lower pole. CT scans have dramatically decreased the need for arteriography in evaluating renal lesions. *(Kasper, pp. 541–542)*

24. **(A)** Renal ultrasound is an important test in the assessment of acute and chronic renal failure. The oliguria suggests that obstruction is a possible explanation for the renal failure. Imaging is very sensitive for obstruction, but if bladder obstruction secondary to a large prostate is suspected, bladder catheterization would be the first step. *(Kasper, p. 248)*

25. **(C)** Urinary tract infections (UTIs) are increased in diabetes mellitus as well as in pregnancy, sickle cell disease, polycystic disease, and structural abnormalities of the urinary tract. *(Kasper, p. 2169)*

26. **(A)** Numerous diseases are associated with renal and pulmonary manifestations, including lupus, Goodpasture's syndrome, and Wegener's granulomatosis. Wegener's is typically associated with antineutrophil cytoplasmic antibodies. *(Kasper, p. 2005)*

27. **(E)** In addition to amyloid disease, other conditions associated with nephrotic syndrome are secondary syphilis, malaria, and treatment with gold salts. Minimal change nephrotic syndrome, focal glomerular sclerosis, membranous nephropathy, and membranoproliferative GN are the primary renal diseases that present as nephrotic syndrome. *(Kasper, p. 1689)*

28. **(C)** ATN is a common complication of prolonged hypotension and ischemic injury to the renal tubules. Heme-granular "muddy brown" casts are consistent with ATN. Peritoneal dialysis is preferred with cerebral trauma as well as with severe heart failure because of risk of hemorrhage or hypotension with hemodialysis. In particular, peritoneal dialysis does not require any anticoagulation and is safer if head trauma has occurred. *(Kasper, pp. 1645–1646)*

29. **(E)** Diabetes mellitus, chronic hypertension, multifetal gestation, and prior preeclampsia are associated with preeclampsia. When toxemia occurs in the first trimester, however, hydatidiform mole must be considered. The clinical manifestations of severe preeclampsia include headache, epigastric pain, visual disturbances, and hypertension. HIV is not associated with preeclampsia unless there is a preexisting renal disease. *(Kasper, p. 32)*

30. **(D)** RA is not associated with polycystic kidney disease. It has an autosomal dominant inheritance and about 50% develop renal failure by age 60 years. Cysts are also seen in the liver (more common) and pancreas. Also 5–10% of asymptomatic patients can have cerebral aneurysms. Renal transplantation is utilized in end-stage renal failure (ESRF). The transplanted kidney cannot be affected by the disease. *(Kasper, pp. 1694–1696)*

31. **(A)** Cystinuria is a congenital disorder associated with decreased tubular resorption of cystine, arginine, ornithine, and lysine. Only cystine is insoluble and is the cause of renal calculi. The typical hexagonal crystals are most likely to be seen on an acidic early-morning urine specimen. A positive cyanide-nitroprusside screening test should be confirmed by chromatography. *(Kasper, p. 1714)*

32. **(A)** Increase in neoplasms in renal transplant recipients includes cervical carcinoma, lymphoma, and cutaneous malignancies. Osteoporosis and persistent hyperparathyroidism are other bony complications. Risk of infection is related to degree of immunosuppression. Nevertheless, the most common causes of death are cardiovascular and tend to occur earlier than in the general population. *(Kasper, p. 1673)*

33. **(C)** Amikacin and vancomycin are the other antibiotics that require dose reduction in renal failure. Newer antibiotics are often used instead of aminoglycosides to reduce the risk of renal damage. *(Kasper, p. 795)*

34. **(D)** Red cell casts are not seen in diabetic nephropathy and suggest another acute GN process. Nephrotic range proteinuria, type IV RTA (hyporeninemic hypoaldosteronism), hypertension, and microalbuminuria are all complications of diabetic kidney disease. *(Kasper, pp. 2164–2165)*

35. **(B)** Isolated hematuria is usually of urologic cause (e.g., tumor, trauma, stone) but can also can be glomerular in origin. The finding of red cell casts or dysmorphic red cells (best appreciated by phase microscopy) suggests the source of bleeding is glomerular in origin. *(Kasper, pp. 250–251)*

36. **(A)** Although evidence of volume contraction cannot confirm prerenal ARF, as this can progress into intrinsic renal failure, it suggests that prerenal factors are contributing. In prerenal ARF, specific gravity is usually >1.020 and sodium concentration is <10 mmol/L. The fractional excretion of sodium relates sodium clearance to creatinine clearance and is more sensitive than direct measurements of sodium excretion. In prerenal azotemia, sodium is avidly resorbed from glomerular filtrate, but not in intrinsic renal azotemia because of tubular epithelial cell injury. Creatinine is resorbed less efficiently in both conditions. Therefore, the fractional excretion of sodium is <1% in prerenal azotemia (often much less) whereas it is >1% in intrinsic renal azotemia. Fractional excretion of sodium(%) = UNa/PCr × PNa/UCr × 100. *(Kasper, pp. 247–248)*

37. **(E)** The ratio of BUN/creatinine is usually <10–15 in intrinsic renal disease and >20 in prerenal azotemia. *(Kasper, p. 248)*

38. **(A, D)** Gestational diabetes can result in hyperglycemia and polyuria with subsequent polydipsia (osmotic diuresis). A primary deficiency in vasopressin can result from increased metabolism by a placental enzyme and result in central DI (called gestational DI). It resolves within a few weeks after delivery. *(Kasper, pp. 2098–2099)*

39. **(A)** Head injury can result in central DI from injury to the pituitary or hypothalamus. This can develop abruptly or gradually. *(Kasper, pp. 2098–2099)*

40. **(B)** Nephrogenic DI can be inherited on the X chromosome. Its X-linked recessive nature means that males are predominantly affected. Only women who are homozygous are affected. *(Kasper, pp. 2098–2099)*

41. **(B)** Lithium is one of the drugs that cause nephrogenic DI. Hypercalcemia and hypokalemia can also cause the syndrome. *(Kasper, pp. 2098–2099)*

42. **(A)** She has a nonanion gap metabolic acidosis because of bicarbonate loss from the diarrhea. The anion gap is calculated as the sodium concentration minus the chloride plus the bicarbonate concentration. Other causes of bicarbonate loss with normal anion gap include proximal RTA and primary hyperparathyroidism. *(Kasper, p. 267)*

43. **(C)** Causes of acute respiratory acidosis include narcotic overdose, myasthenia gravis, airway obstruction, and trauma to the chest. Acute increases in Pa_{CO_2} result in carbon dioxide narcosis. This starts with somnolence and confusion and can lead to coma. Asterixis may be present. Cerebral vasodilation may result in frank papilledema. *(Kasper, p. 269)*

44. **(B)** Diuretics are a common cause of metabolic alkalosis. The disorder can occur in volume expanded patients in whom the alkalosis is unresponsive to sodium chloride loading, as in primary hyperaldosteronism or volume contraction with secondary hyperaldosteronism, as in this case. *(Kasper, p. 268)*

45. **(A)** INH can result in impaired oxygen utilization, leading to lactic acidosis (type B), accumulation of lactate, and increased anion gap. *(Kasper, p. 266)*

46. **(D)** Chronic salicylate use can cause respiratory alkalosis. Severe salicylate toxicity results in an anion gap metabolic acidosis such as during an overdose. During acute hyperventilation, plasma bicarbonate concentrations fall by approximately 3 mEq/L when the arterial pressure of CO_2 falls to about 25 mm Hg. Acute respiratory alkalosis can be caused by anxiety, central nervous system (CNS) disorders, drugs, or fever. Chronic respiratory alkalosis occurs in pregnancy and liver disease as well. *(Kasper, p. 270)*

47. **(E)** The diuretic phase of ATN is characterized by large losses of sodium and water. *(Kasper, p. 251)*

48. **(C)** Primary polydipsia can cause greater medullary washout than either nephrogenic or central DI because primary polydipsia tends to cause expansion of the ECF volume. This tends to increase total delivery of sodium chloride and water to the inner medulla. It also increases renal blood flow, and increased flow through the vasa recta reduces ability to trap solutes in the medulla. *(Kasper, p. 2098)*

49. **(A)** Nephrogenic DI can be caused by hypokalemia as well as hypercalcemia. *(Kasper, p. 2099)*

50. **(C)** Both thioridazine and chlorpromazine have been associated with primary polydipsia. *(Kasper, p. 251)*

51. **(A)** There is little or no response to vasopressin after fluid deprivation in complete nephrogenic DI. Incomplete nephrogenic DI will show some response. *(Kasper, p. 2099)*

52. **(D)** High protein tube feeds may cause a solute diuresis because of excessive excretion of urea. Other causes of solute diuresis include glucosuria, mannitol, radiographic contrast media, and chronic renal failure. *(Kasper, p. 251)*

53. **(H)** The combination of ECF volume contraction with high urinary sodium (20 mmol/L) suggests renal fluid loss. This is commonly caused by diuretics or glucosuria. *(Kasper, pp. 254–256)*

54. **(C)** SIADH is associated with many CNS diseases including meningitis, encephalitis, tumors, trauma, stroke, and acute porphyria. It is assumed that antidiuretic hormone (ADH) in these patients is secreted in response to direct stimulation of the hypothalamic osmoreceptors. *(Kasper, pp. 254–256)*

55. **(C)** Amitriptyline is one of the psychoactive drugs that cause SIADH. Others include phenothiazines, serotonin reuptake inhibitors, and monoamine oxidase inhibitors (MAOIs). Antineoplastic drugs such as vincristine and cyclophosphamide also cause SIADH, as does the hypoglycemic agent chlorpropamide. *(Kasper, p. 2099)*

56. **(B)** The combination of ECF volume contraction and low urinary sodium (<10 mmol/L) suggests extrarenal sodium loss. Common causes are vomiting, diarrhea, or excessive sweating. *(Kasper, pp. 254–256)*

57. **(A)** Hyponatremia associated with nephrotic syndrome, cirrhosis, or CHF is characterized by edema. It is believed that the hyponatremia is caused by a decrease in "effective" circulating volume secondary to decreased cardiac output or sequestration of fluid. *(Kasper, pp. 254–256)*

58. **(J)** This man has osmotic diuresis and associated hyponatremia. The clue to the extra osmoles in the serum is the increased serum osmolality in the setting of hyponatremia. This situation is frequently seen in Type II diabetes. *(Kasper, pp. 254–256)*

59. **(B)** In patients who have prior diuretic use, resulting in hypokalemia at the time of evaluation, the bicarbonate tends to be elevated and the urine potassium low (<25 mmol/L). *(Kasper, pp. 258–260)*

60. **(G)** Glucocorticoid and licorice ingestion can result in hypertension with low plasma renin and aldosterone levels. *(Kasper, pp. 258–260)*

61. **(C)** RTA types I and II cause hypokalemia with high potassium excretion (>25 mmol/L) and a low bicarbonate in the absence of hypertension. Diabetic ketoacidosis can also result in this constellation of findings. *(Kasper, pp. 258–260)*

62. **(F)** Primary hyperaldosteronism is characterized by hypertension with high plasma aldosterone and low plasma renin. *(Kasper, pp. 258–260)*

63. **(A)** In lower GI loss (diarrhea), the blood pressure is normal, the urine potassium is low (<25 mmol/L), and the bicarbonate is either normal or low. *(Kasper, pp. 258–260)*

64. **(B)** Metabolic acidosis and respiratory alkalosis are seen in salicylate overdose. *(Kasper, p. 265, 270)*

65. **(B)** Sepsis can cause cardiovascular insufficiency with lactic acidosis, whereas fever and endotoxemia stimulate the respiratory center, causing respiratory alkalosis. *(Kasper, pp. 265, 270)*

66. **(C)** Chronic pulmonary disease often causes respiratory acidosis, whereas the steroids frequently used in therapy may cause a metabolic alkalosis. *(Kasper, pp. 268, 269)*

67. **(E)** Renal failure causes metabolic acidosis, whereas the loss of H+ ions in vomiting causes a metabolic alkalosis. *(Kasper, pp. 265, 268)*

68. **(B)** Hepatic cirrhosis frequently results in chronic respiratory alkalosis. ARF with metabolic acidosis is common in patients with cirrhosis. *(Kasper, pp. 265, 270)*

69. **(A)** This is a case of Henoch-Schönlein purpura (HSP). Diffuse proliferative GN is characterized by acute nephritic syndrome: ARF over days to weeks, with hypertension, edema, oliguria, and active urine sediment. Less severe clinical presentation correlates with a more benign biopsy. The pattern of glomerular involvement is similar to IgA nephropathy. *(Kasper, p. 2010)*

70. **(A, C, D, G)** Systemic lupus erythematosus (SLE) can cause a wide variety of renal disorders, and can progress to ESRF. It is difficult to diagnose the type of glomerular involvement in SLE without a biopsy. *(Kasper, pp. 1961, 1963)*

71. **(G)** Gold is one of the drugs causing nephrotic syndrome secondary to membranous GN. Captopril and penicillamine have also been implicated. Signs and symptoms of nephrotic syndrome (low albumin, edema, hyperlipidemia) are common, and membranous GN is also associated with a thrombotic diathesis. *(Kasper, p. 1687)*

72. **(I)** This presentation is typical for an inherited disorder of basement membranes such as Alport's syndrome. It is inherited as an X-linked dominant disorder. It is relatively benign in women but frequently progresses to ESRF in men. It is often associated with sensorineural hearing loss. *(Kasper, p. 1691)*

73. **(E)** Rifampin can cause minimal change disease as well as more severe renal damage. The described case is typical for minimal change GN with nephrotic syndrome. Drug-induced minimal change GN frequently has an associated interstitial nephritis. INH is not usually associated with renal disease. *(Kasper, p. 1685)*

74. **(G, H, I, K)** Rickets and osteomalacia can be secondary to a variety of renal tubular defects. There are also two variants of vitamin D-dependent rickets caused by renal tubular defects. In one variant, there is impaired production of 1,25(OH)2 D3, and in the other, there is renal resistance to the action of the hormone. *(Kasper, pp. 1698–1701)*

75. **(A)** The autosomal dominant form of polycystic kidney disease is often associated with hepatic cysts, intracranial aneurysms, and colonic diverticula. The occurrence of renal failure is usually in the third decade or later. Complications include infection, obstruction by stone or clot, and gross hematuria. *(Kasper, p. 1696)*

76. **(D, E)** Bartter syndrome and Liddle syndrome can be inherited in an autosomal dominant fashion. Patients with Liddle syndrome have hypertension, whereas those with Bartter syndrome do not. In both syndromes, hypokalemia is prominent. *(Kasper, pp. 1697–1698)*

77. **(J)** Many of the listed disorders can cause nephrolithiasis, but cystinuria is the most common cause of stones in childhood. It is a common inborn error of amino acid transport and is inherited as an autosomal recessive trait. The disorder affects transport of all dibasic amino acids (lysine, arginine, ornithine, and cystine) in the kidney and the gut, but symptoms arise from the overexcretion of cystine because it is the least soluble. *(Kasper, p. 1714)*

78. **(A, C)** In prerenal ARF (i.e., no histologic damage), the urinalysis reveals only hyaline casts. The urinary osmolality is high (>500), and the urine sodium is low (<20). The fractional excretion of sodium is <1. *(Kasper, p. 1644)*

79. **(B, D, F)** In renal failure from ATN, the urinalysis can reveal heme-granular casts, and tubular cells. The fractional excretion of sodium is >1, and the urinary sodium is generally >40. *(Kasper, pp. 1647–1649)*

CHAPTER 9

Muscles and Joints
Questions

DIRECTIONS (Questions 1 through 24): Each of the numbered items in this section is followed by answers. Select the ONE lettered answer that is BEST in each case.

1. A 42-year-old man of Eastern European Jewish descent develops aseptic necrosis of the femoral head. The other femur shows evidence of osteopenia, and there is diffuse osteopenia of the spine with some collapse. Review of medical records reveals he has had splenomegaly and mild pancytopenia for years. A bone marrow examination is abnormal for infiltration with lipid-laden macrophages called "Gaucher cells." Which of the following is the most likely mechanism for this condition?

    (A) insulin deficiency
    (B) abnormal elastic tissue
    (C) excess iron in tissue
    (D) homocystinuria
    (E) abnormal lysosomal enzymes

2. A 26-year-old woman develops a red rash over her cheeks and pain, and swelling in both wrists as well as several small joints in her hands. The rash gets worse on sun exposure and involves her cheeks, nose, ears, and chin. Medical evaluation reveals oral ulceration and 3+ proteinuria. Which of the following is the most specific test for diagnosis of this condition?

    (A) lupus erythematosus (LE) cells
    (B) antinuclear antibody (ANA)
    (C) anti-Sm antibody
    (D) anti-Ro antibody
    (E) antiphospholipid antibody

3. An 18-year-old man has had fever for several weeks. The fever occurs on an almost daily basis and is associated with an evanescent salmon-colored truncal rash. He has diffuse arthralgias, and an extensive investigation for infections and malignancy is negative. Which of the following is diagnostic of this condition?

    (A) high-titer rheumatoid factor (RF)
    (B) positive ANA
    (C) response to steroid therapy
    (D) response to nonsteroidal anti-inflammatory drug (NSAID) therapy
    (E) lymph node biopsy

4. A 32-year-old woman develops symptoms secondary to a dry mouth and dry eyes. She has enlarged salivary glands. Studies for autoantibodies to Ro (SS-A) are positive. A salivary gland biopsy reveals lymphocytic infiltration. Which of the following is the most likely diagnosis?

    (A) sarcoidosis
    (B) primary Sjögren's syndrome
    (C) human immunodeficiency virus (HIV) infection
    (D) lymphoma
    (E) amyloidosis

5. A young woman presents with a facial rash, arthralgias, and fatigue. The rash on her face is erythematous and raised, her heart and lungs are normal, and wrists are swollen and tender on palpation. She has mild thrombocytopenia (90,000/mL). Which of the following is the most appropriate initial autoantibody test?

   (A) anti-double-stranded (ds) deoxyribonucleic acid (DNA)
   (B) anti-Sm
   (C) anti-Ro or La
   (D) ANA
   (E) antiphospholipid antibodies (lupus anticoagulant)

6. A 39-year-old woman complains of developing painful pale fingers on cold exposure for the past 5 years. Recently, she has noticed swollen fingers and tight skin, which limit flexion and extension. She also has new abdominal symptoms that are bothersome. On examination, the skin on the fingers is smooth and shiny with associated edema. The rest of the examination is normal. Which part of the gastrointestinal (GI) tract is most frequently involved in this condition?

   (A) esophagus
   (B) stomach
   (C) duodenum
   (D) ileum
   (E) colon

7. A 57-year-old woman is complaining of frequent headaches and scalp tenderness. She also has arthralgias, fatigue, and discomfort in her jaw when she chews. On examination, her head and neck is normal, but the right temporal artery is tender on palpation. Her erythrocyte sedimentation rate (ESR) is 50 mm/h and hemoglobin 10.5 g/dL. A temporal artery biopsy is obtained for diagnostic confirmation. Which of the following is the most appropriate next step in management?

   (A) intravenous high-dose steroids
   (B) acetylsalicylic acid
   (C) indomethacin

   (D) low-dose (prednisone 40 mg/day) steroids by mouth
   (E) topical steroid creams

8. A 57-year-old man has pain in his left hand and right knee, which is interfering with his work. The pain came on gradually, first in his hand 6 months ago and now in his knee. It is usually fine when he wakes up, but gets worse as the day progresses. There is no history of any trauma, and he is otherwise well. Taking over-the-counter NSAIDs usually relieves the pain. On examination, there is bony soft tissue swelling of his second and third distal interphalangeal (DIP) joints in the left hand and crepitus over the right knee with flexion. There is no erythema or joint effusion. Which of the following is the initial change noticed in the pathogenesis of osteoarthritis?

   (A) abnormal chondrocyte function
   (B) a defect in the extracellular matrix of cartilage
   (C) inflammatory changes in subchondral bone
   (D) ligament inflammation
   (E) synovial inflammation

9. A 22-year-old woman develops color change in her fingers with cold exposure. The fingers turn white, then blue, and finally red. Which of the following statements regarding this condition is incorrect?

   (A) may lead to gangrene of the fingers
   (B) may precede the onset of scleroderma
   (C) symptoms can be brought on by vibration or stress
   (D) pallor (white color) associated with coldness and numbness while rubor (red color) associated with pain and tingling
   (E) affects the sexes equally

10. A 63-year-old man develops pain and swelling in his knee. It appears warm, red, and swollen with decreased range of movement. A diagnostic aspiration is performed. Which of the

following will most likely distinguish pseudo-gout from gout?

(A) positive birefringent crystals

(B) acute onset

(C) involvement of single joints

(D) involvement of large joints

(E) association with diabetes

11. A 54-year-old woman with rheumatoid arthritis (RA) presents with fatigue and low white count (white blood cells [WBC] 2500/mL) on routine blood work. She has no active joint symptoms and her RA is controlled on low-dose methotrexate and NSAIDs. On examination, she has chronic joint deformities of her hands and a palpable spleen, which is a new finding. Which of the following is the most likely diagnosis for her low white count?

(A) methotrexate therapy

(B) rheumatoid nodules disrupting bone marrow architecture

(C) Felty's syndrome

(D) normal variation

(E) myelofibrosis

12. A 74-year-old woman has pain in her left hand and right knee, which started months ago, and is now interfering with her activities. The pain gets worse as the day progresses. There is no history of any trauma, and she is otherwise well. Taking over-the-counter acetaminophen usually relieves the pain. On examination, there is bony soft tissue swelling of her second and third DIP joints in the left hand and crepitus over the right knee with flexion. There is no erythema or joint effusion. Which of the following is the most likely explanation for the joint pain of osteoarthritis?

(A) synovial inflammation is not the cause

(B) ligament inflammation is a common cause

(C) clinically visible (via plain x-ray) fractures are a common cause of pain

(D) osteophytes can cause pain

(E) muscles are not involved

13. A 10-year-old child has recurrent signs and symptoms of palpable purpura on the buttocks, arthralgias, colicky abdominal pain, diarrhea, and microscopic hematuria. Which of the following is the most likely diagnosis?

(A) influenza

(B) immune complex vasculitis

(C) juvenile RA

(D) systemic lupus erythematosus (SLE)

(E) Wegener's granulomatosis

14. A 75-year-old woman has abrupt onset of soreness, and severe stiffness of the shoulders and upper thighs with low grade fever. Physical examination is entirely normal, but ESR is over 100 mm/h. Which of the following is the most likely diagnosis?

(A) dermatomyositis (DM)

(B) osteoarthritis

(C) polymyalgia rheumatica (PMR)

(D) midline granuloma

(E) sarcoidosis

15. A 63-year-old man presents with weakness and hemoptysis, but no fever, cough, or sputum. He has a 60-pack-per-year history of smoking. The chest x-ray (CXR) reveals a lung mass with mediastinal widening. On examination, there is a blue purple discoloration of the upper eyelids and erythema on his knuckles. He has proximal muscle weakness rated 4+/5, normal reflexes, and sensation. Which of the following is the most likely diagnosis for his muscle weakness?

(A) SLE

(B) scleroderma

(C) dermatomyositis (DM)

(D) polyarteritis

(E) Weber-Christian disease

16. A 27-year-old man has a history of low back pain and stiffness. After several months of mild symptoms, he notes more severe stiffness at night and hip pain. On physical examination, there is paravertebral muscle tenderness and limited flexion of the lumbar spine. X-ray of the lumbar spine shows sacroiliitis. In addition to recommending physiotherapy and exercise, which of the following is the most appropriate next step in management?

(A) NSAID therapy
(B) phenylbutazone
(C) azathioprine
(D) acetaminophen
(E) prednisone

17. A 24-year-old woman notices pain in her left arm, made worse with use. She also has fatigue, fever, night sweats, and arthralgias. On examination, there are no palpable lymph nodes, and the joints and muscle strength are normal. The left radial pulse is absent, and there is a bruit over the left subclavian and common carotid arteries. Preliminary laboratory investigations reveal an elevated ESR and mild anemia. Which of the following vascular findings is most likely to be found in her?

(A) high pressure in the legs and low pressure in the arms
(B) low pressure in the legs and high pressure in the arms
(C) high-pitched diastolic murmur
(D) a relentless course to death
(E) hypotension

18. Figure 9–1 shows an x-ray of a 40-year-old Caucasian man with symptoms of sinusitis and an incidental finding in the skull. Which of the following is the most likely diagnosis?

(A) normal variant
(B) osteomyelitis
(C) Paget's disease
(D) hemangioma
(E) metastatic disease

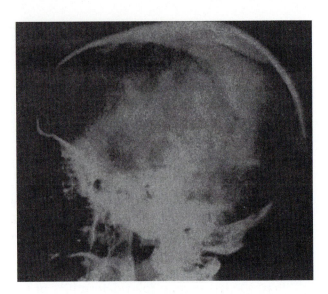

Figure 9–1.

19. A 34-year-old woman develops a red rash over her cheeks, frequent oral ulcers, and pain and swelling in both wrists as well as in several small joints in her hands. Medical evaluation reveals a positive ANA, and 3+ proteinuria. Which of the following organ involvement will cause the most symptoms during the course of this disease?

(A) renal pathology
(B) cardiopulmonary pathology
(C) musculoskeletal pathology
(D) thrombotic events
(E) skin changes

20. A 29-year-old woman develops painful swelling of both hands. She is also very stiff in the morning. Physical examination reveals involvement of the proximal interphalangeal joints and metacarpophalangeal (MCP) joints. Her RF is positive and ANA is negative. Which of the following medications is most likely to improve her joint pain symptoms?

(A) D-penicillamine
(B) an antimalarial
(C) methotrexate
(D) NSAID or aspirin
(E) gold

21. A 55-year-old woman has had several weeks of fever, abdominal pain, weight loss, and lack of energy. Three days prior to the assessment, she developed a left foot drop. Her blood pressure is 160/90 mm Hg, pulse 80/min, and physical examination confirms left peroneal nerve damage and a bilateral sensory peripheral neuropathy in both legs. There are no skin rashes. Laboratory evaluation reveals ESR of 105 mm/h, WBC of 14,000/mL, and negative serologic tests for antineutrophil cytoplasmic antibody (ANCA) and ANA. The eosinophil count is normal, and urinalysis is negative for casts, protein, and red cells. Which of the following is the most likely mechanism for renal injury in this condition?

(A) nephrotic syndrome

(B) diffuse glomerulonephritis

(C) granuloma formation

(D) necrotizing vasculitis of vessels

(E) exclusively small vessel involvement

22. A 20-year-old man with Marfan syndrome is having back pain. On examination, there is a curvature of his thoracic spine to the left. Which of the following is the most appropriate next step in management?

(A) a vigorous exercise program

(B) bisphosphate therapy

(C) mechanical back bracing

(D) a prophylactic surgical procedure

(E) appropriate footwear

23. A 27-year-old man has a history of low back pain and stiffness. Recently, he has noticed more severe stiffness at night and hip pain. The symptoms improve in the morning after doing some "stretching" exercises. On physical examination, there is paravertebral muscle and sacroiliac joint tenderness with limited flexion of the lumbar spine. A 2/6 diastolic murmur is also heard at the left sternal border radiating to the apex. Which of the following is the most likely diagnosis for the diastolic murmur?

(A) mitral stenosis

(B) tricuspid stenosis

(C) aortic insufficiency

(D) pulmonic insufficiency

(E) tetralogy of Fallot

24. A 35-year-old woman notices a red rash over her cheeks, and pain and swelling in both knees as well as several small joints in her hands. She has a history of hypertension and 2 months ago was started on a new medication to control her blood pressure. Her ANA and antihistone antibodies are positive. Which of the following medications is most likely to cause her condition?

(A) hydralazine

(B) hydrochlorothiazide

(C) ramipril

(D) nifedipine

(E) methyldopa

DIRECTIONS (Questions 25 and 26): Each set of matching questions in this section consists of a list of lettered options followed by several numbered items. For each numbered item, select the appropriate lettered option(s). Each lettered option may be selected once, more than once, or not at all. EACH ITEM WILL STATE THE NUMBER OF OPTIONS TO SELECT. CHOOSE EXACTLY THIS NUMBER.

Questions 25 and 26

(A) normal synovial fluid

(B) noninflammatory effusion

(C) inflammatory effusion

(D) septic arthritis

(E) hemorrhagic effusion

For each patient with monoarthritis, select the most likely interpretation of the synovial fluid analysis.

25. A 57-year-old man presents with a swollen, painful left knee. He fell on the knee 3 days ago while hurrying up the stairs. On examination, there is a swollen knee with palpable effusion and decreased range of motion. A diagnostic tap is preformed and 5 cc of transparent fluid is removed. The WBC count is 1000/mL (20% polymorphonuclear neutrophils [PMNs]), glucose is equal to plasma, viscosity is high, and lactate dehydrogenase (LDH) is low. (SELECT ONE)

26. A 77-year-old woman presents with a swollen, painful right knee. She fell on the knee 3 days ago while hurrying up the stairs. On examination, there is a swollen knee with palpable effusion and decreased range of motion. A diagnostic tap is preformed and 5 cc of opaque fluid is removed. The WBC count is 20,000/mL (50% PMNs), glucose is lower than plasma, viscosity is low, and the LDH is high. (SELECT ONE)

DIRECTIONS (Questions 27 through 64): Each of the numbered items in this section is followed by answers. Select the ONE lettered answer that is BEST in each case.

27. A 27-year-old woman presents with a red rash over her cheeks, and pain and swelling in both knees as well as several small joints in her hands. She notes that the rash is worse with sun exposure. Medical evaluation reveals oral ulceration, positive ANA, and 3+ proteinuria. Which of the following is the most likely mechanism for the renal damage in this condition?

    (A) vasculitis
    (B) microemboli
    (C) antibasement membrane antibodies
    (D) deposition of circulating immune complexes
    (E) primary tubular atrophy

28. A 50-year-old man develops fatigue and painful swelling of both hands. He is also very stiff in the morning and requires longer time to get ready for work. Physical examination reveals erythema, swelling, and tenderness on palpation of the proximal interphalangeal joints and MCP joints. Plain x-rays of the hand are taken. Which of the following x-ray findings is characteristic of this condition?

    (A) loss of articular cartilage and bone erosion
    (B) normal
    (C) osteolytic changes
    (D) osteosclerotic changes
    (E) osteolytic and osteosclerotic changes together

29. A 23-year-old man notices new low back pain, stiffness, and left eye discomfort. Sunlight also bothers his eyes. The back pain is worse at night and described as a dull ache in the back and buttock area. On physical examination, there is paravertebral muscle, iliac crest, and ischial tuberosity tenderness with limited flexion of the lumbar spine. His eye is inflamed and the pupil is constricted. Pelvic x-rays show sacroiliitis. Which of the following is the most likely diagnosis for his eye symptoms (it is the most common extra-articular manifestation of this condition)?

    (A) glaucoma
    (B) acute anterior uveitis
    (C) keratitis
    (D) conjunctivitis
    (E) episcleritis

30. A 24-year-old man presents with shortness of breath on exertion. He is tall and thin (Fig. 9–2), visual acuity is poor with his glasses off, the jugular venous pressure (JVP) is 4 cm, first heart sound is normal, second sound is soft, a 3/6 early diastolic murmur is heard at the right second intercostal space radiating to the apex. The pulses are bounding, lungs are clear, and his arms are quite long in comparison to his total length. Which of the following is the most likely diagnosis for his cardiac murmur?

    (A) aortic root dilatation and aortic stenosis
    (B) left ventricular dilatation and mitral valve prolapse
    (C) aortic root dilatation and aortic regurgitation
    (D) aortic dissection
    (E) mitral stenosis

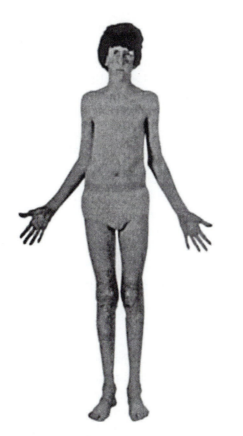

Figure 9–2.

31. A 40-year-old woman complains of being very "stiff" in the morning, in addition to having sore hands and wrists. The symptoms have come on very gradually and she can not recall exactly when they started. Her only other complaint is that of being fatigued. Physical examination reveals involvement of the proximal interphalangeal joints, MCP joints, and wrist joints in a symmetrical fashion. She also has nodules over both elbows. Which of the following is predictive of developing extra-articular features of her condition?

(A) her knees are involved early
(B) there is a poor articular response to disease-suppressing medication
(C) humoral immunity is suppressed
(D) cellular immunity is suppressed
(E) she develops an antibody to her own immunoglobulin (RF)

32. A 24-year-old is referred for assessment of a low white cell count. She has no past medical history and is not on any medications. Her only symptoms are of joint discomfort in her hands, and occasional sharp chest pains that change with breathing. On examination, there is inflammation of some MCP and DIP joints in both hands, and the rest of the examination is normal. Her WBC is 3500/mL and the lymphocytes are low (15%) and PMNs are normal. Which of the following is the most likely diagnosis?

(A) periarteritis nodosa
(B) SLE
(C) scleroderma
(D) DM
(E) osteoarthritis

33. A 69-year-old man develops clubbing of his fingers. Which of the following is most likely associated with this condition?

(A) RF
(B) aortic stenosis
(C) periosteal inflammation
(D) crystal-induced arthritis
(E) diffuse osteoarthritis

34. A 30-year-old woman develops painful swelling of her hands, pleuritic chest pain, and shortness of breath on exertion. She is also very stiff in the morning. Physical examination reveals involvement of the proximal interphalangeal joints and MCP joints. Air entry is decreased to the right lower lobe and the area is dull on percussion. Her RF is elevated and a CXR reveals a pleural effusion. A diagnostic tap is performed, and 500 cc of a straw-colored fluid is removed. Which of the following biochemical patterns is consistent with a pleural effusion due to her primary condition?

(A) exudate protein and LDH ratios with low glucose
(B) exudate protein and LDH ratios with high glucose
(C) transudate protein and LDH ratios with high glucose
(D) transudate protein and LDH ratios with low glucose
(E) normal pleural fluid

35. A 67-year-old man has a long history of symmetrical small joint arthritis with deformities. He now develops shortness of breath on exertion with a dry cough, but no sputum or chest discomfort. His heart sounds have a loud P_2, and the lungs have fine bibasilar crackles. Which of the following is the most likely diagnosis of the pulmonary condition associated with his arthritis?

(A) pleuritis
(B) cavitating lesions
(C) intrapulmonary nodules
(D) interstitial fibrosis
(E) diffuse pneumonitis

36. A 71-year-old woman comes to the office with a history of headaches, fatigue, and weight loss for 3 months. The headaches are new for her, and usually not very severe. Her jaw also hurts when she is chewing food. Two days prior, she had briefly lost partial vision in her left eye. There were no other neurologic symptoms at the time. On examination, her neck is supple to flexion, fundi and neurologic examinations are normal. She is started on prednisone 60 mg/day and a biopsy is performed to confirm the diagnosis. Which of the following is the most likely change seen on the biopsy to confirm the diagnosis?

(A) immune complex deposition
(B) arteritis with giant cells
(C) lymphocytic infiltration
(D) type II muscle fiber atrophy
(E) polyphasic potentials on electromyography (EMG)

37. A 30-year-old woman develops a rash over her cheeks, nose, and ears. She also has pain and swelling in her wrists as well as several small joints in her hands. Medical evaluation reveals oral ulceration and 3+ proteinuria. Her ANA is positive. Which of the following is the most likely cardiac manifestation of her disease?

(A) pericarditis
(B) myocarditis
(C) aortic regurgitation
(D) nonbacterial endocarditis
(E) myocardial vasculitis with infarction

38. A 32-year-old woman has a long history of intermittent bloody diarrhea and crampy abdominal pain. Recently, her bowel symptoms have increased and she is having 4–6 bowel movements a day with mucus and blood in the stool. She now has a low-grade fever, loss of appetite, and new musculoskeletal symptoms. Which of the following is the best description of this patient's accompanying arthritis?

(A) asymmetric migratory polyarthritis involving the large joints of the arms and legs
(B) not usually associated with disease flares
(C) a progressive, crippling course
(D) symmetrical small joint involvement
(E) seropositive

39. A 42-year-old woman has had several weeks of fever, abdominal pain, weight loss, and lack of energy. Three days prior to assessment, she developed a left foot drop and rash on her legs. Her blood pressure is 160/90 mm Hg, pulse 80/min, and physical examination confirms left peroneal nerve damage and a bilateral sensory peripheral neuropathy in both legs. The rash looks like livedo reticularis. Laboratory evaluation reveals ESR of 105 mm/h, WBC of 14,000/mL, and negative serologic tests for ANCA and ANA. Eosinophil count is normal, and urinalysis is negative for casts, protein, and red cells. Biopsy of the skin rash shows inflammation of the small blood vessels. Which of the following is the most appropriate next step in management?

(A) plasmapheresis
(B) steroid therapy alone
(C) combination therapy with steroids and cyclophosphamide
(D) cyclophosphamide therapy alone
(E) combination therapy with steroids and methotrexate

40. A 67-year-old man complains of frequent headaches that are new for him. They are usually not very severe, and relieved with acetaminophen. He also has some back, shoulder, and hip discomfort, which is worse in the

morning as well he feels quite fatigued and does not have his usual energy level. On examination, his neck is supple to flexion, fundi and thyroid examination are normal. Range of motion in the shoulders and hips is reduced because of discomfort but there is no active inflammation. There are no focal deficits on screening neurologic examination. Which of the following is the most appropriate initial diagnostic test?

(A) immunoelectrophoresis
(B) c-ANCA levels
(C) ESR
(D) creatine phosphokinase (CPK)
(E) hemoglobin and red cell indices

41. A 45-year-old man has had several weeks of fever, abdominal pain, weight loss, and lack of energy. Three days prior to assessment, he developed a left foot drop. His blood pressure is 160/90 mm Hg, pulse 80/min, and physical examination confirms left peroneal nerve damage and a bilateral sensory peripheral neuropathy in both legs. There are no skin rashes. Laboratory evaluation reveals ESR of 105 mm/h, WBC of 14,000/mL, and negative serologic tests for ANCA and ANA. Eosinophil count is normal. Which of the following chronic viral infections is sometimes associated with this condition?

(A) high cytomegalovirus (CMV) titers
(B) herpesvirus material in circulating immune complexes
(C) hepatitis B material in circulating immune complexes
(D) epidemiologic relationship to Coxsackie B virus
(E) triggering of symptoms following viral gastroenteritis secondary to rotavirus infection

42. A 19-year-old man has a chronic papulosquamous skin disorder involving his knees and elbows. He now has dull low back pain and morning stiffness that lasts a few hours. On examination, forward flexion at the lumbar spine is reduced but neck movements are normal. There is stress tenderness of both sacroiliac joints. Which of the following is the most likely diagnosis?

(A) RA
(B) ankylosing spondylitis (AS)
(C) psoriatic arthritis
(D) reactive arthritis
(E) PMR

43. A 63-year-old man is worried that he has RA because his RF serology is positive in a low titer. He has pain in his left hand and right knee, which usually bother him in the evening. He has not noticed any inflammation or swelling and there is no history of morning stiffness. On examination, there are no active joints. Which of the following statements regarding the presence of RF is correct?

(A) is positive in 10–20% of people over age 65
(B) is positive in almost 100% of "classical" RA
(C) is seen only in RA
(D) is always abnormal
(E) is frequently present in osteoarthritis

44. A 45-year-old man has had intermittent swelling and pain in the superior part of his auricles for several years. Mild arthritis usually accompanies these episodes. Last year he also had redness, pain, and swelling over the bridge of his nose. Which of the following is the most likely diagnosis?

(A) psoriatic arthritis
(B) Behçet's syndrome
(C) Wegener's granulomatosis
(D) relapsing polychondritis
(E) rheumatoid arthritis

45. Which of the following features is a characteristic of Ehlers-Danlos syndrome?

(A) thickening of the skin
(B) mental retardation
(C) an increased incidence of skin carcinoma
(D) thrombocytopenia
(E) habitual dislocation of joints

46. A 72-year-old man injures his right knee in a car accident, and now it is swollen and extremely painful to bend the knee. X-rays of the knee rule out a fracture, and joint fluid aspiration reveals an opaque-colored fluid containing rhomboid crystals with weak-positive birefringence. Which of the following is the most appropriate next step in management?

    (A) oral prednisone
    (B) intravenous antibiotics
    (C) oral NSAIDs
    (D) acetaminophen
    (E) allopurinol

47. A 64-year-old man is having difficulty getting out of a chair. He has lost 15 lb and feels tired all the time. On examination, there is a blue purple rash on his eyelids and knuckles, and muscle strength in his proximal muscles is rated 4 out of 5. His creatinine kinase (CK) level is elevated and he is started on prednisone. Which of the following is the most important in monitoring response to therapy?

    (A) testing of muscle strength
    (B) sedimentation rates
    (C) urine transaminase enzymes
    (D) EMG
    (E) alkaline phosphatase

48. A 25-year-old woman with SLE notices increasing fatigue and shortness of breath on exertion. Her usual SLE symptoms of joint discomfort, chest pain, and fevers are not present. On examination, there are no active joints, but she is jaundiced. Laboratory studies show hemoglobin 9 g/dL, WBC 5000/mL, platelets 150,000/mL, reticulocyte count 4%, direct antiglobulin test: positive, total bilirubin 4 g/dL, direct 0.5 mg/dL, aspartate amino transferase (AST) 20 U/L, alanine amino transferase (ALT) 15 U/L, LDH 300 U/L. Which of the following is the most likely diagnosis?

    (A) autoimmune hepatitis
    (B) hemolytic anemia
    (C) viral hepatitis
    (D) acute blood loss
    (E) Gilbert syndrome

49. A 38-year-old man has had 3 months of intermittent joint pain and swelling in both knees. The symptoms last weeks at a time and then improve spontaneously. His only past medical history is that of an oval-shaped, red pruritic skin lesion in his right axilla 4 months earlier, which appeared shortly after a camping trip. His immunoglobulin G (IgG) serology for *Borrelia burgdorferi* is positive. Which of the following is the most appropriate next step in management?

    (A) high-dose glucocorticoids
    (B) low-dose glucocorticoids
    (C) high-dose NSAID therapy
    (D) long-term penicillin
    (E) long-term doxycycline

50. A 26-year-old man has had a year of intermittent joint pain and swelling in both knees. The symptoms last weeks at a time and then improve. He has always been healthy. His only past medical history is that of a round, pruritic skin lesion in his left groin 2 years earlier, which appeared shortly after a camping trip. Which of the following is the most appropriate initial diagnostic test?

    (A) positive serologic studies only
    (B) synovial fluid analysis
    (C) skin biopsy
    (D) positive serology and clinical symptoms
    (E) synovial biopsy

51. Which of the following statements concerning the articular manifestations of RA is correct?

    (A) wrists are rarely involved
    (B) involvement of hands is characteristically asymmetric
    (C) fever up to 104°F is common with joint involvement
    (D) ulnar deviation at the wrist is common
    (E) absence of morning stiffness makes RA an unlikely cause of articular symptoms

52. A 22-year-old man has symptoms of low back pain and stiffness. After several months of mild symptoms, he notes more severe stiffness at night and hip pain. On physical examination, there is paravertebral muscle tenderness and

limited flexion of the lumbar spine. Figure 9–3 shows an x-ray of the lumbar spine. Which of the following is the most likely diagnosis?

(A) Reiter syndrome

(B) Marfan syndrome

(C) ankylosing spondylitis (AS)

(D) RA

(E) pseudogout

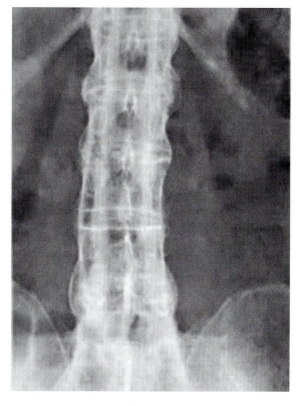

Figure 9–3.

53. A 64-year-old woman presents with fatigue, and musculoskeletal symptoms. She reports of no headache, jaw discomfort, or visual disturbance. Her physical examination is normal, and laboratory testing reveals an elevated ESR of 75 mm/h. She is started on prednisone 10 mg/day and notices a dramatic improvement in her symptoms after 1 week. Which of the following are the most typical symptoms of this disorder?

(A) heliotrope rash

(B) proximal muscle weakness

(C) painful peripheral neuropathies

(D) stiffness and pain of proximal muscles

(E) hematuria

54. A 69-year-old man comes to the office complaining of fatigue, and weight loss for 3 months. He also reports having frequent headaches, which are new for him. There are no other constitutional symptoms of fever, chills or night sweats. He does have chronic lower back pain but lately he has noticed pain in his shoulder, and hip as well. The muscle and joint symptoms are worse in the morning, and the stiffness lasts for 1 hour. His jaw also hurts when he is chewing food. Head and neck examination is normal, there is no lymphadenopathy and fundoscopy is normal. Range of motion in the shoulders and hips is reduced because of discomfort but there is no active inflammation. Which of the following is the most feared complication in patients with this condition?

(A) blindness

(B) cortical stroke

(C) limb claudication

(D) renal infarction

(E) aortic aneurysm

55. A 67-year-old woman has pain in her left hand and right knee, which is interfering with her activities. The pain came on gradually, first in her hand 6 months ago and now in her knee. It is usually fine when she wakes up, but gets worse as the day progresses. There is no history of any trauma, and she is otherwise well. Taking over-the-counter NSAIDs usually relieves the pain. On examination, there is bony soft tissue swelling of his second and third DIP joints in the left hand and crepitus over the right knee with flexion. There is no erythema or joint effusion. Which of the following best describes this disease condition?

(A) disease of the synovial membrane

(B) disease of the articular cartilage

(C) disease of the entire joint

(D) disease of the subchondral bone

(E) disease of the ligaments

56. A very tall, slender 16-year-old boy is referred for evaluation. Physical examination reveals long fingers, pectus excavatum, and a high arched palate. Which of the following is most likely to be seen on his CXR?

(A) dextrocardia

(B) aortic dilatation

(C) pneumothorax

(D) apical interstitial fibrosis

(E) rib notching

57. A 29-year-old woman develops symptoms of painful swelling, and stiffness of both hands. Physical examination reveals involvement of the proximal interphalangeal joints and MCP joints. A clinical diagnosis of rheumatoid arthritis is made. Which of the following is the most likely cause of the inflammation in her joints?

(A) activated T cells

(B) antineutrophil antibodies

(C) microvascular injury

(D) interleukin-4 (IL-4)

(E) precipitated RF

58. A 25-year-old woman develops painful swelling of both hands and wrists. She is also very stiff in the morning. Physical examination reveals erythema, swelling and joint line tenderness of the proximal interphalangeal, MCP, and wrists joints. Her RF is positive, ANA is negative, and x-rays of the hands show early erosive joint changes. Which of the following medications is most likely to prevent progression of disease?

(A) D-penicillamine

(B) antimalarial

(C) methotrexate

(D) NSAID or aspirin

(E) gold

59. A 22-year-old woman develops a red rash over her cheeks, and pain and swelling in both knees as well as several small joints in her hands. Medical evaluation reveals oral ulceration and 3+ proteinuria. Which of the following is the most sensitive test for the diagnosis of this condition?

(A) LE cells

(B) ANAs

(C) anti-Sm

(D) anti-Ro

(E) antiphospholipid

60. A 39-year-old man has had several weeks of fever, abdominal pain, weight loss, and lack of energy. Three days prior to assessment, he developed a left foot drop. Physical examination confirms left peroneal nerve damage and a bilateral sensory peripheral neuropathy in both legs. Laboratory evaluation reveals ESR of 105 mm/h, WBC of 14,000/mL, and a negative serologic test for ANCA. The eosinophil count is normal. Which of the following is a reasonable method of establishing a diagnosis?

(A) testicular biopsy

(B) skin biopsy

(C) spiral computerized tomography (CT) of chest

(D) further serologic testing

(E) abdominal angiography

61. A 32-year-old woman complains of having intermittent arthralgias of multiple joints and occasional swelling in both knees. The symptoms started about 6 months ago and usually last for weeks at a time and then improve spontaneously. She reports no morning stiffness or any constitutional symptoms. About 1 year ago, she recalls having a round, red, pruritic skin lesion along her belt line, which resolved on its own. Serologic tests confirm a clinical diagnosis of Lyme disease. Which of the following mechanisms is the most likely cause of this syndrome?

(A) autoimmune

(B) viral infection

(C) spirochetal infection

(D) circulating immune complexes

(E) metabolic (abnormal crystal metabolism)

62. A 74-year-old man presents with a history of increasing frequency of headaches, fatigue, and weight loss for 3 months. He has had migraine headaches in the past, but these are different from them. He is also experiencing back, shoulder, and hip discomfort, which is worse in the morning. His head and neck examination is normal. Range of motion in the shoulders and hips is reduced because of discomfort but there is no active inflammation. Which of the following signs or symptoms is most helpful in the diagnosis?

(A) throat pain on swallowing

(B) pain in the jaw when chewing

(C) malaise

(D) fatigue

(E) sweating

63. A 60-year-old man has pain in his left hand and right knee, which is interfering with his work. The pain came on gradually, first in his hand 6 months ago and now in his knee. It is usually fine when he wakes up, but gets worse as the day progresses. There is no history of any trauma, and he is otherwise well. Taking over-the-counter NSAIDs usually relieves the pain. On examination, there is bony soft tissue swelling of his second and third DIP joints in the left hand and crepitus over the right knee with flexion. There is no erythema or joint effusion. Which of the following characteristics is a risk factor for this condition?

(A) being Chinese

(B) being African

(C) being male

(D) being overweight

(E) hyperthyroidism

64. Which of the following is the most common location for osteoarthritis?

(A) hip

(B) base of thumb

(C) knee

(D) spine

(E) DIP joints of hand

DIRECTIONS (Questions 65 through 74): Each set of matching questions in this section consists of a list of lettered options followed by several numbered items. For each numbered item, select the

appropriate lettered option(s). Each lettered option may be selected once, more than once, or not at all. **EACH ITEM WILL STATE THE NUMBER OF OPTIONS TO SELECT. CHOOSE EXACTLY THIS NUMBER.**

Questions 65 through 69

(A) associated with hemolysis

(B) seen in mixed connective tissue disease

(C) most sensitive test for SLE

(D) most sensitive test for drug-induced lupus

(E) causes false-positive VDRL (Venereal Disease Research Laboratory)

(F) relatively disease specific

For each autoantibody, select the most likely clinical manifestation.

65. ANA (SELECT ONE)

66. Anti-dsDNA (SELECT ONE)

67. Antiphospholipid (SELECT ONE)

68. Antihistone (SELECT ONE)

69. Anti-ribosomal nuclear protein (RNP) (SELECT ONE)

Questions 70 through 74

(A) Felty's syndrome

(B) rheumatoid vasculitis

(C) episcleritis

(D) Sjögren's syndrome

(E) rheumatoid nodules

(F) rheumatoid pleural involvement

(G) Caplan's syndrome

(H) pericardial disease

For each extra-articular manifestation of RA, select the most likely diagnosis.

70. May present as small brown spots in the nail folds (SELECT ONE)

71. Most common form of eye involvement (SELECT ONE)

72. Associated with increased frequency of infections (SELECT ONE)

73. Found in association with occupational lung disease (SELECT ONE)

74. Commonly involves Achillis tendon (SELECT ONE)

DIRECTIONS (Questions 75 through 83): Each of the numbered items in this section is followed by answers. Select the ONE lettered answer that is BEST in each case.

75. A 67-year-old woman develops symptoms of cough and sputum production after an upper respiratory tract infection. A CXR does not show any signs of pneumonia but the report mentions a "pseudofracture" sign (Looser zones) seen in the left scapula compatible with osteomalacia. She has no pain in the scapula. Which of the following best differentiates rickets and osteomalacia?

(A) the mineralization defect is less severe in osteomalacia

(B) osteomalacia is only produced by vitamin D deficiency, unlike rickets

(C) the skeleton is at a different stage when affected

(D) parathyroid hormone levels are only routinely elevated in rickets

(E) rickets always is characterized by hypocalcemia

76. A 72-year-old man is recently found to have hypocalcemia and osteomalacia is suspected based on the decrease in the cortical bone thickness and osteopenia is seen on x-rays. Which of the following is the most likely mechanism of the resistance to the effects of vitamin D?

(A) excess parathyroid hormone secretion

(B) insufficient parathyroid hormone secretion

(C) defective receptors for 25(OH) vitamin D

(D) defective receptors for 1,25(OH)2 vitamin D

(E) mineralocorticoid excess

77. A 66-year-old woman complains of pain in her left hip when walking. Three days ago, she tripped and fell in her apartment. On examination, there is decreased range of motion in the hip, no leg length discrepancy. X-rays of the hip reveal osteopenia. Which of the following is the primary defect in vitamin D metabolism that causes osteopenia associated with aging?

(A) impaired intestinal absorption of vitamin D

(B) impaired liver hydroxylation of vitamin D

(C) impaired renal hydroxylation of 1(OH) vitamin D

(D) low parathyroid hormone levels

(E) low phosphate levels

78. Which of the following clinical findings is characteristic of both osteomalacia and rickets?

(A) frontal bossing in the skull

(B) muscle weakness

(C) prominent costochondral junctions

(D) defects in tooth enamel

(E) knock-knees

79. An 84-year-old man, previously well except for chronic osteoarthritis, develops a hot, red, painful knee. Physical examination reveals an exquisitely tender, swollen knee. Which of the following is the most likely finding on synovial fluid analysis?

(A) staphylococcal infection

(B) gonococcal infection

(C) calcium hydroxyapatite crystals

(D) calcium pyrophosphate crystal deposition

(E) calcium oxalate

80. A 74-year-old man has recurrent attacks of pain, swelling, and redness in his left knee. He has background osteoarthritis of both knees, which require him to take acetaminophen on a regular basis. Joint fluid was removed during one acute episode of knee pain, and synovial fluid analysis revealed calcium pyrophosphate deposition disease crystals (CPPD). Which of the following methods is the most effective prophylaxis for this condition?

(A) allopurinol

(B) continuous NSAIDs

(C) low-dose glucocorticoids

(D) continuous antibiotic therapy

(E) colchicine

81. A 79-year-old woman on chronic hemodialysis presents with severe pain in her left knee. On examination, the knee is warm, swollen, and painful to move. Diagnostic joint aspiration is performed. Which of the following is the most likely finding in her joint fluid?

(A) uric acid crystals

(B) calcium pyrophosphate crystals (CPPD)

(C) calcium hydroxyapatite crystals

(D) calcium oxalate crystals

(E) crystallized urea

82. An 81-year-old woman develops progressive pain and immobility of her right shoulder. A series of x-rays over 8 months reveals destruction of the shoulder joint and an aspiration reveals blood in the effusion. Her only other articular manifestations are mild episodes of pain in her knees. Which of the following is the most likely diagnosis?

(A) a chronic bacterial infection

(B) uric acid deposition

(C) CPPD disease

(D) calcium oxalate deposition

(E) calcium hydroxyapatite deposition

83. A 59-year-old woman with RA, under reasonable control with methotrexate, develops a hot, swollen, red knee. Joint aspiration removes 10 cc of an opaque yellow-colored fluid with a white count of 100,000/μL, predominantly neutrophils. The joint fluid protein is high and glucose is much lower than blood. Which of the following is the most likely diagnosis?

(A) uric acid deposition

(B) CPPD deposition

(C) septic arthritis

(D) reactivation of RA

(E) calcium hydroxyapatite deposition

DIRECTIONS (Questions 84 through 88): Each set of matching questions in this section consists of a list of lettered options followed by several numbered items. For each numbered item, select the appropriate lettered option(s). Each lettered option may be selected once, more than once, or not at all. EACH ITEM WILL STATE THE NUMBER OF OPTIONS TO SELECT. CHOOSE EXACTLY THIS NUMBER.

(A) polyarteritis nodosa (PAN)

(B) Churg-Strauss disease

(C) Henoch-Schönlein purpura

(D) vasculitis associated with infectious diseases

(E) vasculitis associated with connective tissue diseases

(F) Wegener's granulomatosis

(G) giant cell arteritis

(H) Kawasaki disease

(I) Behçet's syndrome

For each patient with vasculitis syndrome, select the most likely diagnosis.

84. A 48-year-old man presents with 3 weeks of fever, fatigue, and shortness of breath. He has a history of "nasal allergies" and asthma, which have been poorly controlled in the past month. Two days prior to presentation, he developed weakness in his left foot and it now "drags" when he walks. On examination, his blood pressure is 165/90 mm Hg, pulse 100/min, respirations 20/min, and lungs have bilateral expiratory wheezes. There is left foot drop, and the rest of the neurologic examination is normal. Laboratory evaluation reveals ESR of 90 mm/h, WBC of 14,000/mL with 10% eosinophils, and 1+ proteinuria. A CXR shows bilateral pulmonary infiltrates. (SELECT ONE)

85. A 39-year-old man has had several weeks of fever, weight loss, and lack of energy. Three days prior to the assessment, he developed a left foot drop. Physical examination confirms left peroneal nerve damage and a bilateral sensory peripheral neuropathy in both legs. Laboratory evaluation reveals ESR of 105 mm/h, neutrophilia of 14,000, and a negative serologic test for ANCA. Eosinophil count is normal. Angiography reveals small aneurysms of the celiac and renal arteries. (SELECT ONE)

86. A 40-year old man complains of cough, shortness of breath, and nasal ulcers. He was previously well until 1 month ago. He noticed some blood in his sputum on the day of presentation. On examination, his blood pressure is 170/90 mm Hg, pulse 90/min, respirations 22/min, and there are bilateral inspiratory crackles. The oral cavity is normal, but there is a 1-cm nasal septal ulcer. Investigations reveal a positive c-ANCA, 3+ proteinuria with red cell casts, and pulmonary infiltrates on the CXR. His ESR is 110 mm/h and WBC 12,000/mL with normal eosinophils. (SELECT ONE)

87. A 24-year-old woman presents with abdominal pain, joint discomfort, and lower limb rash. She was well until 1 week before presentation. On examination, she has a palpable purpuric rash on her legs, nonspecific abdominal discomfort, and no active joints. She has 3+ proteinuria, normal WBC, no eosinophils, and elevated creatinine of 1.6 mg/dL. Biopsy of the rash confirms vasculitis with immunoglobulin A (IgA) and C3 (complement 3) deposition on immunofluorescence. (SELECT ONE)

88. A 34-year-old man has recurrent painful oral and genital ulcers. Recently, he has noticed multiple painful joints and a decrease in his vision. Last year he had deep vein thrombosis that required treatment. On examination, he has multiple small shallow oral ulcers and similar lesions on his scrotum. The left eye is red and tearing, while his left wrist and right knee are warm and inflamed. Laboratory investigations including complete blood count (CBC), biochemistry, and ANCA are all normal. His ESR and C-reactive protein are elevated. (SELECT ONE)

Answers and Explanations

1. **(E)** Each syndrome in the lysosomal storage diseases is caused by a mutation-produced deficiency in the activity of a lysosomal enzyme. For example, Tay-Sachs disease is caused by a deficiency of hexosaminidase A, resulting in accumulation of GM2 ganglioside. Gaucher's disease is caused by a deficiency of beta-glucocerebrosidase, resulting in an accumulation of glucosylceramide. It has several forms and, as in this case, is most common in Ashkenazi (Eastern European) Jews. Type I Gaucher's disease, as described in this case, is the most common type. Severe bone disease and hepatosplenomegaly is characteristic. Lipid-laden macrophages (Gaucher cells) are found in the bone marrow. *(Kasper, p. 2317)*

2. **(C)** Anti-Sm detects a protein complexed to six species of small nuclear ribonucleic acid (RNA). It is believed to be very specific for SLE. However, only 30% of patients have a positive test. In the case presented, there are enough clinical criteria (four) to confirm the diagnosis of SLE with 98% specificity and 97% sensitivity. *(Kasper, p. 1964)*

3. **(D)** Still's disease (juvenile RA) in an adult may present as fever of unknown origin. Unfortunately, RF is often negative, and a response to NSAIDs along with exclusion of other diseases confirms the diagnosis. *(Kasper, p. 109)*

4. **(B)** The sicca syndrome is a recognized feature of Sjögren's syndrome. It can be primary or secondary to other autoimmune disorders such as RA, SLE, scleroderma, or vasculitis. Primary Sjögren's syndrome is most common in middle-aged women; sicca symptoms can also occur as a complication of HIV infection or in sarcoidosis. Sjögren's syndrome is more likely to have positive serology, while the serology in sarcoid or HIV is negative. Both HIV and Sjögren can have lymphocytic infiltration, but in HIV it is predominantly by CD8+ lymphocytes, whereas in Sjögren's syndrome, the infiltration is by CD4+ lymphocytes. In sarcoidosis, biopsy reveals granulomas. *(Kasper, p. 1991)*

5. **(D)** ANA is the most important diagnostic autoantibodies in patients being evaluated for SLE. It is rare to have ANA negative SLE. The other antibodies can occur in SLE but not as sensitive for the diagnosis as ANA. Anti-dsDNA and anti-SM are specific for SLE but not sensitive. *(Kasper, p. 1964)*

6. **(A)** This patient has scleroderma and esophageal symptoms are present in more than 50% of patients. They are due to the reduced tone of the gastroesophageal sphincter and dilation of the distal esophagus. Gastric and small intestinal motility problems can also occur. Vascular ectasia in the GI tract can result in bleeding. *(Kasper, p. 1984)*

7. **(D)** The response of pain, stiffness, and headaches to 40–60 mg of prednisone is dramatic in giant cell arteritis. The duration of treatment is not known but most patients require treatment for more than 2 years. ESR is used to monitor response to therapy. Patients need treatment and evaluation for the complications of long-term steroid use such as osteoporosis and diabetes. *(Kasper, p. 2009)*

8. **(B)** It is most likely that the primary change in osteoarthritis occurs in the cartilage. It is possible that there is a disruption of the collagen network of the cartilage, specifically a disruption of the "glue" holding together adjacent fibers. *(Kasper, pp. 2038–2039)*

9. **(E)** Raynaud's phenomenon may lead to gangrene of the fingers. It can be primary (Raynaud's disease) or secondary to other diseases, especially scleroderma, in which it can be the presenting symptom. In women, the primary form is common (over 50%), and the phenomenon is generally much more frequent in women. Digital infarction is much more common in relationship to scleroderma than it is in primary Raynaud's disease. *(Kasper, p. 1983)*

10. **(A)** Pseudogout (calcium pyrophosphate crystals—CPPD) is distinguishable from gout by positive birefringent crystals. CPPD are short, blunt rhomboids, and urate crystals (seen in gout) are needle-shaped with negative birefringence. *(Kasper, p. 2046)*

11. **(C)** The triad of chronic RA, splenomegaly, and neutropenia is called Felty's syndrome. It is associated with high titers of RF and extra-articular disease. The increased susceptibility to infections is secondary to both decreased neutrophil number and function. Felty's syndrome is rare in African Americans. *(Kasper, p. 1972)*

12. **(D)** Osteophytes can cause pain by stretching periosteal nerve endings. Synovial inflammation is frequently seen in osteoarthritis, but not in ligament inflammation. Microfractures, but not macrofractures, commonly cause pain. Muscle spasm can be an important factor in the joint pain. *(Kasper, p. 2038)*

13. **(B)** The child most likely has Henoch-Schönlein purpura, an immune complex vasculitis affecting the skin, GI tract, and renal glomeruli. Inciting antigens include upper respiratory tract infections, drugs, foods, and insect bites. *(Kasper, p. 2010)*

14. **(C)** This patient has PMR. Proximal arm and hip muscle/joint discomfort is the hallmark of this disorder. Difficulty in getting out of bed or rising from a chair may suggest polymyositis, but the muscles are normal when muscle strength is assessed. In general, PMR causes painful muscles, not weak muscles. However, pain may lead to profound disuse atrophy and apparent muscle weakness. In these cases, normal CK and non-specific muscle biopsy still allow accurate differentiation from polymyositis. *(Kasper, p. 2009)*

15. **(C)** This man has dermatomyositis, a paraneoplastic phenomenon of many cancers. The most common tumors associated with DM have been bronchogenic carcinomas, ovarian cancers, breast cancers, and melanoma but many others have occurred. The malignancy may antedate or postdate the myositis. Older age makes malignancy more likely. The extent of the workup for malignancy, if DM is the presentation, depends on clinical circumstances, but history and physical examination, not x-rays, are the cornerstones of evaluation. *(Kasper, p. 2540)*

16. **(A)** All NSAIDs are probably equally effective in the treatment of this man's ankylosing spondylitis. Options include indomethacin or naproxen, but not phenylbutazone since it can cause aplastic anemia. Exercise and maintaining proper posture are very important. *(Kasper, pp. 1995–1996)*

17. **(A)** High pressure in the legs and low pressure in the arms characterize Takayasu's syndrome. Clinical manifestations include easy fatigability of the arms and atrophy of the soft tissues of the face. The course is variable, and spontaneous remissions can occur. The disease predominantly affects young women. *(Kasper, pp. 2009–2010)*

18. **(C)** This is a rarefied area involving the frontal and parietal bones, and it is an early stage of Paget's disease in which calvarial thickening and foci or radiopacity are not present within the radiolucent area. At this stage of the disease, a cross-section through the margin of the lesion reveals a compact inner and outer table

in the normal portion, whereas the diploe widens and extends to the outer and inner surfaces of the calvarium without a change in the calvarial thickness in the lesion. *(Kasper, p. 2279)*

19. **(C)** About 95% of patients will develop musculoskeletal symptoms during the course of SLE. Arthralgias and myalgias predominate, but arthritis, hand deformities, myopathy, and avascular necrosis of bone also occur. About 85% of patients will have hematologic disease and 80% will have skin manifestations. *(Kasper, p. 1962)*

20. **(D)** This patient has RA and aspirin or other nonsteroidal agents are effective medications for relieving the signs and symptoms of disease. They do little to modify the course of the disease, however. The new generation of NSAIDs that are more specific inhibitors of cyclooxygenase 2 cause less GI toxicity. Glucocorticoids are very powerful at suppressing signs and symptoms of disease and may alter disease progression. Methotrexate is an important disease modifying drug (DMRD) used to prevent joint destruction. Gold and antimalarials were important DMRDs in the past before the use of methotrexate and newer "biological" agents. *(Kasper, p. 1974)*

21. **(D)** This patient has polyarteritis nodosa (PAN) and in classic PAN, unlike microscopic polyangiitis, both small and medium vessels are involved. The renal lesions are ischemic secondary to fibrinoid necrosis of the vessels. In microscopic polyangiitis, a diffuse glomerulonephritis is frequently present. The most common organ systems involved are the kidneys, musculoskeletal system, and peripheral nervous system. *(Kasper, p. 2008)*

22. **(C)** The major musculoskeletal issue is progressive scoliosis, which is usually treated with physiotherapy and mechanical bracing. Only severe scoliosis is treated with surgery. Vigorous exercise and pregnancy are felt by some experts to increase the rate of aortic root dilatation. *(Kasper, p. 2330)*

23. **(C)** The frequency of aortic insufficiency has been about 4% in ankylosing spondylitis (AS).

Other cardiac valve anomalies are not increased in incidence. Rarely, congestive heart failure or third degree heart block can occur as well. *(Kasper, p. 1994)*

24. **(A)** Hydralazine can cause drug-induced lupus (defined by positive ANA and antihistone antibodies). About 25–30 % of patients treated chronically with hydralazine will develop ANA positivity and about 10–20% of patients with ANA positivity will develop systemic symptoms compatible with lupus, particularly arthralgias. Genetic variation in drug acetylation rates might be a predisposing factor. *(Kasper, p. 1967)*

25. **(B)** This man has a noninflammatory effusion likely from the trauma caused by the fall. In the noninflammatory category, the fluid is transparent, WBC 200–2000/mL (<25% PMNs), glucose is normal, and LDH is low. Another cause for a noninflammatory effusion is osteoarthritis. *(Kasper, p. 2032)*

26. **(C)** This woman has an inflammatory category of effusion in view of the opaque color, high WBC 2000–10,000 (>50% PMNs), low glucose, and high LDH. Common causes for this include crystal induced arthritis, SLE, and RA. In septic arthritis, WBC is usually 50,000/mL or more and often >100,000/mL with >75% PMNs. Other important tests on synovial fluid include Gram stain and culture when an inflammatory effusion is suspected clinically. *(Kasper, p. 2032)*

27. **(D)** Renal disease is usually secondary to deposition of circulating immune complex. Although most patients with SLE have such deposits, only half have clinical nephritis as defined by proteinuria. Renal biopsy can provide both prognostic and therapeutic information. *(Kasper, p. 1963)*

28. **(A)** This patient has features of rheumatoid arthritis, and early in RA there may not be any bony changes seen, except nonspecific findings of soft tissue swelling and joint effusions. With longer active inflammation of the joints, loss of cartilage and bony erosions can be seen. The value of x-rays is to determine the extent of bone and cartilage damage. *(Kasper, p. 1973)*

29. **(B)** Acute anterior uveitis is the most common extra-articular manifestation of ankylosing spondylitis (AS). Pain, photophobia, and increased lacrimation are the usual symptoms. Attacks are unilateral and tend to recur, often in the other eye. Cataracts and secondary glaucoma are not uncommon sequelae. The iritis is usually managed with local glucocorticoid administration in association with a mydriatic agent. *(Kasper, p. 1994)*

30. **(C)** The patient has Marfan syndrome (triad of long thin extremities, lens dislocation, and aortic aneurysms). Aortic involvement occurs in about 80%, with degenerative changes predominating. Aortic root dilatation can cause aortic regurgitation or aortic aneurysm and rupture. *(Kasper, pp. 2329–2330)*

31. **(E)** Extra-articular manifestations of RA generally develop in patients with high titers of autoantibody to the Fc component of IgG (also known as rheumatoid factor (RF)). *(Kasper, p. 1971)*

32. **(B)** Leukopenia occurs in almost two-thirds of the SLE patients, and the differential count is usually normal. Lymphocytes and platelets can also be reduced. *(Kasper, p. 1964)*

33. **(C)** Mononuclear cell infiltration and edema develop in the periosteum, synovial membrane, and joint capsule. Secondary hypertrophic osteoarthropathy (HOA) (e.g., lung cancer) is more common than primary HOA. *(Kasper, p. 2061)*

34. **(A)** Pleuritis is common at autopsy in patients with RA but is not usually symptomatic. Typically, the pleural fluid shows increased pleural fluid: serum protein and LDH ratios (exudate pattern), and low glucose and low complement levels. Pleuropulmonary manifestations are more common in men with RA. *(Kasper, p. 1972)*

35. **(D)** In RA, pleural involvement is very common at autopsy but infrequently causes symptoms. Interstitial lung disease (ILD) is the most common manifestation of rheumatoid lung disease. RA associated interstitial lung disease (RA-ILD) is usually similar to idiopathic pulmonary fibrosis (IPF) in terms of its clinical presentation, pathology, disease spectrum, and pathogenesis. Presentation is more common at age 50–60 years, in men (M:F = 2–3:1), and in association with seropositive and erosive joint disease. If pleural fluid is present, glucose levels are very low. *(Kasper, pp. 1971–1972)*

36. **(B)** Temporal artery biopsy is required for definitive diagnosis of giant cell arteritis, because of the relatively nonspecific nature of the presenting symptoms, signs, and routine laboratory tests. The arteritis can be segmental, however, and great care must be taken in the pathologic assessment. *(Kasper, p. 2009)*

37. **(A)** This patient has SLE and pericarditis, sometimes leading to tamponade, is the most common manifestation of cardiac disease. Myocarditis does occur and can cause arrhythmias, sudden death, or heart failure. Libman-Sacks endocarditis is associated with thrombotic events or, less commonly, valvular regurgitation. Myocardial infarction is more commonly a result of atherosclerotic disease than vasculitis. *(Kasper, p. 1964)*

38. **(A)** In inflammatory bowel disease, there are two common types of arthritis involvement. The first is an asymmetric, migratory polyarthritis that affects the large joints of the lower and upper extremities and is closely related to the activity of bowel disease. Spondylitis is also common (though not always symptomatic) and is not always related to activity of bowel disease. *(Kasper, p. 1784)*

39. **(C)** Current treatment for polyarteritis nodosa (PAN) mimics that of Wegener's granulomatosis in the initial treatment with combination steroid and cyclophosphamide therapy. This will result in up to a 90% long-term remission rate even after discontinuation of therapy. In cases associated with hepatitis B infection, plasmapheresis is sometimes used as initial therapy. *(Kasper, p. 2008)*

40. **(C)** Almost all patients with temporal arteritis will have an elevated ESR. Although a high

ESR cannot make the diagnosis, a normal ESR helps in excluding the diagnosis. C-ANCA is a diagnostic tool for Wegener's granulomatosis. Elevated CPK is not seen in temporal arteritis, even with associated PMR. Normochromic, or slightly hypochromic, anemia often seen in temporal arteritis is too nonspecific to be of much diagnostic help. *(Kasper, p. 2009)*

41. **(C)** About 20–30% of patients with PAN have hepatitis B antigenemia. Circulating immune complexes containing hepatitis B antigen and immunoglobulin have been detected, and immunofluorescence of blood vessel walls have also demonstrated hepatitis B antigen. Antiviral therapy has been used in these cases. *(Kasper, p. 2007)*

42. **(C)** This patient has a sacroiliac form of arthritis seen in patients with psoriasis. Patients with psoriasis can develop five different patterns of musculoskeletal symptoms. These include arthritis of the DIP joints; asymmetric oligoarthritis; symmetric polyarthritis similar to RA; spine and sacroiliac type; and arthritis mutilans, a highly destructive form. Most patients with psoriatic arthritis also have nail involvement. Only about a quarter actually develop a progressive, destructive disease. Uric acid may be elevated because of high tissue turnover but is not part of the pathogenesis of joint disease. *(Kasper, p. 1998)*

43. **(A)** The presence of RF has little predictive power in determining the diagnosis of RA. However, it is useful in determining prognosis, as high titers of RF are associated with more severe and progressive disease, as well as with extra-articular manifestations. *(Kasper, p. 1972)*

44. **(D)** The disease is relapsing polychondritis and is characterized by frequent remissions and exacerbations of lesions and is rarely fatal. Auricular chondritis and nasal chondritis are the most common manifestations. It can also be secondary to SLE, RA, Sjögren's syndrome, and vasculitis. *(Kasper, pp. 2015–2016)*

45. **(E)** In Ehlers-Danlos syndrome, skin hyperextensibility, fragility, and bruisability are marked, and this condition may create difficulties at operation. Habitual dislocation of joints is also a characteristic of this syndrome. *(Kasper, p. 2328)*

46. **(C)** In traumatic arthritis, swellings, ecchymoses, muscular spasms, and tenderness tend to be present, but fractures must be excluded. This man has calcium pyrophosphate (CPPD) crystal-induced monoarthritis, so called "pseudogout." It is most common in the elderly and can be precipitated by minor trauma. The crystals have a rhomboid shape, and the clinical presentation can mimic that of gout. It can be associated with metabolic abnormalities such as hyperparathyroidism or hemochromatosis. Treatment is with an NSAID for 7–10 days. If there are multiple joints involved, then steroids can be considered. An alternative to oral NSAIDs is intra-articular steroids for single joint disease. Allopurinol is not effective in CPPD. Synovial fluid is bloody, but the fluid is of normal viscosity, so a "string" test is usually positive. *(Kasper, pp. 2047–2048)*

47. **(A)** The course of muscle necrosis in dermatomyositis can be best followed by repeated CK determinations. Repeated muscle biopsies are rarely required. However, the goal of therapy is to increase muscle strength and function, so following muscle strength is the key clinical assessment of response to therapy. *(Kasper, p. 2544)*

48. **(B)** This patient with SLE has developed autoimmune hemolytic anemia. Treatment consists of high-dose oral steroids. The positive Coombs' test (direct antiglobulin test), high indirect bilirubin, high LDH, and high retic count are all supportive of hemolytic anemia. A normal AST and ALT rule out hepatitis. *(Kasper, p. 1964)*

49. **(E)** This story is typical of Lyme disease. The spirochete involved (*B. burgdorferi*) is transmitted by ixodic ticks and is most common in the Northeastern and Midwestern parts of the United States. The host animal varies depending on the exact type of tick. Treatment is briefer and more effective earlier in the course of the disease. The treatment of choice is doxycycline 100 mg bid for 1–2 months. Amoxicillin is a second choice drug. *(Kasper, pp. 997–998)*

50. **(D)** This story is typical of Lyme disease. The spirochete involved *(B. burgdorferi)* is transmitted by ixodic ticks and is most common in the Northeastern and Midwestern parts of the United States. The host animal varies depending on the exact type of tick. Because antibody studies cannot differentiate between active and inactive disease, the appropriate constellation of symptoms is also required for diagnosis. *(Kasper, p. 997)*

51. **(E)** As in most inflammatory arthritides, the patient with RA generally has morning stiffness for more than 1 hour. Wrist involvement is nearly universal and is associated with radial deviation (unlike the ulnar deviation of the digits) and carpal tunnel syndrome. Hand involvement characteristically involves the proximal interphalangeal and MCP joints in a symmetric involvement. High fever (>100.4°F), even with active synovitis, should suggest an intercurrent problem such as infection. *(Kasper, pp. 1970–1971)*

52. **(C)** AS occurs in 1–6% of adults inheriting human lymphocyte antigen B27 (HLA-B27). However, the prevalence in B27-positive relatives of patients with AS is up to 30%. Men are three times more likely to be affected. *(Kasper, p. 1993)*

53. **(D)** This patient has PMR. It is characterized by stiffness, aching, and pain in proximal muscle groups in the neck, shoulders, back, hips, and thighs. It is considerably more common than temporal arteritis. Both diseases are almost exclusively seen in the over 50 age group. *(Kasper, p. 2009)*

54. **(A)** Although all these complications have been reported in giant cell arteritis, the only one with a significant likelihood is blindness secondary to ischemic optic neuropathy. Thus, if the disease is suspected, urgent diagnosis and treatment is required. *(Kasper, p. 2009)*

55. **(C)** Although the hallmark of osteoarthritis is the progressive loss of articular cartilage, it is best considered as a disease of the entire organ, the synovial joint, rather than of any of its component tissues. In fact, all areas of the joint, bone, cartilage, synovium, meniscus, and ligaments are involved. *(Kasper, p. 2038)*

56. **(B)** In Marfan syndrome, inheritance is autosomal dominant, and the aortic lesion is a cystic medial necrosis with loss of elastic tissue, resulting in aneurysm formation. Pneumothorax can occur but is not as characteristic. Mitral valve prolapse can also be part of the syndrome. Dislocation of the lens is the most apparent eye abnormality. Severe chest deformities and long limbs are characteristic. High, arched palate; high pedal arches; and pes planus are common. *(Kasper, p. 2330)*

57. **(A)** Numerous mediators of inflammation are found in the synovium of patients with rheumatoid arthritis (RA). The evidence favoring activated T cells as the initiators of the inflammation include the predominance of CD4+ T cells in the synovium, the increase in soluble interleukin-2 (IL-2) receptors (a product of T-cell activation), and amelioration of symptoms by T-cell removal. *(Kasper, p. 1969)*

58. **(C)** Methotrexate, 7.5–20 mg once weekly, is the most commonly recommended disease modifying drug, because its effect is more rapid and patients are able to tolerate it for longer periods of time. Maximum improvement with methotrexate occurs after 6 months of therapy. Toxicity includes GI upset, oral ulceration, and liver function abnormalities. GI upset in particular may be ameliorated by concurrent folic acid administration. Pneumonitis has also been reported. *(Kasper, p. 1975)*

59. **(B)** ANAs are present in 98% of patients with SLE. Repeatedly negative tests make the diagnosis of SLE very unlikely. Unfortunately, the test is not specific and may be positive in normal people (especially in older individuals), or secondary to infections, drugs, or other autoimmune disorders. *(Kasper, p. 1964)*

60. **(E)** This patient likely has PAN. ANCA and other serology are usually negative in PAN; positive serology suggests another diagnosis. The optimal diagnostic strategy is the biopsy of

an affected organ. However angiography to look for aneurysms of small- and medium-sized arteries generally has higher yield than blind biopsy of unaffected organs. The lungs are not a characteristic site of involvement. *(Kasper, p. 2008)*

61. **(C)** This story is typical of Lyme disease. The spirochete involved (*B. burgdorferi*) is transmitted by ixodic ticks and is most common in the Northeastern and Midwestern parts of the United States. The host animal varies depending on the exact type of tick. *(Kasper, p. 996)*

62. **(B)** Although malaise, fatigue, and sweating are common in temporal arteritis, they are too nonspecific to help in making the diagnosis. Claudication of the jaw and tongue, while not very sensitive for temporal arteritis, are more specific than the constitutional symptoms. Odynophagia is not a characteristic of this disease. *(Kasper, p. 2009)*

63. **(D)** There are numerous diseases and risk factors associated with the development of osteoarthritis. People of Chinese and African heritage have a lower risk than Caucasians, while Native Americans have a higher risk. Women are more affected than men, and obesity is a significant risk factor. Hyperthyroidism is not one of the many metabolic/endocrine disorders associated with osteoarthritis. *(Kasper, pp. 2039–2040)*

64. **(E)** Heberden's nodes, bony enlargement of the DIP joints of the hand, are the most common type of osteoarthritis. Although they can present acutely with pain and inflammation, they are frequently slow in developing and relatively asymptomatic. *(Kasper, pp. 2039–2040)*

65. **(C)** Although not specific, ANA is positive in 95% of patients with SLE. A repeatedly negative test makes SLE unlikely. *(Kasper, p. 1961)*

66. **(F)** Anti-dsDNA is relatively disease-specific and associated with nephritis and clinical activity. Anti-single-stranded (ss) DNA is not very specific. *(Kasper, p. 1961)*

67. **(E)** The presence of anticardiolipin antibodies is associated with false-positive VDRL, vascular thrombosis, and spontaneous abortion. *(Kasper, p. 1961)*

68. **(D)** Antihistone antibodies are seen in 95% of patients with drug-induced LE and in 70% of those with SLE. *(Kasper, p. 1961)*

69. **(B)** Anti-RNP is found in high titer in syndromes with features of polymyositis, scleroderma, lupus, and mixed connective tissue disease. *(Kasper, p. 1961)*

70. **(B)** Although widespread vasculitis is rare, limited forms of vasculitis are not, particularly in White patients with high titers of RF. Cutaneous vasculitis usually presents as crops of small brown spots in the nail beds, nail folds, and digital pulp. *(Kasper, p. 1971)*

71. **(D)** Direct eye involvement with the rheumatoid process (episcleritis or scleritis) occurs in less than 1% of patients. However, 15–20% may develop Sjögren's syndrome with attendant keratoconjunctivitis sicca. *(Kasper, p. 1972)*

72. **(A)** Felty's syndrome consists of chronic RA, splenomegaly, and neutropenia. The increased frequency of infections is due to both decreased number and function of neutrophils. *(Kasper, p. 1972)*

73. **(G)** Caplan's syndrome is a diffuse, nodular fibrotic process that may result when rheumatoid nodules occur in the lungs of patients with pneumoconiosis. *(Kasper, pp. 1971–1972)*

74. **(E)** Rheumatoid nodules occur in 20–30% of patients with RA. Common locations include the olecranon bursa, the proximal ulna, the Achillis tendon, and the occiput. *(Kasper, p. 1971)*

75. **(C)** Both rickets and osteomalacia are disorders in which mineralization of the organic matrix of the skeleton is defective. Rickets is the name when this disorder occurs in a growing skeleton, whereas osteomalacia occurs after the epiphyseal plates are closed. *(Kasper, p. 2247)*

76. **(D)** Deficient or defective 1,25(OH)2 vitamin D receptors will result in vitamin D resistance. Parathyroid hormone levels increase secondary to decreased vitamin D effect. The 1(OH) vitamin D is an intermediate metabolite. *(Kasper, p. 2247)*

77. **(C)** Aging decreases the responsiveness of the renal 25(OH) D-1-hydroxylase to parathyroid hormone (PTH), thus decreasing circulatory levels of the active metabolite 1,25(OH)2 vitamin D. This results in decreased calcium absorption from the gut. There is not a close relationship of 1(OH) vitamin D levels and osteopenia. *(Kasper, pp. 2246–2247)*

78. **(B)** Muscle weakness is common in both rickets and osteomalacia, and proximal leg muscles are particularly involved. The combination of leg deformity and muscle weakness in rickets can result in an inability to walk. The presentation of osteomalacia is more insidious in the elderly, but proximal myopathy may be severe enough to cause a waddling gait and mimic a primary muscle disorder. The other clinical findings listed are found only in rickets. *(Kasper, p. 2247)*

79. **(D)** The term *pseudogout* refers to crystal deposition disease not due to uric acid (gout). By far the most common cause of pseudogout is calcium pyrophosphate deposition (CPPD). The major predisposing factors are advanced age and preexisting joint disease. The knee is the most common joint involved, and presentation can mimic acute gout. However, in the majority of cases, the deposition of calcium pyrophosphate seems to be asymptomatic. *(Kasper, p. 2047)*

80. **(E)** Unfortunately, there is no medical means to remove the deposits of CPPD. Colchicine does seem to decrease the rate of recurrence. NSAIDs, steroids (systemic or intra-articular), and colchicine are all helpful in acute attacks. *(Kasper, pp. 2048–2049)*

81. **(C)** Although gout and CPPD disease are found in chronic renal failure, hydroxyapatite deposition is characteristic of end-stage renal failure. The crystals are very small, nonbirefringent, and only seen on election microscopy. Treatment is symptomatic, and similar to the treatment of gout or CPPD disease. *(Kasper, p. 2049)*

82. **(E)** "Milwaukee shoulder" represents an unusual manifestation of calcium hydroxyapatite deposition disease. Once destruction changes start occurring, medical management is relatively unsuccessful. The exact reason why destructive arthritis occurs is not understood. The knee is the other joint affected in this manner. *(Kasper, p. 2048)*

83. **(C)** The high white cell count suggests infection. In RA and crystal-induced arthritis, the white cell count is usually less than $50,000/\mu L$. *Staphylococcus aureus* infection is the most common type in RA. *(Kasper, p. 2050)*

84. **(B)** Churg-Strauss is a granulomatous vasculitis. Pulmonary involvement often dominates the clinical presentation with severe asthma attacks and pulmonary infiltrates. Peripheral eosinophilia is present in virtually all cases. *(Kasper, p. 2007)*

85. **(A)** PAN is a multisystem, necrotizing vasculitis of small- and medium-sized muscular arteries. Aneurysmal dilations of the arteries are characteristic. Nonspecific signs and symptoms are the usual method of presentation. Renal involvement is clinically present in 60% of cases and is the most common cause of death in untreated cases. *(Kasper, pp. 2007–2008)*

86. **(F)** A high percentage of patients with Wegener's develop ANCAs. In particular, cytoplasmic or c-ANCAs are both sensitive and specific for Wegener's. However, tissue diagnosis is still required. *(Kasper, pp. 2004–2006)*

87. **(C)** Henoch-Schönlein purpura, characterized by palpable purpura, arthralgias, GI symptoms, and glomerulonephritis, can be seen in any age-group but is most common in children. It can resolve and recur several times over a period of weeks or months and can resolve spontaneously. *(Kasper, p. 2010)*

88. **(I)** Behçet's syndrome is a leukocytoclastic venulitis characterized by episodes of oral ulcers, genital ulcers, iritis, and cutaneous lesions. Eye involvement can rapidly progress to blindness. *(Kasper, pp. 2012, 2014)*

CHAPTER 10

Infection
Questions

DIRECTIONS (Questions 1 through 58): Each of the numbered items in this section is followed by answers. Select the ONE lettered answer that is BEST in each case.

1. A 22-year-old recent immigrant to the United States has never been vaccinated for tetanus. He sustains a minor, but soil-contaminated, injury. Which of the following statements is correct?

    (A) tetanus usually develops within 2 weeks following exposure

    (B) tetanus always develops within 4 hours following exposure in patients who have not been previously immunized

    (C) tetanus may develop many months or years following exposure in susceptible individuals

    (D) the usual incubation period for tetanus is 48 hours

    (E) tetanus may be prevented with penicillin

2. A 19-year-old man has donated blood for the first time. Despite having no risk factors for human immunodeficiency virus (HIV) infection, his blood tests positive for HIV by enzyme immunoassay (EIA). Which of the following statements is correct?

    (A) EIA is currently the most specific test for HIV

    (B) he might have a false-positive secondary to an unsuspected collagen-vascular disease

    (C) he has a 75% chance of truly being infected with HIV

    (D) EIA is an excellent screening test

    (E) a Western blot test would be more sensitive

3. A 27-year-old man presents with symptoms of fever, chills, malaise, and joint discomfort in his hands and knees. He looks unwell, his temperature is 39.4°C, blood pressure 115/70 mm Hg, pulse 110/min, head and neck is normal, and his jugular venous pressure (JVP) has a prominent *c-v* wave. There is also a 3/6 pansystolic murmur heard at the right sternal border that increases with respiration. His lungs are clear, abdomen is soft, and hand joints are normal. He has multiple puncture sites on his forearms from injection drug use. Which of the following is the most likely causative organism?

    (A) *Staphylococcus aureus*

    (B) *Staphylococcus epidermidis*

    (C) *Streptococcus viridans*

    (D) enterococci

    (E) *Candida*

4. A 23-year-old woman develops vesicular lesions on an erythematous base on her vulvar area. She has tender lymphadenopathy and dysuria as well. Which of the following is the most likely causative organism?

    (A) cytomegalovirus (CMV)

    (B) gonococcus

    (C) herpes simplex virus type 2 (HSV-2)

    (D) *Treponema pallidum*

    (E) varicella zoster

5. A 17-year-old man presents with new symptoms of fatigue, malaise, fever, and a sore throat. He has no significant past medical history and is not on any medications. Physical examination is entirely normal except for enlarged, palpable cervical, lymph nodes. He reports no weight loss or night sweats. Laboratory investigations include a normal chest x-ray, negative throat swab, but abnormal blood film with atypical lymphocytes. The hemoglobin is 15.5 g/dL; hematocrit 42%; platelets 290,000/mL; WBC 10500/mL, with 45% segmented neutrophils, 1% eosinophils, and 54% lymphocytes, of which 36% were atypical. Which of the following is the most appropriate initial diagnostic test?

   (A) lymph node biopsy
   (B) bone marrow
   (C) erythrocyte sedimentation rate (ESR)
   (D) heterophil antibody (sheep cell agglutination) test
   (E) hepatic biopsy

6. A 34-year-old man is traveling in Southeast Asia on business. He is staying in Western-style hotels and eating food in large restaurants. He has not eaten from street vendors. One week after arrival, he develops symptoms of anorexia, nausea, and abdominal cramps followed by the sudden onset of watery diarrhea. He has no fever or chills and there is no blood or pus in the stools. Which of the following is the most appropriate therapy for his condition?

   (A) amoxicillin
   (B) symptomatic therapy with loperamide
   (C) doxycycline
   (D) oral rehydration only
   (E) specific antitoxin

7. An 18-year-old woman presents with headache, anorexia, chilly sensations, and discomfort on both sides of her jaw. She has also noticed discomfort in both lower abdominal quadrants. Physical examination reveals bilateral enlarged parotid glands that are doughy, elastic, and slightly tender; with a reddened orifice of Stensen's duct. Her abdomen is soft with bilateral lower quadrant abdominal tenderness; a temperature of 38.5°C; and a pulse rate of 92/min. Laboratory data show hemoglobin 13 g/dL; hematocrit 40%; white blood cells (WBC) 9000/mL, with 35% segmented neutrophils, 7% monocytes, and 58% lymphocytes. Which of the following is the most likely cause for her abdominal pain and tenderness?

   (A) mesenteric lymphadenitis
   (B) oophoritis
   (C) gonorrhea
   (D) peritoneal metastases
   (E) intestinal hyperperistalsis

8. A 32-year-old man, previously well, develops a fever and dry cough. On examination, his chest is clear and heart sounds are normal. A chest x-ray (CXR) reveals a diffuse interstitial infiltrate. Which of the following is the most likely causative organism?

   (A) bacterium
   (B) mycoplasma
   (C) fungus
   (D) rickettsia
   (E) spirochete

9. A 25-year-old man is admitted with fever and rust-colored sputum. He looks unwell, temperature 38.4°C, pulse 100/min, and blood pressure 115/80 mm Hg. On auscultation, there are bronchial breath sounds in the right axilla and inspiratory crackles. The CXR is shown in Fig. 10–1. Which of the following is the most likely diagnosis?

   (A) right middle lobe pneumonia
   (B) loculated pleural effusion
   (C) aspergilloma
   (D) aspiration pneumonia
   (E) right lower lobe pneumonia

10. A 30-year-old man develops a pustular lesion at the site of a cat scratch on his forearm. This is followed 1 week later by malaise, fever, and lymphadenopathy. On examination, he has tender axillary lymph nodes. Which of the following is the most likely causative organism?

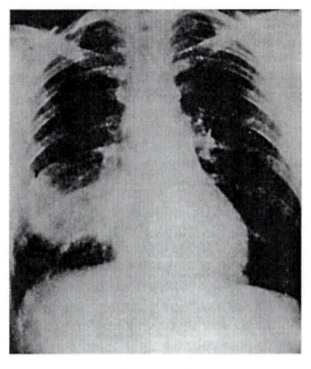

Figure 10–1.

(A) *Bartonella henselae*
(B) *Bartonella bacilliformis*
(C) *Bartonella quintana*
(D) *Coxiella burnetii*
(E) *Borrelia burgdorferi*

11. A 7-year-old child, unvaccinated because of his parents' religious beliefs, develops malaise, cough, coryza, and conjunctivitis with a high fever. Examination of his mouth reveals blue white spots on a red base beside his second molars. The next day he develops an erythematous, nonpruritic, maculopapular rash at his hairline and behind his ears, which spreads over his body. Which of the following is the most likely diagnosis?

(A) hand-foot-and-mouth disease (coxsackievirus)
(B) measles (rubeola)

(C) rubella (German measles)
(D) mumps
(E) pertussis

12. A 60-year-old man presents with fever and malaise 6 weeks after mitral valve replacement. On examination, his temperature is 38°C, blood pressure 130/80 mm Hg, pulse 80/min, and a loud pansystolic murmur at the apex, which radiates to the axilla. He has no skin or neurologic findings. Which of the following is the most likely causative organism?

(A) *Staphylococcus aureus*
(B) a fungus
(C) *Staphylococcus saprophyticus*
(D) pneumococcus
(E) *Staphylococcus epidermidis*

13. A 73-year-old man from a nursing home develops headache, fever, cough, sore throat, malaise, and severe myalgia during a community outbreak affecting numerous other residents at the home. The symptoms gradually resolve after 3 days, and he starts feeling better but then there is a reappearance of his fever, with cough and yellow sputum production. On examination, his temperature is 38.5°C, pulse 100/min, respiration 24/min, oxygen saturation 88% and crackles in the right lower lung base, bronchial breath sounds and dullness on percussion. CXR reveals a new infiltrate in the right lower lobe. Which of the following is the most likely causative organism?

(A) primary viral pneumonia
(B) an autoimmune reaction
(C) *Mycoplasma pneumoniae*
(D) *Streptococcus pneumoniae*
(E) *Neisseria catarrhalis*

14. A 56-year-old man is having intermittent fevers and malaise for the past 2 weeks. He has no other localizing symptoms. Two months ago, he had valve replacement surgery for a bicuspid aortic valve. A mechanical valve was inserted and his postoperative course was uncomplicated. On examination, his temperature is 38°C, blood pressure 124/80 mm Hg, pulse 72/min, and head and neck are normal. There is a 3/6 systolic ejection murmur, the second heart sound is mechanical, and a 2/6 early diastolic murmur is heard. The lungs are clear and the skin examination is normal. Three sets of blood cultures are drawn and an urgent echocardiogram is ordered. Which of the following is the most likely causative organism?

    (A) *Staphylococcus aureus*
    (B) *S. epidermidis*
    (C) *S. viridans*
    (D) enterococci
    (E) *Candida*

15. Two students from a university dormitory building have contracted meningitis due to *Neisseria meningitides*. Which of the following students in the dormitory are most likely to benefit from chemoprophylaxis?

    (A) everybody in the dormitory, with oral amoxicillin
    (B) close contacts only, with oral amoxicillin
    (C) everybody in the dormitory, with oral rifampin
    (D) close contacts only, with oral rifampin
    (E) everybody in the dormitory, with meningococcal vaccine

16. A 21-year-old woman visits her physician because of 3 weeks of a "flu-like" illness. She reports symptoms of malaise, fever, fatigue, and a sore throat. There is no weight loss or night sweats, and she has not traveled out of country. Her past medical history is not significant and she is not taking any medications. Physical examination is normal except for enlarged cervical lymph nodes. Laboratory data show hemoglobin 13.2 g/dL; hematocrit 42%; platelets 380,000/mL; WBC 8500/mL, with 35% segmented neutrophils, 1% eosinophils, and 64% lymphocytes, of which 36% were atypical. A heterophil antibody (sheep cell agglutination) test is negative. Which of the following is the most likely causative organism?

    (A) herpes simplex
    (B) echovirus
    (C) CMV
    (D) coxsackievirus
    (E) reovirus

17. A 23-year-old woman visits your office because of headache, malaise, anorexia, pain in both sides of her jaw, and discomfort in both lower abdominal quadrants. Physical examination reveals enlarged parotid glands; bilateral lower quadrant abdominal tenderness; a temperature of 38.7°C; and a pulse rate of 92/min. Serologic testing (IgM) confirms the diagnosis of mumps. Which of the following is the most appropriate treatment for this condition?

    (A) symptomatic
    (B) immunization
    (C) broad-spectrum antibiotics
    (D) sulfonamides
    (E) steroids

18. A 10-year-old boy presents with fever, headache, photophobia, and neck discomfort in the middle of summer. He is alert and oriented, but has neck pain with flexion and extension of the head. His fundi are normal, and there are no focal neurologic findings or skin changes. A lumbar puncture reveals normal protein and glucose with a cell count of 240/mL (90% lymphocytes). Which of the following is the most likely causative organism?

    (A) enterovirus (coxsackievirus or echovirus)
    (B) *Streptococcus pneumoniae*
    (C) *Neisseria meningitides*
    (D) *Listeria monocytogenes*
    (E) HSV-1

19. An 18-year-old woman has eaten homemade preserves. Eighteen hours later, she develops diplopia, dysarthria, and dysphagia. Which of

the following is the most likely causative organism?

(A) *Clostridium botulinum* toxin
(B) staphylococcal toxin
(C) salmonellosis
(D) brucellosis
(E) shigellosis

20. A previously healthy 19-year-old female university student develops myalgia, headache, fever, and malaise. Blood tests reveal lymphocytosis, with 20% of the lymphocytes being atypical. She remains tired and unwell for 6 weeks, but repeated tests for heterophil antibody are negative. Which of the following is the most likely diagnosis?

(A) Epstein-Barr virus (EBV) infection
(B) primary HIV infection
(C) human herpes virus type 7 (HHV-7)
(D) CMV infection
(E) toxoplasmosis

21. A 43-year-old man developed a cough shortly after returning from a 1-month hiking trip in California. While there, he was hiking in the central California valleys. During his trip, he had developed a "flu-like" illness consisting of fever, cough, and muscle pains, which resolved spontaneously. A CXR shows a thin-walled cavity in the right upper lobe, and the sputum reveals fungal elements. Which of the following is the most likely causative organism?

(A) ringworm
(B) *Cryptococcus neoformans*
(C) *Candida albicans*
(D) mycobacteria
(E) coccidioidomycosis

22. An 8-year-old boy from an impoverished inner-city area has never been vaccinated appropriately. He develops fever, cough, and coryza. The next day, blue white spots develop on the buccal mucosa. On the third day, an erythematous, nonpruritic maculopapular rash develops on the face and spreads over the entire

body. Which of the following is the most likely complication?

(A) pneumonia
(B) encephalitis
(C) otitis media
(D) bronchitis
(E) mastoiditis

23. A 6-year-old boy develops symptoms of cough, fever, and malaise followed by a generalized maculopapular rash that has spread from the head downwards. A clinical diagnosis of measles is made. A few days after the onset of the rash he is drowsy, lethargic, and complaining of headache. A lumbar puncture, electroencephalogram (EEG), and computerized tomography (CT) of the brain exclude other etiologies and confirm the diagnosis of encephalitis. Which of the following is the most likely delayed neurologic complication of measles virus encephalitis?

(A) meningitis
(B) pure motor paralysis
(C) autonomic neuropathy
(D) mental retardation or epilepsy
(E) "stocking-glove" peripheral neuropathy

24. A 27-year-old man presents with diarrhea. He returned 3 weeks ago from a trip to rural South America. Over the past few days, he has gradually developed lower abdominal pain and diarrhea. Now the symptoms are much worse with eight stools a day consisting mostly of mucus and blood. He is afebrile, the abdomen is tender in left lower quadrant, and the remaining examination is normal. His stool is mostly comprised of blood and mucus. Which of the following is the most appropriate initial diagnostic test?

(A) stool culture
(B) stool toxin assay
(C) examination of a dried stool specimen
(D) immunofluorescence of stool specimen
(E) examination of a wet stool specimen

25. A 4-year-old boy is sent to the emergency room because of clinical suspicion of meningitis. He has been ill for 2 days with fever and lethargy. On examination, he is febrile, the neck is stiff, and papilledema is present. There is no rash, the lungs are clear, and heart sounds normal. Which of the following is the most likely causative organism?

    (A) *Neisseria meningitidis*
    (B) *Streptococcus pneumoniae*
    (C) *Haemophilus influenzae*
    (D) *Staphylococcus*
    (E) *Listeria* species

26. Which of the following is a contraindication to receiving the live rubella vaccine?

    (A) children between 1 year old and puberty
    (B) infants <1 year old
    (C) all adults
    (D) pregnant women
    (E) all exposed patients

27. A 24-year-old woman presents with chills and rigors. She looks unwell, and her temperature is 39.4°C, blood pressure 100/60 mm Hg, pulse 110/min, and oxygen saturation 95%. There is a 3/6 pansystolic murmur at the right sternal border, which increases with inspiration. Her arms have multiple tattoos and needle marks from injection drug use. Blood cultures (2/2 sets) are positive for *S. aureus*, and she is started on appropriate antibiotics. Her renal function is mildly impaired and her urinalysis is positive for protein, and microscopy reveals red cell casts. Which of the following mechanisms is the most likely explanation for her renal abnormalities?

    (A) septic emboli
    (B) cardiac failure with prerenal azotemia
    (C) a high level of circulating immune complexes
    (D) fungal disease
    (E) inevitable progression to renal failure

28. A 22-year-old university student complains of fatigue and malaise for the past 2 weeks. She also reports feeling feverish, and recently had a sore throat. Physical examination reveals enlarged tonsils and palpable cervical lymph nodes. There is also tenderness in the right upper quadrant on deep palpation, and minimal splenomegaly. Laboratory data show hemoglobin 13 g/dL; hematocrit 40%; platelets 340,000/mL; WBC 9400/mL, with 35% segmented neutrophils, 1% eosinophils, and 64% lymphocytes, of which 36% were atypical. A heterophil antibody (sheep cell agglutination) test is positive. Which of the following is the most appropriate initial treatment for this condition?

    (A) gamma-globulin
    (B) adequate rest
    (C) chlorambucil
    (D) chloramphenicol
    (E) radiation therapy

29. A 23-year-old woman presents with a painless chronic vulvar ulcer. She recently arrived to study in the United States from Southern India. The lesion began as a papule and then ulcerated. It has persisted for several months. Currently, physical examination reveals a painless elevated area of beefy red, friable granulation tissue. She has been sexually active for several years. Which of the following is the most likely causative organism?

    (A) spirochete
    (B) Gram-positive coccus
    (C) intracellular Gram-negative bacteria
    (D) chronic viral infection
    (E) fungus

30. A 20-year-old woman presents with headache, fever, and neck stiffness. On examination, her blood pressure is 100/70 mm Hg, pulse 100/min, temperature 38.6°C, and the neck is stiff and painful to flex and extend. The ears, throat, and sinuses are normal, there are no focal neurologic signs, and the remaining examination is normal. There are no reported similar cases in the community. Which of the following is the most likely source of her infection?

(A) an infected heart valve

(B) nasopharynx

(C) skin

(D) oral ingestion

(E) bowel

31. A 44-year-old renal transplant patient develops severe cough and shortness of breath on exertion. On examination, he appears dyspneic, respirations 24/min, pulse 110/min, and oxygen saturation 88%. His lungs are clear on auscultation and heart sounds are normal. CXR shows bilateral diffuse perihilar infiltrates. Bronchoscopy and bronchial brushings show clusters of cysts that stain with methenamine silver. Which of the following is the most appropriate next step in management?

(A) amphotericin B

(B) cephalosporins

(C) trimethoprim-sulfamethoxazole

(D) aminoglycosides

(E) penicillins

32. A 34-year-old man presents with diarrhea 3 weeks after returning from a trip to rural South America. Over the past few days, he has gradually developed lower abdominal pain and diarrhea. Now the symptoms are much worse with eight stools a day consisting mostly of mucus and blood. He is afebrile, the abdomen is tender in left lower quadrant, and the remaining examination is normal. His stool is mostly comprised of blood and mucus, and stools tests show trophozoites of *Entamoeba histolytica*. Which of the following is the most likely site of extraintestinal involvement?

(A) genitals

(B) pleura

(C) pericardium

(D) liver

(E) cerebral cortex

33. A 20-year-old woman complains of headache and discomfort in both sides of her jaw. Physical examination reveals enlarged parotid glands that are slightly tender on palpation. There is reddening of the orifice of Stensen's duct on intra oral examination; her temperature is 38.3°C, and the pulse rate is 80/min. Laboratory data show hemoglobin 14 g/dL; hematocrit 40%; WBC 11000/mL, with 33% segmented neutrophils, 7% monocytes, and 60% lymphocytes. Which of the following diagnostic tests will help to confirm the diagnosis of epidemic parotitis?

(A) single blood sample for a specific immunoglobulin G (IgG)

(B) blood cell count

(C) blood culture

(D) single blood test for a specific immunoglobulin M (IgM)

(E) serum amylase

34. Three hours after a church social, eight people develop severe diarrhea. Other symptoms included nausea, vomiting, and abdominal cramps. Food served included chicken salad and cream-filled pastries. All affected individuals had the chicken salad. Which of the following is the most likely causative organism?

(A) staphylococcal enterotoxin

(B) *C. botulinum*

(C) *Clostridium perfringens*

(D) *Salmonella* species

(E) ptomaine poisoning

35. A young woman complains of hair loss, loss of hair luster, and intense scalp irritation. Examination reveals patches of hair loss with tiny little black dots where the hair shaft has broken off. A Wood's light examination is positive. Which of the following is the most likely diagnosis?

(A) seborrheic dermatitis

(B) *Aspergillus* infection

(C) *Trichophyton* infection

(D) neurosis

(E) excess androgen levels

36. A 9-year-old boy has a severe sore throat with fever and dysphagia. On examination, there are grayish-white papulovesicular lesions on an erythematous base that ulcerate. They are located on the soft palate, anterior pillars of the tonsils and uvula. There are no lesions on the gingiva, tongue, or lips. A clinical diagnosis of herpangina is made. Which of the following is the most likely causative organism?

    (A) measles (Morbillivirus)
    (B) rubella (rubivirus)
    (C) coxsackievirus A
    (D) HSV-1
    (E) HSV-2

37. A young man has recently been bitten by a stray dog. He has a penetrating wound to the right forearm. The dog is nowhere to be found. In the emergency room, the wound is cleaned with water and povidone-iodine solution. Which of the following is the most appropriate next step in management?

    (A) start postexposure prophylaxis
    (B) contact the local public health professional for further advice
    (C) treat with oral doxycycline
    (D) treat with IV ceftriaxone
    (E) start IV acyclovir

38. Which of the following malignancies in the United States is most likely to contain EBV deoxyribonucleic acid (DNA) in a non-HIV patient?

    (A) gastric cancer
    (B) well-differentiated thyroid cancer
    (C) anaplastic nasopharyngeal carcinoma
    (D) Burkitt's lymphoma
    (E) Hodgkin's disease

39. A 24-year-old man complains of fatigue, malaise, fever, and a sore throat. He was previously well, but now feels tired all the time and has to rest multiple times a day. Physical examination shows enlarged tonsils and palpable anterior and posterior cervical, axillary, and inguinal lymph nodes. There is also tenderness in the right upper quadrant with a liver

span of 10 cm. Laboratory data is significant for a heterophil antibody (sheep cell agglutination) test that is positive. Which of the following rare complications can be associated with this condition?

    (A) retinitis
    (B) esophagitis
    (C) splenic rupture
    (D) Kaposi sarcoma
    (E) hemorrhage

40. A 40-year-old man develops erythema nodosum, conjunctivitis, and a pleural effusion. Over several weeks, pulmonary lesions lead to cavitation and a large, thin-walled cavity. He was traveling in Arizona before becoming ill. Sputum samples reveal mature spherules. Which of the following is the most likely diagnosis?

    (A) *Streptococcus*
    (B) coccidioidomycosis
    (C) candidiasis
    (D) *Staphylococcus*
    (E) *Pneumocystis carinii*

41. A patient undergoing emergency surgery for trauma receives 20 blood transfusions during the operation. Four weeks later, she develops a syndrome resembling infectious mononucleosis. Which of the following is the most likely causative organism?

    (A) EBV
    (B) hepatitis C virus
    (C) delayed hemolysis
    (D) CMV
    (E) serum sickness

42. A 32-year-old woman acutely develops high fever, hypotension, and rash. This is followed by vomiting, diarrhea, confusion, and abdominal pain. In the hospital, evidence of multiorgan failure develops. Desquamation of the skin occurs 1 week after the acute illness. On further history, the illness started 3 days after the onset of menstruation. Which of the following is the most likely diagnosis?

(A) *S. aureus* toxic shock syndrome (TSS)

(B) streptococcal infection (scarlet fever)

(C) clostridial infection

(D) RMSF

(E) staphylococcal scaled skin syndrome

43. An 18-year-old man develops fever, neck stiffness, and headache. On examination, his blood pressure is 105/80 mm Hg, pulse 100/min, temperature 38.7°C, and neck flexion is very painful. The ears, throat, and sinuses are normal; there are no focal neurologic signs, and the remaining examination is normal. His is the second case of meningitis in his university dormitory building. Which of the following is the most likely causative organism?

(A) *Neisseria meningitidis*

(B) *Streptococcus pneumoniae*

(C) *Haemophilus influenzae*

(D) *Staphylococcus*

(E) *Listeria* species

44. A 45-year-old woman is undergoing chemotherapy for breast cancer. She presents 10 days after her last chemotherapy with fever (temperature >38.5°C), but no other symptoms except a sore throat and mouth. On examination, she looks well, there is oral mucositis, ears are normal, lungs are clear, and the central line site is clean. The CXR, urinalysis, and biochemistry are normal. Her WBC is 800/mL and the absolute neutrophil count is low (<500). Which of the following is the most appropriate next step in management?

(A) start empiric bacterial antibiotics

(B) start empiric antifungal and bacterial antibiotics

(C) acetaminophen alone until culture results are available

(D) start antiviral medications for HSV-1

(E) start antiviral and bacterial antibiotics

45. An elderly bedridden patient in the hospital develops cough, fever, and shortness of breath. On examination, the JVP is 4 cm, heart sounds are normal, and there are crackles on inspiration in the right lower lobe. A CXR reveals a new right lower lobe infiltrate and his WBC is 15,000/mL. He was admitted to the hospital 7 days ago for the treatment of congestive heart failure. Which of the following is the most likely diagnosis?

(A) hospital-acquired pneumonia

(B) atelectasis

(C) pulmonary embolism

(D) community-acquired pneumonia

(E) asymmetric congestive heart failure

46. A 74-year-old man residing in a nursing home develops symptoms of high fever, diarrhea, chest pain, and nonproductive cough. His temperature is 40°C, blood pressure 120/80 mm Hg, respiration 24/min, and oxygen saturation 90%. He has bibasilar crackles, normal heart sounds, and a soft nontender abdomen. His CXR reveals bilateral lower lobe infiltrates. He is not able to provide any sputum, and the urine is positive for legionella antigen. Which of the following is the most appropriate antibiotic choice?

(A) trimethoprim-sulfamethoxazole

(B) azithromycin

(C) ceftriaxone

(D) cefuroxime

(E) gentamicin

47. A businesswoman needs to make frequent trips to South America, but every time she is there, she develops traveler's diarrhea, which requires her to change her business schedule. To prevent future episodes during business trips, she is inquiring about prophylaxis methods. Which of the following is the most helpful advice for her?

(A) take loperamide for symptoms

(B) take trimethoprim-sulfamethoxazole every day

(C) take azithromycin every day

(D) take doxycycline every day

(E) take ciprofloxacin only if moderate or severe symptoms develop

48. The dental condition illustrated in Fig. 10–2 is usually associated with a congenital infectious disease. The teeth are characterized by centrally notched, widely spaced, peg-shaped upper central incisors and molars that have poorly developed cusps. Which of the following is the most likely diagnosis?

    (A) congenital rubella
    (B) congenital syphilis
    (C) congenital toxoplasmosis
    (D) congenital HIV
    (E) congenital measles

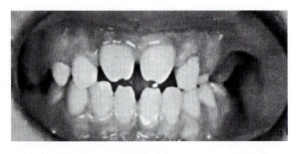

Figure 10–2.

49. A 53-year-old man with alcoholic cirrhosis presents with increasing jaundice and abdominal discomfort. He reports no fevers or chills. On examination, his blood pressure is 100/60 mm Hg, pulse 100/min, temperature 38.1°C. He has a distended abdomen, peripheral edema, and shifting dullness. The abdomen is tender and bowel sounds are present. A diagnostic paracentesis is performed; the total cell count is 940/mL with polymorphonuclear neutrophils (PMNs) equal to 550/mL, Gram stain is negative, and cultures are pending. Which of the following is the most likely diagnosis?

    (A) pancreatic ascites
    (B) malignant ascites
    (C) spontaneous bacterial peritonitis (SBP)
    (D) secondary peritonitis
    (E) tuberculous ascites

50. A 20-year-old woman presents with headache, anorexia, chilly sensations, pain, and drawing sensations in both sides of her jaw. She has also noticed discomfort in both lower abdominal quadrants. Physical examination reveals bilateral enlarged parotid glands that are doughy, elastic, and slightly tender; with a reddened orifice of Stensen's duct. Her abdomen is soft with bilateral lower quadrant abdominal tenderness, a temperature of 38.5°C, and a pulse rate of 92/min. Laboratory data show hemoglobin 13 g/dL; hematocrit 40%; WBC 9000/mL, with 35% segmented neutrophils, 7% monocytes, and 58% lymphocytes. Which of the following is the most likely diagnosis?

    (A) cervical lymphadenitis
    (B) Mikulicz's syndrome
    (C) parotid gland tumor
    (D) uveoparotid fever
    (E) mumps

51. Which of the following statements concerning Lyme disease is correct?

    (A) the incubation period is 3 months
    (B) after an initial brisk immune response, immunity wanes with continuous infection
    (C) the disease is caused by a spirochete
    (D) the disease is caused by a tick
    (E) the characteristic skin lesion of erythema migrans is found in over 95% of cases

52. An 18-year-old woman visits her physician because of 3 weeks of malaise, 2 weeks of fever, and a sore throat. Physical examination shows pharyngeal infection with enlarged tonsils and a patchy, white exudate; enlarged, palpable anterior and posterior cervical, axillary, and inguinal lymph nodes; tenderness in the right upper quadrant; and minimal splenomegaly. Laboratory data show hemoglobin 14 g/dL; hematocrit 42%; platelets 380,000/mL; WBC 8500/mL, with 35% segmented neutrophils, 1% eosinophils, and 64% lymphocytes, of which 36% were atypical. Which of the following is the most likely diagnosis?

    (A) infectious hepatitis
    (B) lymphocytic leukemia
    (C) infectious mononucleosis
    (D) Hodgkin's disease
    (E) cat-scratch fever

53. A 19-year-old woman was traveling in a rural area of South America. She returned 3 weeks ago and, over the past few days, has gradually developed lower abdominal pain and diarrhea. Now the symptoms are much worse with 10 stools a day consisting mostly of mucus and blood. She is afebrile, the abdomen is tender in left lower quadrant, and the remaining examination is normal. Her stool is mostly comprised of blood and mucus. Which of the following is the most likely causative organism?

(A) *Escherichia coli* infection
(B) *Salmonella* infection
(C) *Shigella* infection
(D) *Vibrio parahaemolyticus* infection
(E) *E. histolytica* infection

54. An 18-year-old man develops fever, neck stiffness, and headache. On examination, his blood pressure is 110/80 mm Hg, pulse 100/min, temperature 38.7°C, and neck flexion is very painful. The ears, throat, and sinuses are normal; there are no focal neurologic signs; and the remaining examination is normal. There are no reported similar cases in the community. Which of the following is the most likely causative organism?

(A) *Neisseria meningitides*
(B) *Streptococcus pneumoniae*
(C) *Haemophilus influenzae*
(D) *Staphylococcus*
(E) *Listeria* species

55. A 21-year-old man presents with symptoms of headache, fever, chills, and discomfort in both sides of his jaw. He has also noticed discomfort in his testes, but no dysuria or urethral discharge. Physical examination reveals bilateral enlargement of the parotid glands, as well as bilateral testicular enlargement and tenderness on palpation. His temperature is 38.5°C pulse rate of 92/min, and the remaining examination is normal. Laboratory data show hemoglobin 15 g/dL; hematocrit 40%; WBC 12000/mL, with 30% segmented neutrophils, 8% monocytes, and 62% lymphocytes. Which of the following statements concerning this disease is true?

(A) the disease is caused by a herpesvirus
(B) the incubation period is 3–5 days
(C) the most common complication of this disease in postpubertal boys and men is orchitis
(D) recurrent infections may occur
(E) an increased serum amylase is proof of the existence of pancreatitis as a complication

56. A 43-year-old businesswoman is developing a new enterprise in Mexico. On her most recent trip, she developed diffuse watery diarrhea with severe cramps 1 week after arriving. The illness resolved after about 2 days with no further complications. Which of the following is the most likely causative organism?

(A) *Campylobacter*
(B) *E. coli*
(C) *Salmonella*
(D) *Shigella*
(E) rotavirus

57. A 22-year-old man is an avid spelunker (cave explorer) and has recently been exploring several caves. A routine CXR taken for a new job reveals hilar adenopathy and two patches of pneumonitis. His physical examination is completely normal. Careful questioning reveals he has just gotten over a "cold" with mild fever, cough, and malaise. Which of the following is the most likely diagnosis?

(A) tuberculosis (TB)
(B) sarcoidosis
(C) candidiasis
(D) histoplasmosis
(E) coccidioidomycosis

58. A previously well 28-year-old female has developed gradual onset of fever and malaise over 2–3 weeks. She also complains of arthralgias and myalgias. Repeated measurement of her temperature reveals a low grade fever between 38°C and 39°C. Physical examination reveals an oval retinal hemorrhage with a clear, pale center; a pansystolic cardiac murmur heard best at the apex; and small, tender nodules on her fingertips. Which of the following is the most likely causative organism?

   (A) *Staphylococcus aureus*

   (B) *S. epidermidis*

   (C) *Viridans streptococci*

   (D) *enterococcus*

   (E) *Candida*

DIRECTIONS (Questions 59 through 68): Each set of matching questions in this section consists of a list of lettered options followed by several numbered items. For each numbered item, select the appropriate lettered option(s). Each lettered option may be selected once, more than once, or not at all. EACH ITEM WILL STATE THE NUMBER OF OPTIONS TO SELECT. CHOOSE EXACTLY THIS NUMBER.

Questions 59 through 63

   (A) *Staphylococcus aureus*

   (B) *Candida*

   (C) *P. carinii*

   (D) *Streptococcus pneumoniae*

   (E) Gram-negative enteric bacilli

   (F) *Haemophilus influenzae*

   (G) *Neisseria* species

   (H) *Nocardia* species

   (I) *Salmonella*

   (J) rubella virus

For each patient with impaired immunity, select the most likely pathogen causing infection.

59. A 55-year-old man is receiving chemotherapy for colon cancer. His last dose was 2 weeks ago, and he now has symptoms of fevers and chills but no other localizing symptoms. His

examination is normal except that he is pale. Investigations reveal that he is neutropenic (absolute neutrophil count <500/mL), and his CXR is normal. (SELECT ONE)

60. An 18-year-old man of European decent with selective immunoglobulin A (IgA) deficiency presents with another respiratory tract infection. He has had two episodes of pneumonia in the past year requiring antibiotic therapy. He now has symptoms of fever, cough, and sputum production. His CXR reveals a right lower lobe infiltrate. (SELECT ONE)

61. A 4-year-old boy is diagnosed with an inherited disorder of the complement system after having recurrent sinopulmonary infections. (SELECT THREE)

62. A 24-year-old woman complains of pain in the upper chest every time she eats or drinks anything. She is HIV positive, but currently not on any antiretroviral therapy. Her last CD4 count was 400/mL. (SELECT ONE)

63. A 67-year-old man has back pain and newly discovered hypercalcemia. Further investigations determine that he has multiple lytic lesions, anemia, and a monoclonal protein in his serum. A bone marrow aspirate confirms the diagnosis of multiple myeloma. (SELECT ONE)

Questions 64 through 68

   (A) *Staphylococcus aureus*

   (B) *C. perfringens*

   (C) *Vibrio cholerae*

   (D) enterotoxigenic *E. coli*

   (E) *Salmonella*

   (F) *Shigella*

   (G) *Vibrio parahaemolyticus*

   (H) *Bacillus cereus*

For each patient with foodborne illness, select the most likely pathogen.

64. A 34-year-old woman is at a family picnic where she has a ham sandwich and potato

salad. Three hours after the meal, she feels nauseous and throws up. (SELECT ONE)

65. A 22-year-old university student is backpacking in South America. Ten days after arriving, she develops symptoms of anorexia, malaise, and abdominal cramps followed by a sudden onset of watery diarrhea. There are no symptoms of fever or chills, and the stools are nonbloody. (SELECT ONE)

66. A 24-year-old man is traveling in Southeast Asia. He is eating at local restaurants and from street vendors. He now develops high fevers, anorexia, and frequent passage of small-volume stools containing blood, pus, and mucus. This is associated with severe abdominal cramps and painful straining when having bowel movements. (SELECT ONE)

67. A 27-year-old woman is on holiday on the East coast of the United States. She is at a seafood restaurant and has fresh shellfish for dinner. Twenty-four hours later, she develops symptoms of nausea, vomiting, abdominal cramps, and watery diarrhea. (SELECT ONE)

68. A family of four has dinner at a local Asian restaurant, where multiple dishes are ordered and shared amongst the group. Three hours after the meal, all members develop stomach symptoms consisting of nausea and vomiting. (SELECT ONE)

DIRECTIONS (Questions 69 through 85): This section consists of clinical situations, each followed by a series of questions. Study each situation, and select the ONE best answer to each question following it.

69. A 19-year-old man is seen in the office 9 days after a hiking trip in Colorado. Five days ago, he developed a fever, headache, myalgia, and nausea. Two days later, he noticed the start of a nonitchy rash on his wrists and ankles. He presents today because of light-headedness while standing and progression of the rash on to his body. He reports that he had numerous insect bites during his hike. On examination,

his blood pressure is 90/60 mm Hg, pulse 100/min, and respirations 20/min. There are multiple 1–5 mm macules on his body and some of them have a hemorrhagic center consistent with petechia. His heart sounds are normal, lungs clear, and legs are edematous. Which of the following is the most likely diagnosis?

(A) circulating immune complex disease
(B) a drug reaction
(C) infective endocarditis
(D) Rocky mountain spotted fever (RMSF)
(E) *S. aureus* sepsis

70. A 22-year-old sexually active man presents with painful urination. He reports no joint symptoms, rash, fever, or penile discharge. Examination of the prostate, testes, and penis are normal, and there is no visible discharge that can be expressed from the urethra. Which of the following is the most appropriate initial diagnostic test?

(A) history alone
(B) anterior urethral swab
(C) routine urinalysis
(D) Gram stain of a midstream urine specimen
(E) urine culture

71. A 25-year-old woman has new symptoms of fever, headache, myalgia, and macular rash. She recently went on a camping trip with friends to the South-Central United States. She endured many "bug bites" during the trip but does not specifically recall any tick bites. The rash consists of macules 3 mm in size on her hands and feet. A clinical diagnosis of RMSF is made and she is started on treatment. Serology is drawn to confirm the diagnosis. Which of the following is the most appropriate treatment choice for this condition?

(A) plasmapheresis plus glucocorticoids
(B) ampicillin
(C) vancomycin
(D) erythromycin
(E) doxycycline

72. A 21-year-old man presents with cough, headache, malaise, and fever. He reports minimal whitish sputum production and now has chest soreness from coughing so much. He has no other past medical history and no risk factors for HIV. On examination, his temperature is 38.3°C, pharynx is normal, and lungs are clear. CXR reveals diffuse bilateral infiltrates. Mycoplasma pneumonia is considered in the possible differential diagnosis of his pneumonia. Which of the following skin manifestations is most likely seen in mycoplasma pneumonia?

    (A) erythema nodosum
    (B) erythema multiforme
    (C) maculopapular rash
    (D) vesicular rash
    (E) urticaria

73. A 23-year-old university student presents with painful urination and penile discharge. He is sexually active, and reports no joint symptoms, rash, or fever. Examination of the prostate, testes, and penis are normal, and there is a visible discharge that can be expressed from the urethra. Which of the following is the most likely causative organism?

    (A) *Neisseria gonorrhoeae*
    (B) *Chlamydia trachomatis*
    (C) herpes simplex virus (HSV)
    (D) *Ureaplasma ureolyticum*
    (E) *Mycoplasma genitalium*

74. A 22-year-old woman complains of vulvar itching, burning, and pain when voiding urine. She has no other symptoms of fever, vaginal discharge, or urinary frequency. Physical examination reveals some vulvar ulceration but no vaginal discharge. The ulcers are small 2–3-mm lesions with an erythematous base. Which of the following is the most likely diagnosis?

    (A) HSV infection
    (B) *Trichomonas vaginalis* infection
    (C) *N. gonorrhoeae* infection
    (D) *C. trachomatis* infection
    (E) *M. genitalium* infection

75. A 34-year-old woman presents with symptoms of fever, headache, and myalgia. She recently returned from a camping trip to the South-Central United States. She endured many insect bites during the trip but does not specifically recall any tick bites. On examination her neck is supple, heart sounds are normal, and lungs are clear. She does have a rash consisting of macules 3 mm in size on her hands, feet, and upper body. A clinical diagnosis of RMSF is made and treatment is started. Serology is drawn to confirm the diagnosis. Which of the following sites is the major target for intracellular injury by this infectious agent?

    (A) microcirculation
    (B) liver
    (C) heart
    (D) brain
    (E) kidney

76. A 29-year-old sexually active man presents with painful urination and penile discharge. He reports no joint symptoms, rash, or fever. Examination of the prostate, testes, and penis are normal, and there is a visible discharge that can be expressed from the urethra. Microscopic examination of the appropriate specimens is not possible in this clinic. Which of the following is the most appropriate next step in management?

    (A) send the patient to another clinic for cultures
    (B) treat for *C. trachomatis* with azithromycin
    (C) treat for *N. gonorrhoeae* infection with ceftriaxone
    (D) treat for *N. gonorrhoeae* infection with penicillin
    (E) treat for *C. trachomatis* and *N. gonorrhoeae* with azithromycin and ceftriaxone

77. A 56-year-old previously healthy man is admitted to the hospital for community-acquired pneumonia. He is started on empiric antibiotics. Two days later, his blood cultures are positive of *S. pneumoniae*. Which of the following

statements concerning the epidemiology of *S. pneumoniae* is correct?

(A) most children are nasopharyngeal carriers

(B) most adults are nasopharyngeal carriers

(C) bacteremia is not common in people over 55

(D) in adults, bacteremia is most common in midwinter

(E) bacteremia always occurs with pneumonia

78. A 62-year-old woman presents with fever, cough, sputum production, and pleuritic chest pain. CXR reveals a right middle lobe infiltrate, and she is started on antibiotics for the treatment of pneumonia. Her sputum Gram stain is positive for *S. pneumoniae*. Which of the following immunologic mechanisms is the most specific host defense against pneumococcal infection?

(A) intact splenic function

(B) intact complement function

(C) IgG antibody directed against capsular antigens

(D) alveolar macrophages

(E) liver macrophages

79. A 5-year-old boy presents with ear pain and fever. The left eardrum is inflamed with a small perforation in it and pus is seen in the external canal. A swab of the area grows *S. pneumoniae*. Which of the following is the most likely mechanism for *S. pneumoniae* to cause otitis media?

(A) hematogenous spread

(B) direct extension from the nasopharynx

(C) direct inoculation on the ear

(D) spread through lymphatic tissue

(E) associated dental disease

80. A 31-year-old woman presents with symptoms of vulvar itching and burning made worse by urinating. She has no fever or frequency, but has noticed a recent whitish vaginal discharge. Clinical examination reveals vulvar erythema, edema, and fissures. On speculum examination, there is a white discharge with small white plaques loosely adherent to the vaginal wall. Which of the following treatments is appropriate for her asymptomatic male sexual partner?

(A) azole cream to the penis

(B) oral fluconazole

(C) standard urethritis investigation

(D) no investigation or treatment

(E) azithromycin plus cefixime

81. A 29-year-old man is seen in the office after returning from a hiking trip in Colorado. He complains of feeling unwell and reports symptoms of fever, myalgia, headache, and nausea. Two days ago, he noticed a rash on his wrists and ankles that has now spread to his body. He recalls having had numerous insect bites during his trip. On examination, his blood pressure is 90/60 mm Hg, pulse 100/min, and respirations 20/min. There are multiple 1–5 mm macules on his body and some of them have a hemorrhagic center consistent with a petechia. His neck is supple and fundi are normal. The heart sounds are normal, lungs clear, and legs are edematous. Cranial nerve, motor and sensory examination is normal. A clinical diagnosis of RMSF is made and he is started on appropriate therapy. Which of the following is the most common type of central nervous system (CNS) presentation in this condition?

(A) hemiplegia

(B) cranial nerve abnormalities

(C) paraplegia

(D) encephalitis

(E) ataxia

82. Three individuals living on the same floor in a university dormitory residence develop symptoms and signs of pneumonia. The diagnosis is confirmed by CXR, and sputum samples are positive for *S. pneumoniae*. In an outbreak, which of the following conditions most likely predisposed these three individuals to developing pneumococcal pneumonia?

    (A) immotile cilia syndrome
    (B) previous viral infection
    (C) asthma
    (D) cigarette-induced chronic lung disease
    (E) allergies

83. A 78-year-old woman with a prior stroke is not feeling well. Her appetite is poor, and today her family noticed that she is confused so they sent her to the emergency room. She reports no cough, fever, or sputum production but her CXR reveals a left lower lobe infiltrate. Blood cultures are drawn, and she is started on antibiotics. The next day the cultures are positive for *S. pneumoniae* sensitive to penicillin. Which of the following is the most likely complication of pneumococcal pneumonia?

    (A) peritonitis
    (B) empyema
    (C) pericarditis
    (D) endocarditis
    (E) osteomyelitis

84. A 23-year-old woman presents with cough, malaise, and fever. She reports minimal whitish sputum production and now has chest soreness from coughing so much. She has no other past medical history and no risk factors for HIV. On examination, her temperature is 38.3°C, pharynx is normal, and lungs are clear. CXR reveals diffuse bilateral infiltrates. Mycoplasma pneumonia is considered in the possible differential diagnosis of her pneumonia. Which other symptom besides cough is also prominent in patients with mycoplasma pneumonia?

    (A) sputum
    (B) shortness of breath
    (C) headache

    (D) shaking chills
    (E) pleuritic chest pain

85 A 24-year-old woman has new symptoms of fever, headache, myalgia, and macular rash. She recently went on a camping trip with friends to the South-Central United States. She endured many "bug bites" during the trip but does not specifically recall any tick bites. The rash consists of macules 3 mm in size on her hands and feet. A clinical diagnosis of RMSF is made and she is started on treatment. Serology is drawn to confirm the diagnosis. Which of the following is the most likely causative organism?

    (A) Gram-positive bacterium
    (B) Gram-negative bacterium
    (C) virus
    (D) type of rickettsia
    (E) type of chlamydia

DIRECTIONS (Questions 86 through 105): Each set of matching questions in this section consists of a list of lettered options followed by several numbered items. For each numbered item, select the appropriate lettered option(s). Each lettered option may be selected once, more than once, or not at all. EACH ITEM WILL STATE THE NUMBER OF OPTIONS TO SELECT. CHOOSE EXACTLY THIS NUMBER.

Questions 86 through 90

    (A) beta-lactams (penicillins and cephalosporins)
    (B) vancomycin
    (C) erythromycin
    (D) sulfonamides and trimethoprim
    (E) ciprofloxacin

For each mechanism of antibiotic action, select the most likely drug.

86. Major cellular target is interference with cell metabolism (SELECT ONE)

87. Work by inhibiting DNA synthesis (SELECT ONE)

88. Resistance can be caused by drug inactivation (SELECT ONE)

89. Work by inhibiting protein synthesis (SELECT ONE)

90. Decreased intracellular accumulation can result in resistance (SELECT ONE)

Questions 91 through 95

    (A) erythromycin

    (B) ciprofloxacin

    (C) tetracycline

    (D) sulfonamides

    (E) metronidazole

    (F) rifampin

For each antibiotic side effect, select the most likely drug.

91. Can cause unwanted pregnancy (SELECT ONE)

92. Can contribute to hypoglycemia in non-insulin-dependent diabetes mellitus (NIDDM) (SELECT ONE)

93. Can cause severe reaction to alcohol (SELECT ONE)

94. Drug interaction can result in rejection for transplant recipients (SELECT ONE)

95. Can result in phenytoin toxicity (SELECT ONE)

Questions 96 through 100

    (A) brucellosis

    (B) coccidioidomycosis

    (C) histoplasmosis

    (D) leprosy

    (E) leptospirosis

    (F) infectious mononucleosis

    (G) TB

    (H) tularemia

For each of the following patients, select the most likely diagnosis.

96. A previously healthy 43-year-old man presents with symptoms of cough, fever, weight loss, and lymphadenopathy for the past 2 months. His physical examination reveals multiple axillary and cervical lymph nodes and oropharyngeal ulcerations. His CXR reveals fibronodular pulmonary infiltrates in the apex, his sputum is negative for TB, and the HIV test is negative. A bronchoalveolar lavage (BAL) confirms the diagnosis. (SELECT ONE)

97. A 34-year-old man presents with fever, cough, and sputum production. The CXR reveals a thin-walled pulmonary cavity. His tests for TB and HIV are negative. Four weeks ago, he was traveling in southern California, including visiting the San Joaquin valley. While there he did experience a "flu-like" illness, which slowly improved but then his symptoms of cough and sputum started. A BAL confirmed the diagnosis. (SELECT ONE)

98. A 42-year-old man presents with symptoms of cough, sputum, fever, and weight loss. His CXR reveals upper lobe pulmonary infiltrates and his Mantoux test (purified protein derivative [PPD]) is positive. He emigrated from Southeast Asia 3 years ago. (SELECT ONE)

99. A 25-year-old woman presents with fever, night sweats, and muscles aches for the past 1 month. She was previously well. On examination, she has axillary and cervical lymph nodes, but no active joints or hepatosplenomegaly. She currently works on a hog farm. Her investigations are negative for EBV, CMV, and HIV. Serologic tests for the infecting agent confirm the diagnosis in her. (SELECT ONE)

100. A 42-year-old man presents with sudden-onset fever, chills, headaches, myalgias, and arthralgias. He has no prior medical history, but noticed a new ulcer on his hand 1 week ago. On examination, there is a small "punched out" ulcer, which is erythematous and indurated on his hand, as well as epitrochlear and axillary lymph nodes that are tender. As a hobby, he keeps rabbits in a large pen outside his house and recalls being bitten by one 2 weeks ago. Serologic testing for the organism confirms the diagnosis. (SELECT ONE)

Questions 101 through 105

    (A) toxoplasmosis

    (B) tetanus

    (C) syphilis

    (D) *Streptococcus*

    (E) *Staphylococcus*

    (F) smallpox

    (G) salmonellosis

For each of the following patients, select the most likely infecting organism.

101. A 28-year-old man presents with a new genital ulcer on his penis that is painless. He is sexually active and noticed the lesion 1 week ago. The ulcer is 1 cm in size, has an eroded base, and an indurated margin. Dark-field examination of the ulcer fluid confirmed the diagnosis. (SELECT ONE)

102. Infection with this organism during pregnancy can cause congenital hydrocephalus. (SELECT ONE)

103. A 35-year-old woman develops nausea, vomiting, abdominal pain, and diarrhea 1 day after attending an outdoor picnic. Other people who attended the picnic have similar gastrointestinal symptoms. Most symptomatic individuals recall having egg salad sandwiches. (SELECT ONE)

104. For this infectious disease, preventive measures are no longer used since it has been effectively eradicated. (SELECT ONE)

105. A 34-year-old man who works as a carpenter presents with symptoms of jaw discomfort, dysphagia, and pain as well as stiffness in his neck, back, and shoulders. On examination, he is unable to open his jaw, his proximal limb muscles are stiff as is his abdomen and back, but the hands and feet are relatively spared. He occasionally has violent generalized muscles spasms that cause him to stop breathing, but there is no loss of consciousness. A clinical diagnosis is made and he is treated with antibiotics, antitoxin, and diazepam as well as muscle relaxants for the spasms. (SELECT ONE)

Answers and Explanations

1. **(A)** In tetanus, an acute onset is usual. The median onset is 7 days, and 90% present within 14 days of injury. The organism is an anaerobic, motile Gram-positive rod. It has the ability to survive for years in the form of spores, which are resistant to disinfectants and heat. Tetanus can occur in nonimmunized individuals, or those who have neglected their booster shots. Penicillin, or metronidazole, is used in treatment, but their efficacy is not clear. *(Kasper, p. 842)*

2. **(D)** EIA is an excellent screening test for HIV infection as it is positive in over 99.5% of cases. However, it lacks specificity, and in low risk populations, only about 10% of EIA positive results are true positives. Recent influenza vaccination, acute viral infections, and liver disease are common causes for false positives. The Western blot test is more specific and is the usual confirmatory test, although even more specific tests are now available. *(Kasper, pp. 1100–1101)*

3. **(A)** *S. aureus* causes more than 50% of cases of native valve endocarditis in drug abusers. The onset is usually acute, and the tricuspid valve is the most commonly affected. In staphylococcal tricuspid endocarditis, septic pulmonary emboli are common. Frequently, no murmur is heard. *(Kasper, p. 732)*

4. **(C)** HSV-2 genital infections may be associated with fever, malaise, and anorexia. Vesicular lesions usually ulcerate rapidly and become covered with exudate. There is a 90% chance of recurrent symptoms in the first year following a primary infection. HSV-1 genital infections are similar, but the chance of recurrence is less. *(Kasper, p. 1037)*

5. **(D)** The presence of IgG antibodies by the indirect immunofluorescence test indicates recent or prior EBV infection. IgM antibodies indicate recent infection only. Heterophil antibodies are present in 50% of children and 90–95% of adolescents and adults with infectious mononucleosis. Monospot tests are the best diagnostic tools but may not turn positive until the second or third week of the illness. Specific EBV antibodies and cultures are rarely used. *(Kasper, p. 1047)*

6. **(B)** Current recommendations suggest that mild diarrhea be treated with oral rehydration alone, but when enteric symptoms such as cramps are bothersome, treatment with loperamide or bismuth subsalicylate is warranted. More severe infections with severe diarrhea, severe pain, or fever should be treated with antibiotics such as fluoroquinolones or trimethoprim-sulfamethoxazole. *(Kasper, p. 728)*

7. **(B)** Pain referring to either or both lower quadrants is common when oophoritis is present. Fever usually accompanies oophoritis. Sterility is not a consequence of mumps oophoritis. *(Kasper, p. 1154)*

8. **(B)** Mycoplasmas have no cell walls and have filtration characteristics of viruses, but morphologically are closer to bacteria. The typical *M. pneumoniae* infection produces an influenza-like respiratory illness characterized by headache, malaise, fever, and cough. If pneumonia occurs, physical examination can be

relatively benign despite a grossly abnormal CXR. *(Kasper, p. 1008)*

9. **(A)** The x-ray shows a silhouette sign indicating right middle lobe pneumonia. The organism is most likely to be pneumococcus, but care must be taken to consider blockage of the right middle lobe bronchus. *(Kasper, p. 1533)*

10. **(A)** The cause of cat-scratch fever is a tiny Gram-negative bacillus, *B. henselae.* Cats acquire the organism from the soil and inoculate humans via scratches or bites. The disease is generally benign and self-limited, and is treated with analgesics and antipyretics. Encephalitis, seizures, coma, meningitis, and transverse myelitis can occasionally occur even in immunocompetent patients. A variety of antibiotics have been used when severe disease is present but an optimal regimen has not been identified. *(Kasper, p. 930)*

11. **(B)** This is a typical case of measles. The Koplik's spots in the mouth are easily missed with poor illumination. They are white blue spots of 1 mm on a red background and are not seen in any other infectious disease. The rash of measles becomes confluent while that of rubella does not. Pneumonia is an infrequent complication but accounts for many measles deaths. Giant cell pneumonia is also seen, most commonly in children suffering with a severe disease such as leukemia or immunodeficiency. Aerosolized ribavirin has been used to treat severe pneumonia secondary to measles, but its efficacy is still unclear. The other potentially lethal complication of measles is encephalitis. *(Kasper, p. 1149)*

12. **(E)** About half of all early-onset (<60 days after surgery) prosthetic endocarditis is caused by staphylococcal infection, with *S. epidermidis* predominating. Early-onset prosthetic endocarditis is generally the result of intraoperative contamination of the prosthesis or a bacteremic postoperative complication. *(Kasper, p. 732)*

13. **(D)** This man has a complication of viral influenza; a secondary bacterial pneumonia has developed. This usually occurs 2–3 days after the initial viral symptoms resolve. Primary viral pneumonia with influenza is not common. *S. pneumoniae, Staphylococcus,* and *H. influenzae* are the most common bacterial invaders in pulmonary complications of influenza. Pneumonia is the leading cause of death and may also be due to *S. pneumoniae* and *H. influenzae.* Mixed viral and bacterial pneumonia is common; pure viral pneumonia in influenza is uncommon (but can be very severe). *(Kasper, p. 1068)*

14. **(B)** *S. epidermidis* is still the leading cause of prosthetic valve endocarditis in the early postoperative period (usually defined <2 months). It is usually the consequence of intraoperative contamination or postoperative bacteremia. Endocarditis occurring 12 months after surgery is usually due to the same organisms that cause native valve endocarditis. *(Kasper, p. 736)*

15. **(D)** Although only close contacts need chemoprophylaxis, it is sometimes given more widely than recommended because of community concern. Meningococcal vaccine is effective against serotype A and C, and will prevent late secondary infection in close contacts. Ciprofloxacin or ofloxacin are alternatives to rifampin. *(Kasper, p. 854)*

16. **(C)** The most common cause of non-EBV mononucleosis-type syndrome is CMV. It is the most common presentation of CMV in non-neonates with normal immune function. *(Kasper, p. 1048)*

17. **(A)** Antibiotics, sulfas, steroids, and mumps convalescent sera are of no value. Mouth care, analgesics, and a bland diet are usually recommended. Glucocorticoids are usually prescribed for orchitis, although definite evidence of their effectiveness is lacking. Prevention via vaccination is the preferred strategy for mumps. *(Kasper, p. 1155)*

18. **(A)** The cerebrospinal fluid (CSF) picture in this individual is consistent with viral meningitis rather than a bacterial process. Enteroviruses are a prominent cause of viral meningitis in the summer and fall months. They received

their name because they multiply in the GI tract. Fever, sometimes associated with respiratory symptoms, is the most common sequela of enterovirus infection. There are about 70 enteroviruses that affect humans. These include polioviruses, coxsackieviruses, echoviruses, and others. The spectrum of disease includes paralytic disease, encephalitis, aseptic meningitis, pleurodynia, exanthems, pericarditis, myocarditis, and nonspecific febrile illnesses. They can on occasion cause fulminant disease in a newborn. The most important enteroviruses are the three poliovirus serotypes. *(Kasper, p. 1144)*

19. **(A)** The incubation period of *C. botulinum* toxin is 18–36 hours but ranges from a few hours to days. There are no sensory symptoms. Foodborne botulinum is associated primarily with home-canned food. Severe foodborne botulinum can produce diplopia, dysarthria, and dysphagia; weakness then can progress rapidly to involve the neck, arms, thorax, and legs. There is usually no fever. Nausea, vomiting, and abdominal pain can precede the paralysis or come afterward. *(Kasper, p. 842)*

20. **(D)** Heterophil antibody-negative mononucleosis syndrome is the most common manifestation of CMV infection in immunocompetent adults and is more common than the similar syndrome caused by toxoplasmosis. As of yet, no syndromes caused by HHV-7 have been identified in adults. *(Kasper, p. 1050)*

21. **(E)** Coccidioidomycosis is the usual cause of pulmonary cavitation resulting from fungal infection. A rarefaction may be demonstrable in a pneumonic lesion within 10 days of onset. In the United States, most cases are acquired in California, Arizona, and western Texas. *(Kasper, p. 1181)*

22. **(C)** The most common complication of measles is otitis media, other complications include mastoiditis, pneumonia, bronchitis, encephalitis, and lymphadenitis. Otitis media is usually a bacterial superinfection, and should be treated with antibiotics. *(Kasper, p. 1149)*

23. **(D)** Subacute sclerosing panencephalitis causes involuntary spasmodic movements and progressive mental deterioration, frequently ending in death within a year. It usually occurs in children whose measles occurred at an early age (= 2 years). It occurs 6–8 years after the primary infection. It presents with nonspecific symptoms such as poor school performance or mood and personality changes. It then progresses to intellectual decline, seizures, myoclonus, ataxia, and visual disturbances. Continued deterioration results in inevitable death. *(Kasper, p. 1150)*

24. **(E)** Demonstration of hematophagous trophozoites of *E. histolytica* in stool confirms the diagnosis. The trophozoites are rapidly killed by drying, so wet mounts of stool should be examined. *(Kasper, p. 1216)*

25. **(B)** Since the introduction of *H. influenzae* type B vaccine, *S. pneumoniae* has become the most common type of meningitis in infants and toddlers. *(Kasper, p. 810)*

26. **(D)** Pregnancy or anticipated pregnancy within 4 weeks of vaccination is a contraindication to receiving the rubella vaccine. There is a theoretical concern that fetus might develop congenital rubella syndrome from the live attenuated virus used for the vaccine. Vaccination is usually given to children combined with measles and mumps vaccine between 12 and 15 months of age, and then repeated during childhood at age 4–6 years. It is given even to children with HIV infection. Infants <1 year old can be given the vaccine but may not develop adequate immunity and should still be given the recommended two doses. *(Kasper, p. 1152)*

27. **(C)** The clinical manifestations of infective endocarditis are a result of three factors: (1) direct infection in the heart, (2) septic emboli, and (3) high levels of circulating immune complexes. Glomerulonephritis, arthritis, and many of the mucocutaneous lesions are secondary to circulating immune complexes. Renal emboli cause hematuria and flank pain, but rarely impair renal function. *(Kasper, p.734)*

28. (B) Adequate rest is the treatment of choice, but forced bed rest is not necessary. Glucocorticoids hasten defervescence and resolution of pharyngitis but are not routinely used. Acyclovir halts oropharyngeal shedding of EBV but has minimal effect on the clinical disease. Similarly alpha-interferon and ganciclovir have antiviral efficacy but have no role to play in uncomplicated infectious mononucleosis. Antibiotics are not helpful, and ampicillin is likely to cause a pruritic maculopapular rash in most patients. (*Kasper, p. 1048*)

29. (C) Donovanosis, or granuloma inguinale, is a mildly contagious, chronic, indolent disease that can be sexually transmitted. *Calymmatobacterium granulomatis*, a Gram-negative intracellular bacterium, is felt to be the cause. It is endemic in many tropical areas. Daily doxycycline or weekly azithromycin until the lesions are healed are the usual treatments. Erythromycin is used in pregnant patients. (*Kasper, pp. 932–933*)

30. (B) *S. pneumoniae* colonizes the nasopharynx of 5–10% of healthy adults and up to 20–40% of children. The source of pneumococcal meningitis is either direct extension from middle ear or sinus infections, or via seeding from a bacteremia. In the latter circumstance, bacteremia from pneumonia would be more likely than from infective endocarditis. (*Kasper, pp. 807–808*)

31. (C) The patient is infected with *Pneumocystis* organisms invading an immunocompromised host. The treatment of choice is trimethoprim-sulfamethoxazole. Alternate therapies include pentamidine (highly toxic) and trimetrexate plus folinic acid. (*Kasper, p. 1195*)

32. (D) All the sites mentioned can be involved by amebiasis, but the liver is the most common. Most travelers who develop an amebic liver abscess will do so within a few months of their return. Pleuropulmonary and pericardial involvement results from extension from the liver. (*Kasper, p. 1215*)

33. (D) Acute and convalescent titres of specific IgG antibodies will confirm the diagnosis of mumps. A single test revealing a specific IgM antibody can also confirm the disease. Urine, saliva, and throat swabs will grow the mumps virus, but blood does not. Salivary amylase is elevated but is relatively nonspecific. Of course, a typical presentation during an epidemic probably does not require any confirmatory tests. Sporadic cases require more active confirmation. Other causes of parotitis requiring specific treatment include calculi, bacterial infections, and drugs. Tumors, sarcoid, TB, leukemia, Hodgkin's disease, Sjögren's syndrome, and lupus erythematosus can also cause parotid enlargement. (*Kasper, p. 1155*)

34. (A) Staphylococcal enterotoxin food poisoning is characterized by violent GI upset with severe nausea, cramps, vomiting, and diarrhea. It occurs very rapidly after ingestion (1–6 hours) and usually resolves by 12 hours. (*Kasper, p. 819*)

35. (C) The patient has tinea capitis, which may be caused by *Trichophyton* or *Microsporum* species. It may be successfully treated with topical azole drugs (e.g., clotrimazole). More severe infections are usually treated with systemic medications. (*Kasper, p. 1191*)

36. (C) Coxsackie A viruses may cause a number of syndromes, including herpangina, exanthem, aseptic meningitis, common cold, paralysis, pneumonitis, and summer febrile illness. It is distinguished from HSV-1 herpes stomatitis by the fact that most of the lesions are concentrated in the posterior portion of the mouth and that there is no gingivitis. The other virus does not cause oral lesions. HSV-2 can occasionally cause oral lesions. (*Kasper, p. 1145*)

37. (B) Rabies is transmitted through the saliva of infected animals. Once clinical signs develop, the disease is almost 100% fatal. Symptoms of rabies may include apathy as well as hyperexcitability. Finding Negri bodies in nerve cells of the brain in infected animals confirms the diagnosis. Polymerase chain reaction for detection of viral material is another method of confirming the diagnosis. In cats and dogs that are not available for observation (lasting 10 days) to determine if they have signs of rabies, public health authorities should be consulted to determine the potential risk of rabies in the animal based on local rates of rabies in wild animals. Alternatively if there is a high risk the animal is infected, then postexposure prophylaxis should be started with rabies vaccination on days 0, 3, 7, 14, and 28 as well as one dose of rabies immune globulin on day 0. *(Kasper, p. 1156)*

38. **(C)** EBV genetic material has been found in association with many malignancies. In Africa, about 90% of patients with Burkitt's lymphoma have an association with EBV, but in the United States, only 15% of cases are associated with EBV. In contrast, almost all cases of anaplastic nasopharyngeal carcinoma and also HIV-related CNS lymphomas are associated with EBV genetic material. *(Kasper, p. 1047)*

39. **(C)** Splenic rupture occurs during the second or third week of the illness and can be insidious or abrupt in presentation. Surgery is required. Hemorrhage is not a usual complication of infectious mononucleosis. Over 90% of cases are benign and uncomplicated, but liver involvement is clinical in 5–10%. Over 85% of EBV-associated neurologic problems resolve spontaneously. Although hemorrhage does not occur, autoimmune hemolytic anemia can occur. It is usually mediated by IgM antibodies with anti-i specificity. *(Kasper, p. 1047)*

40. **(B)** Coccidioidomycosis may present with a syndrome of erythema nodosum, fever, and conjunctivitis. Serious complications include cavitating lung lesions or meningitis. *(Kasper, p. 1181)*

41. **(D)** CMV is probably transmitted in the leukocyte component of transfusions. The syndromes include fever and lymphocytosis. Screening donors for this virus reduces the incidence of transmission. *(Kasper, p. 1050)*

42. **(A)** TSS is most characteristically seen in females using vaginal tampons and is secondary to staphylococcal enterotoxins called TSS toxin 1 (TSST-1). Abrupt onset is characteristic. The clinical criteria for diagnosis include high fever, a diffuse rash that desquamates on the

palms and soles over the subsequent 1–2 weeks, hypotension, and involvement in three or more organ systems. This involvement can include GI dysfunction (vomiting and diarrhea), renal insufficiency, hepatic insufficiency, thrombocytopenia, myalgias with elevated creatine kinase (CK) levels, and delirium. Staphylococcal scaled skin syndrome most often affects newborns and children. It results in localized or quite extensive fluid-filled blisters that easily rupture to expose denuded skin. It is caused by an exfoliative toxin. *(Kasper, p. 819)*

43. **(A)** In epidemics, *N. meningitidis* is usually the cause, generally serotype A (sub-Saharan Africa) or C (North America). Serotype B is more common in sporadic outbreaks. *(Kasper, p. 849)*

44. **(A)** Several antibiotic combinations could be used and may vary with the indigenous organisms. Aminoglycoside and cephalosporin are commonly used in combination. The antibiotic combination must cover both Gram-positive and Gram-negative organisms. Antifungal or viral agents are not empirically started unless there is an appropriate clinical fungal or viral infection. In some centers, empiric antifungal agents are started if the patient remains febrile on antibiotics after 5 days. Observation alone is not an option, since these individuals usually have some form of bacteremia causing the fever. *(Kasper, p. 479)*

45. **(A)** Hospital-acquired pneumonia is defined as pneumonia occurring >48 hours after admission and not incubating at the time of admission. It is caused by *S. aureus, Gram-negative bacilli,* or *Streptococcus* pneumoniae. Mixed aerobic and anaerobic infections are also common. Pulmonary embolism is always a consideration in the diagnosis based on clinical probability. The elevated WBC makes atelectasis unlikely and the normal JVP rules out congestive heart failure. *(Kasper, p. 1538)*

46. **(B)** Legionnaires' disease is transmitted via infectious aerosols and may cause severe disease characterized by dry cough and fevers. Mild infections and asymptomatic seroconversion also occur. Natural reservoirs for the

organisms include streams, hot springs, and stagnant lakes. Amplifiers are man-made water supplies that favor growth of *legionellae*. Common amplifiers are hot water systems and heat exchange units. Treatment of choice is either a newer generation macrolide-like azithromycin, or a respiratory quinolone-like levofloxacin or moxifloxacin. Erythromycin is also an option but the newer macrolides are better tolerated. Tetracyclines or TMP/SMX are second line options, and the cephalosporins are not effective for legionella. *(Kasper, p. 872)*

47. **(E)** Prophylactic antibiotics can prevent enteric bacterial infections, but at the cost of drug side effects (rash, *Clostridium difficile* colitis) and the possibility of developing an infection with a drug-resistant organism. Most experts recommend against taking daily prophylaxis unless the consequences of traveler's diarrhea outweigh the risks of the side effects. Such individuals include patients with inflammatory bowel disease (IBD), or immunocompromised states like transplant recipients. Bismuth subsalicylate at a dosage of two tablets (525 mg) four times a day is safe and effective for up to 3 weeks, but can be difficult to take because of the large quantity required. It is also only 60% effective in preventing symptoms. Improving food and drink selection and appropriate caution are the best advice, and medications are only indicated if moderate or severe symptoms develop, including taking loperamide for severe diarrhea. *(Kasper, p. 728)*

48. **(B)** Figure 10–2 illustrates Hutchinson's teeth, which is a manifestation of late congenital syphilis. This may be associated with cardiovascular and neurologic manifestations as well as "saddle nose" and "saber shins." *(Kasper, p. 981)*

49. **(C)** The findings of SBP can be subtle and not as dramatic as that of secondary peritonitis (when bacteria contaminate the peritoneum). As many as 80% of patients with SBP will present with fever. Preexisting ascites is almost always present, but only 10% of cirrhotics at most will develop SBP. The microbiology is characteristically that of a single organism (*E. coli* most commonly). Polymicrobial

infection should suggest the possibility of peritonitis secondary to a perforation. More than 300 PMNs/μL of ascitic fluid is said to be diagnostic. *(Kasper, p. 750)*

50. **(E)** Mumps is an acute, communicable infection with localized swelling of one or more salivary glands. At times, gonads, meninges, pancreas, and other organs can be involved. Up to 25% of infections are inapparent clinically. The virus is transmitted in saliva but is also found in urine, and this might be another source of transmission. *(Kasper, p. 1154)*

51. **(C)** Lyme disease is caused by the spirochete *B. burgdorferi*, a fastidious microaerophilic bacterium. It is a tick-transmitted disease but is not caused by the tick. The incubation period is 3–32 days and is associated, initially, with minimal immune response. Perhaps as many as 25% of patients lack the characteristic skin lesion. *(Kasper, p. 996)*

52. **(C)** Infectious mononucleosis is an acute, self-limited infection of the lymphatic system by the EBV. Typical infectious mononucleosis has an incubation period of 4–8 weeks. The prodrome includes malaise, anorexia, and chills, and then the classic symptoms of pharyngitis, fever, and lymphadenopathy develop. Headache is also common. *(Kasper, p. 1046)*

53. **(E)** The time course, clinical features, and stool examination are characteristic of intestinal amebiasis. It is very common in most developing countries in the tropics and infects about 10% of the world's population. It is the third most common cause of death from parasitic disease. *(Kasper, p. 1215)*

54. **(B)** In adults (age >15 years), *S. pneumoniae* is the single most common organism, accounting for one-third to one-half of all cases. This pneumococcal predominance is even more pronounced in sporadic cases. *(Kasper, p. 2471)*

55. **(C)** Orchitis occurs in about 20% of males, but is usually unilateral, thus sterility is rare. The disease is caused by a paramyxovirus and one infection confers lifelong immunity. The incubation

period is 14–18 days. Serum amylase is elevated in most cases of mumps because of parotitis, not pancreatitis. Other complications include thyroiditis, myocarditis, and polyarthritis. *(Kasper, p. 1154)*

56. **(B)** The most common cause of traveler's diarrhea worldwide is toxigenic *E. coli*. In North Africa and Southeast Asia, *Campylobacter* infections predominate. Other causative organisms include *Salmonella*, *Shigella*, rotavirus, and the Norwalk agent. The most common parasite causing traveler's diarrhea is *Giardia lamblia*. *(Kasper, p. 728)*

57. **(D)** *Histoplasma capsulatum* is a dimorphic fungus with worldwide distribution. In the United States, it is particularly common in Southeastern, mid-Atlantic, and Central states. It is frequently found in soil enriched by droppings of certain birds and bats. Caves are common sites of infection. Most infections are asymptomatic or mild and require no therapy. Acute disseminated infection usually occurs in patients with HIV infection or other immunocompromised states, but chronic dissemination can occur in immunocompetent patients. Findings may include hepatosplenomegaly, lymphadenopathy, anemia, and Addison's disease. Mediastinal fibrosis can result in superior vena cava compression. Fibrosis can also involve the pulmonary arteries, esophagus, and pulmonary veins. Only rare nonviable organisms are found on pathologic examination in such cases. The prognosis is generally poor. *(Kasper p. 1179)*

58. **(C)** This woman likely has native valve endocarditis, probably in the setting of a previous valvular abnormality. Streptococci cause over half the cases of native valve endocarditis in nonintravenous drug abusers. Of these, 75% are viridans streptococci. *Streptococcus bovis* is the most common nonviridans streptococcus causing endocarditis and is usually found in the older population (60 years), particularly if bowel lesions are present. Staphylococcal endocarditis is the next most common type, but it is usually associated with a more acute

presentation. Enterococci cause about 6% of cases in native valve endocarditis, but fungi are rare causes. *(Kasper, p. 732)*

59. **(E)** Cytotoxic chemotherapy frequently results in neutropenia and subsequently Gram-negative bacillary infection. *Pseudomonas*, *Staphylococcus*, *Candida*, and *Aspergillus* infections are also common. *(Kasper, p. 479)*

60. **(D)** Selective immunoglobulin A (IgA) deficiency predisposes to *G. lamblia* infection, hepatitis virus, and *S. pneumoniae*. *H. influenzae* infection occurs, but this is not as characteristic as *Giardia*. *(Kasper, p. 1944)*

61. **(D, F, G)** Defects in the complement pathway predisposes individuals to recurrent infections with encapsulated organisms such as *H. influenzae*, *Neisseria* species, or *S. pneumonia*. *(Kasper, p. 1928)*

62. **(B)** All forms of T-lymphocyte deficiency/dysfunction are characterized by candidal infections. *Candida* species can cause thrush, skin lesions, esophagitis, and cystitis. Hematogenous spread can occur and disseminate the organism widely in individuals with low CD4 counts. *(Kasper, pp. 1940–1941)*

63. **(D)** Patients with myeloma have defects in humoral immunity and are prone to recurrent pneumonias due to *S. pneumoniae*. Lung infections with *S. aureus* and *Klebsiella pneumoniae* are also frequent. *E. coli* and other Gram-negatives cause recurrent urinary tract infections. *(Kasper, p. 657)*

64. **(A)** The preformed toxin of *Staphylococcus* causes nausea within 1–6 hours of ingestion. Ham, poultry, potato and egg salad, mayonnaise, and cream pastries are common food sources. *(Kasper, p. 819)*

65. **(D)** Enterotoxigenic *E. coli* causes 15–50% of traveler's diarrhea, depending on geographic location. The incubation period is more than 16 hours, and water and many foods can be the source. *(Kasper, p. 728)*

66. **(F)** *Shigella* causes an invasive diarrhea with blood and has an incubation period of more than 16 hours. Potato and egg salad, lettuce, and raw vegetables are common food sources. *(Kasper, p. 904)*

67. **(C)** *Vibrio cholerae* causes profuse watery diarrhea with an incubation period of more than 16 hours. Shellfish are a common source. *(Kasper, p. 912)*

68. **(H)** *B. cereus* causes an early onset of food poisoning when found in fried rice. This occurs within 1–6 hours and, like staphylococcal food poisoning, is characterized by vomiting. The enteric form of *B. cereus* food poisoning is characterized by watery diarrhea and occurs 8–16 hours after ingestion of contaminated food such as meat, vegetables, dried beans, or cereals. *(Kasper, p. 758)*

69. **(D)** The location of infection, the possibility of tick exposure, and the nonspecific nature of the presentation are consistent with a rickettsial infection, likely RMSF. *(Kasper, p. 1000)*

70. **(B)** The diagnosis is usually made by proximal to distal "milking of the urethra" and showing evidence of a purulent or mucopurulent discharge. Other methods include examining a urethral swab or the sediment from the first 20–30 mL of voided urine (after the patient has not voided for several hours). Dysuria without inflammation may represent a functional problem and usually does not benefit from antibiotics. *(Kasper, p. 764)*

71. **(E)** Doxycycline is the treatment of choice, with tetracycline as the second choice. There is insufficient evidence to determine the exact role of fluoroquinolones in RMSF. Beta-lactam antibiotics, erythromycin, and aminoglycosides are of no value. Sulfa-containing drugs may actually exacerbate the condition. Glucocorticoids have not been shown to be helpful, but meticulous control of volume status is important. *(Kasper, p. 1001)*

72. **(B)** Although all the skin problems listed have been described with *M. pneumoniae* infection, the only clearly linked entity is erythema multiforme. *(Kasper, p. 1009)*

73. **(B)** *C. trachomatis* causes 30–40% of cases in the United States. The exact prevalence depends on the effectiveness of *Chlamydial* control programs in the population. The other organisms can all cause urethritis in men. *(Kasper, p. 763)*

74. **(A)** HSV and *C. albicans* are the common causes of vulvar infection. Although they can cause dysuria, it is of the "external" variety (i.e., secondary to urine passing over the inflamed vulvar area). The other infections cause "internal dysuria" and/or vaginal discharge. *(Kasper, p. 765)*

75. **(A)** Pulmonary and systemic microcirculation are the primary targets of the disease. The resultant damage results in increased vascular permeability. This can cause edema, decreased plasma volume, decreased albumin, prerenal azotemia, and even hypotension. Involvement of the pulmonary microcirculation can result in noncardiogenic pulmonary edema. *(Kasper, p. 1000)*

76. **(E)** Empiric treatment should include coverage for both *Chlamydial* infection (with azithromycin) and *N. gonorrhoeae* infection (usually with ceftriaxone). There are numerous alternatives for *N. gonorrhoeae* infection, such as oral cefixime (not available in the United States), oral ciprofloxacin, or intramuscular (IM) ceftriaxone. However, resistance to penicillin is too common to allow the routine use of this drug. *(Kasper, p. 765)*

77. **(D)** There is a definite midwinter spike in bacteremia in adults, but not in children. Invasive disease is highest in children under 2 years of age. Bacteremia is more common in certain groups (e.g., Native Americans, Native Alaskans, African Americans), suggesting a genetic predisposition. Up to 40% of healthy children and 10% of healthy adults are asymptomatic

carriers. In adults, the organism can persist in the nasopharynx for up to 6 months. *(Kasper, p. 806)*

78. **(C)** The most specific immunologic defense is directed at capsular antigens and is serotype specific. Antibodies are not naturally occurring, but are the result of prior colonization, infection, or vaccination. Intact spleen, complement and macrophage function is important in clearance of pneumococci from sterile areas, but specific immunoglobulin G (IgG) antibody coating of a pneumococcal polysaccharide capsule is essential for macrophages to ingest and kill the bacteria. *(Kasper, p. 807)*

79. **(B)** Infections of the middle ear, trachea, sinuses, bronchi, and lungs are caused by direct spread from nasopharyngeal colonization. Disease of the CNS, heart valves, bones, joints, and peritoneal are usually caused by hematogenous dissemination. *(Kasper, p. 808)*

80. **(D)** There is no need to investigate or treat an asymptomatic male partner. If candidal dermatitis of the penis is present, topical azole therapy would be appropriate. *(Kasper, p. 768)*

81. **(D)** Although all these can be manifestations of RMSF, encephalitis as manifested by confusion or lethargy is by far the most common CNS manifestation. It occurs in about one-quarter of cases, and can progress to coma. *(Kasper, p. 1001)*

82. **(B)** It is possible that such outbreaks can occur in people with no predisposing factors, unlike the vast majority of sporadic cases. However, the only common predisposing factor in a young healthy population such as this would be a previous viral respiratory infection. *(Kasper, p. 807)*

83. **(B)** Approximately 2% of cases of pneumococcal pneumonia are complicated by empyema. However, not all pleural effusions in the setting of pneumococcal pneumonia represent pleural infection. Frank pus, a positive Gram stain, or a pH = 7.1 on thoracentesis suggest empyema and the need for aggressive drainage. *(Kasper, p. 810)*

84. **(C)** The most common presentation is with cough and headache. Both can be quite severe. Cough becomes more prominent if a lower respiratory tract infection ensues, but sputum production is not usually prominent. Shaking chills and pleuritic chest pain are quite uncommon. *(Kasper, p. 1009)*

85. **(D)** RMSF is the most severe of the rickettsial diseases and has been documented in 48 American states, Canada, and parts of Central and South America. The specific tick that is the vector for this rickettsial disease varies in different geographical locations. *(Kasper, p. 999)*

86. **(D)** Sulfonamides and trimethoprim competitively inhibit enzymes involved in folic acid biosynthesis. *(Kasper, pp. 789–793)*

87. **(E)** Ciprofloxacin, rifampin, and metronidazole inhibit DNA synthesis, albeit by different mechanisms. *(Kasper, pp. 789–793)*

88. **(A)** Beta-lactams can be inactivated by beta-lactamase. *(Kasper, pp. 789–793)*

89. **(C)** Macrolides (clarithromycin, azithromycin, erythromycin), lincosamides (clindamycin), and chloramphenicol inhibit protein synthesis by binding to the 50S ribosomal subunit. Tetracyclines and aminoglycosides inhibit protein synthesis by binding to the 30S ribosomal subunit. *(Kasper, pp. 789–793)*

90. **(E)** Some Gram-negative bacteria acquire mutations in their outer membrane pori, so they are no longer permeable to ciprofloxacin. Some Gram-positive bacteria develop a mutation that allows them to actively pump the drug out. The most common form of resistance, however, is a mutation in the DNA gyrase, which is the target of ciprofloxacin action. *(Kasper, pp. 789–793)*

91. **(F)** Rifampin is an excellent inducer of many cytochrome P450 enzymes and increases the hepatic clearance of a number of drugs, including oral contraceptives. *(Kasper, p. 789–806)*

92. (D) Sulfonamides potentiate the effects of oral hypoglycemics through reduction in metabolism or displacement from serum protein. *(Kasper, pp. 789–806)*

93. (E) Metronidazole can cause a disulfiram-like syndrome when alcohol is ingested. Instructions to avoid alcohol should be given when this drug is prescribed. *(Kasper, pp. 789–806)*

94. (F) Rifampin's enzyme-induction properties can result in increased metabolism of cyclosporine, with resultant organ rejection. In contrast, erythromycin inhibits the enzyme involved in cyclosporine metabolism and can result in enhanced toxicity. *(Kasper, pp. 789–806)*

95. (D) Sulfonamides may potentiate the effects of phenytoin through reduction in metabolism or displacement from serum protein. *(Kasper, pp. 789–806)*

96. (C) Disseminated histoplasmosis has many features in common with hematogenously disseminated TB. Common findings include fever, weight loss, cough, lymphadenopathy, anemia, abnormal liver enzymes, and hepatosplenomegaly. The chronic pulmonary disease is characterized by cough, increasing sputum production, and apical infiltrates. One-third improve or stabilize spontaneously while the remainder progress slowly to develop cavitation of the upper lobes and altered pulmonary function. In histoplasmosis, oropharyngeal ulcerations begin as solitary indurated plaques with no pain present at first, although eventually pain becomes deep-seated. These oropharyngeal manifestations are usually part of disseminated infection. *(Kasper, p. 1179)*

97. (B) In coccidioidomycosis, hemoptysis may call attention to cavitations, or patients may complain of pain at the cavity site. Only half of the patients with a thin-walled pulmonary cavity secondary to coccidioidomycosis will have symptoms, however. *(Kasper, p. 1180)*

98. (G) The intracutaneous tuberculin test with purified protein derivative (PPD) is read for evidence of delayed hypersensitivity at 48 hours. Although induration >10 mm is felt to be positive, interpretation is really dependent on the population being studied. In an HIV-infected patient, any reaction should be considered significant. When testing household contacts, >5 mm is probably enough to warrant prophylactic treatment. *(Kasper, p. 953)*

99. (A) In the United States, brucellosis is rare and found most commonly among farmers, meat-processing workers, and veterinarians. Transmission is by contact of *Brucella* organisms with abraded skin, through the conjunctiva, or by inhalation. Person-to-person transmission is rare or nonexistent. The disease can be acute, localized, or chronic. It requires prolonged antibiotic treatment. A typical treatment course would be doxycycline plus an aminoglycoside for 4 weeks followed by a further 4 weeks of doxycycline and rifampin. *(Kasper, p. 914)*

100. (H) Tularemia can be acquired through direct contact with an infected rabbit, which may occur in preparation or cooking inadequately. The incubation period is 2–5 days, and the syndrome includes fevers, chills, headaches, myalgias, and tender hepatosplenomegaly. In addition, specific syndromes such as ulceroglandular or oculoglandular tularemia can accompany the nonspecific syndrome. *(Kasper, p. 917)*

101. (C) On dark-field examination, *T. pallidum* (the spirochete that causes syphilis) is a thin, delicate organism with tapering ends and 6–14 spirals. When dark-field examination is not possible, direct fluorescent antibody tests are used. *(Kasper, p. 977)*

102. (A) Congenital toxoplasmosis is initiated in utero usually as a complication of a primary infection. Infants may be asymptomatic at birth but later can present with a multitude of signs and symptoms, including chorioretinitis, strabismus, epilepsy, and psychomotor retardation. The presence of hydrocephalus is a bad prognostic sign. *(Kasper, p. 1243)*

103. **(G)** Salmonellosis is an acute infection resulting from ingestion of food containing bacteria and is characterized by abdominal pain and diarrhea. *Salmonella* gastroenteritis is not usually treated with antibiotics because the length of the illness is not shortened, but the length of time the organism is carried is increased. Antibiotics are used for more serious systemic *Salmonella* infections. *(Kasper, p. 897)*

104. **(F)** Preventive measures are not used because smallpox is thought to be eradicated worldwide, and vaccination may be associated with serious side effects. As humans are the only reservoir for smallpox, there is no longer any risk of infection from natural sources. However, smallpox could be used in bioterrorism. *(Kasper, p. 1284)*

105. **(B)** Patients with tetanus develop hypertonus, seizures, respiratory distress, and asphyxia unless they are treated with diazepam and muscle relaxants. The treatment of tetanus requires diazepam, muscle relaxants, antitoxin, respiratory care, and managing autonomic dysfunction. Antibiotics are given but are probably of little help. *(Kasper, p. 840)*

CHAPTER 11

Immunology and Allergy
Questions

DIRECTIONS (Questions 1 through 20): Each of the numbered items in this section is followed by answers. Select the ONE lettered answer that is BEST in each case.

1. A 29-year-old woman is being treated with penicillin for "strep throat." She develops arthralgia, lymphadenopathy, urticaria, and an active urine sediment 6 days after starting the antibiotics. Which of the following is the most likely mechanism of this drug reaction?

   (A) immunoglobulin E (IgE) release
   (B) mast cell degranulation
   (C) immediate-type hypersensitivity
   (D) macrophage-endothelial cell interaction
   (E) circulating immune complexes

2. A 24-year-old man is diagnosed with disseminated histoplasmosis after developing symptoms of fever, lymphadenopathy, hepatosplenomegaly, and pancytopenia. Which of the following is the body's major immunologic defense against histoplasmosis?

   (A) immunoglobulin G (IgG) antibodies
   (B) mononuclear leukocytes
   (C) complement
   (D) immunoglobulin M (IgM) antibody
   (E) neutrophils

3. Which of the following are large, granular lymphoid cells that are mediators of antibody-dependent cellular cytotoxicity?

   (A) macrophages
   (B) natural killer (NK) cells
   (C) T lymphocytes, suppressor subset
   (D) B lymphocytes
   (E) granulocytes

4. A 9-year-old boy presents with sneezing, runny nose, and nasal congestion. The symptoms are seasonal and worse in the spring time. He is diagnosed with hay fever (allergic rhinitis). Which of the following statements about hay fever is correct?

   (A) sufferers may develop asthma
   (B) symptoms are not improved by moving to different locations
   (C) sufferers are less prone to develop upper respiratory infections (URIs)
   (D) sufferers are severely disturbed emotionally
   (E) hay fever can be improved symptomatically only with steroids

5. A 19-year-old man has recurrent attacks of gastrointestinal colic and swelling of his face and legs. There is no relationship of the attacks to any foods or activity. His father has a similar syndrome. Which of the following is the most likely cause of death in this disease?

   (A) an unrelated condition
   (B) an anaphylactic shock reaction
   (C) edema of the glottis
   (D) overtreatment
   (E) a reaction

6. A 34-year-old woman with human immunodeficiency virus (HIV) has a routine complete blood count performed. She was diagnosed 2 years ago, and is currently doing well with no symptoms and not on any antiretroviral therapy. Which of the following changes is most likely seen on her peripheral blood cell counts?

   (A) granulocytosis
   (B) lymphopenia
   (C) increased helper T cells
   (D) monocytosis
   (E) decreased NK cells

7. A 30-year-old woman with myasthenia gravis is found to have an autoimmune hemolytic anemia. The chest x-ray (CXR) reveals an anterior mediastinal mass. Which of the following is the most likely diagnosis?

   (A) thymoma
   (B) nodular sclerosing Hodgkin's disease
   (C) small cleaved cell non-Hodgkin's lymphoma
   (D) teratoma
   (E) bronchogenic carcinoma, small cell undifferentiated type

8. A 19-year-old man presents with coughing up blood and decreased urine output. On examination, he has normal air entry, and heart sounds. There is no skin rash or lymph nodes and his abdomen is normal. CXR reveals patchy infiltrates in both lower lobes and his creatinine is elevated. Urinalysis is positive for red cells and protein. A renal biopsy reveals autoantibodies to basement membranes. Which of the following is the most likely diagnosis?

   (A) thyroiditis
   (B) myasthenia gravis
   (C) Goodpasture's syndrome
   (D) thrombocytopenia
   (E) hemolytic anemia

9. A 25-year-old woman presents with decreased urine output, new leg edema, and facial swelling. She was previously well with no past medical history. Laboratory investigations reveal acute renal failure and a renal biopsy is performed. Immunofluorescence of the biopsy specimen reveals a granular pattern of immune complex-mediated glomerulonephritis. Which of the following conditions is most likely to cause this pattern of renal injury? (See Fig. 11–1.)

   (A) acute tubular necrosis (ATN)
   (B) Wegener's granulomatosis
   (C) postinfectious glomerulonephritis
   (D) hemolytic uremic syndrome (HUS)
   (E) Goodpasture's syndrome

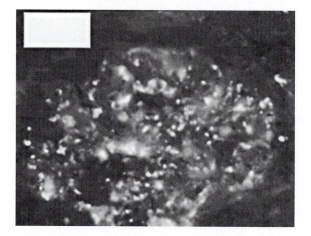

Figure 11–1.

10. A 25-year-old woman has been getting desensitization shots for an allergy for 1 year. Today she developed diffuse urticaria 5 minutes after the injection. Which of the following is the most appropriate next step in management?

   (A) discontinuation of subsequent injections for 3 weeks
   (B) application of a tourniquet distal to the injection site
   (C) administration of steroids prior to the next injection
   (D) administration of aminophylline subcutaneously
   (E) administration of epinephrine (1:1000) subcutaneously

11. A 23-year-old man treated for strep throat with penicillin develops arthralgia, urticaria, and lymphadenopathy. Urinalysis reveals red cell casts. Which of the following is characteristic of the syndrome?

(A) it usually requires corticosteroids

(B) symptoms last several months

(C) it may recur after apparent recovery

(D) it may be transferred by leukocyte infusions

(E) most patients are children

12. A 22-year-old woman has recurrent fungal infections and is suspected of having immunodeficiency secondary to impaired T-cell function. Which of the following is the most cost-effective screening test of cellular immunity?

(A) quantification of serum immunoglobulin A (IgA)

(B) lymphocyte enumeration on a cell sorter

(C) lymphocyte responses to mitogens

(D) nitroblue tetrazolium assay

(E) intradermal skin test with *Candida albicans*

13. A 19-year-old female university student unwittingly eats shrimp in the dormitory dining room. Over the next 20 minutes, acute skin lesions consisting of erythematous, elevated wheals appear. Which of the following is most characteristic of these lesions? (See Fig. 11–2.)

(A) are most common on the palms and soles

(B) are rarely itchy

(C) do not blanch on pressure

(D) are caused by a localized vasculitis

(E) are caused by an ongoing, immediate, hypersensitivity reaction

14. A 27-year-old man develops small (several millimeters) pruritic wheals when he goes jogging and when he takes very hot showers. Which of the following is most appropriate in the management of this condition?

(A) discontinuation of all vigorous exercises

(B) counseling regarding recognition and treatment of anaphylactic reactions

(C) treatment with anticholinergic medications

(D) treatment with hydroxyzine

(E) cool baths rather than hot showers

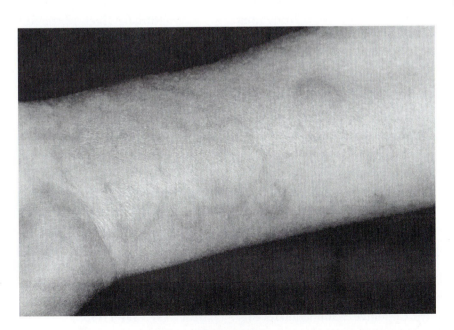

Figure 11–2.

15. A 42-year-old man has an allergy to penicillin. He is given cephalexin for a skin infection on his finger after a cut became infected. He now develops angioedema after drug exposure. Which of the following physical findings is characteristic of this syndrome?

(A) invariably severe itching

(B) prolonged nature of the edema

(C) fluid extravasation from subcutaneous and intradermal postcapillary venules

(D) involvement of lips, tongue, eyelids, genitalia, and dorsum of hands or feet

(E) fluid accumulation in the most dependent areas of the body

16. A 47-year-old woman, with Type I diabetes of 30 years' duration, is in the hospital for assessment of atypical chest pain. While in the hospital, she develops a true anaphylactic reaction. Which of the following is the most likely cause for the reaction?

(A) radiographic contrast media

(B) erythromycin

(C) insulin

(D) folic acid supplement

(E) exposure to nuts

17. A 27-year-old long-time intravenous (IV) drug user has recurrent infections and a low CD4$^+$ count. Which factor is true concerning this immunosuppression?

(A) qualitative defects in T lymphocytes follow quantitative problems

(B) the low CD4 count in advanced disease is secondary to the direct cytotoxic effects of virus infection

(C) B-lymphocyte abnormalities do not occur early in the disease

(D) macrophages are important in viral dissemination

(E) circulating immune complexes are rarely present

18. A 24-year-old man with known HIV infection presents with a right hemiparesis that developed over several days. Cognitive examination reveals global impairment, and a computed tomography (CT) scan reveals multiple cortical lesions that are spherical and ring enhancing. Which of the following is the most likely diagnosis?

(A) glioblastoma multiforme

(B) toxoplasmosis

(C) lymphoma

(D) progressive multifocal leukoencephalopathy

(E) cytomegalovirus (CMV)

19. A 23-year-old woman has had several episodes of severe wheezing over the past 3 years. She is a nonsmoker and feels well in between episodes. She has no personal or family history of atopy. The wheezing episodes are most likely to occur in spring. Which of the following is the most likely mechanism of wheezing in this woman?

(A) elevated IgE levels

(B) mast cell instability

(C) nonspecific hyperirritability of the tracheobronchial tree

(D) disordered immediate hypersensitivity

(E) disordered delayed hypersensitivity

20. A 45-year-old man with severe asthma is doing well after a recent exacerbation requiring hospital admission. He is interested in avoiding any potential agents that might trigger his asthma. Which of the following foods is most likely to precipitate an asthmatic reaction in this man?

(A) red meat

(B) egg whites

(C) green salad

(D) gluten

(E) mayonnaise

DIRECTIONS (Questions 21 through 36): Each set of matching questions in this section consists of a list of lettered options followed by several numbered items. For each numbered item, select the appropriate lettered option(s). Each lettered option may be selected once, more than once, or not at all. EACH ITEM WILL STATE THE NUMBER OF OPTIONS TO SELECT. CHOOSE EXACTLY THIS NUMBER.

Questions 21 through 23

    (A) allergic reaction caused by sensitized mast cells

    (B) may be mediated by drug effect on kinin system

    (C) final mediator of symptoms are leukotrienes

For each patient with symptoms after taking a new medication, select the most likely mechanism.

21. A 23-year-old man has a reaction after being given oral penicillin for a sore throat. (SELECT ONE)

22. A 56-year-old woman is given an angiotensin-converting enzyme (ACE) inhibitor for control of hypertension and develops a reaction consisting of urticaria. (SELECT ONE)

23. A 23-year-old man has an exacerbation of asthma when he takes aspirin for a headache. (SELECT ONE)

Questions 24 through 30

    (A) human lymphocyte antigen (HLA) B27

    (B) HLA DR4

    (C) HLA DR3

    (D) HLA B17

    (E) HLA B8

    (F) multigenic disorder

Match the following diseases with the appropriate HLA.

24. A 29-year-old man presents with severe back pain and a red eye. The pain is located in his lower back and gluteal area, and is associated with morning stiffness that improves after several hours. On examination, he has limited forward flexion and tenderness of the ischial tuberosities. (SELECT ONE)

25. A 24-year-old woman has a facial skin lesion, thrombocytopenia, arthralgia, and pericarditis. (SELECT ONE)

26. A 12-year-old child has severe deforming arthritis of the hands. (SELECT ONE)

27. A 14-year-old girl presents with weight loss, increased thirst, and urination. Her laboratory tests reveal hyperglycemia and a mildly increased anion gap metabolic acidosis. (SELECT ONE)

28. A 22-year-old man with iritis, balanitis, urethritis, and arthritis. (SELECT ONE)

29. A 27-year-old woman has severe symmetrical small joint arthritis. She notices 1 hour of morning stiffness and swelling with redness in her wrists and hand joints. The distal finger joints are spared. X-rays of the hands reveal early bone erosion in some of the joints. (SELECT ONE)

30. A 33-year-old policeman develops acute asymmetric arthritis involving his left knee and ankle and right ankle. The pain in the feet prevents him from walking. He recalls having a diarrheal illness 3 weeks ago. (SELECT ONE)

Questions 31 through 36

    (A) B-cell deficiency/dysfunction

    (B) mixed T- and B-cell deficiency/dysfunction

    (C) T-lymphocyte deficiency/dysfunction

    (D) neutropenia

    (E) chemotaxis

    (F) C3 (complement 3) deficiency

For each patient with a medical condition, select the most likely immune dysfunction.

31. A 73-year-old man has a history of recurrent pneumonias. He now complains of bone discomfort in his back and chest. X-rays reveal multiple lytic lesions and his serum protein electrophoresis has an IgG spike of 12 g/dL. (SELECT ONE)

32. A 22-year-old woman notices multiple lymph nodes in her neck. They are nontender on palpation and mobile. A monospot test is negative and a biopsy of the node reveals Hodgkin's disease. (SELECT ONE)

33. A 73-year-old man has 30,000/mL mature lymphocytes on his blood film. This is an incidental finding and he is clinically feeling well. (SELECT ONE)

34. A 24-year-old woman with malar rash, thrombocytopenia, and arthralgia. (SELECT ONE)

35. A 69-year-old man is receiving chemotherapy for acute myeloid leukemia. (SELECT ONE)

36. A young woman with ataxia-telangiectasia syndrome. (SELECT ONE)

Answers and Explanations

1. **(E)** Drug hypersensitivity is the most common cause of serum sickness. It is believed that the drug acts as a hapten binding to a plasma protein. The resultant drug-protein complex induces an immune response. Common signs and symptoms include fever, skin rash (urticarial or morbilliform), arthralgias, lymphadenopathy, and albuminuria. Arthritis, nephritis, neuropathy, and vasculitis are less common. Primary sensitization requires 1–3 weeks, but symptoms can occur rapidly on reexposure. *(Kasper, p. 319)*

2. **(B)** The major reaction to fungal infections such as histoplasmosis is delayed-type hypersensitivity. This is a reaction of T cells, which have been stimulated by antigen to react against infectious agents, grafts, and tumors. A classic example is the response to the tuberculin skin test in a person previously exposed to *Mycobacterium tuberculosis* organisms which occurs between 48 and 72 hours after antigen exposure. *(Kasper, pp. 1179, 1940–1941)*

3. **(B)** NK cells may be of T-cell lineage or monocyte-macrophage lineage. They appear to play an important role in surveillance mechanisms. *(Braunwald, pp. 1911–1913)*

4. **(A)** Allergic asthma is often associated with a personal and/or family history of allergic diseases. It is dependent on an IgE response controlled by T and B lymphocytes and activated when antigens interact with mast cell-bound IgE molecules. Most provoking allergens are airborne. Allergic asthma can be seasonal. *(Kasper, pp. 1954–1955)*

5. **(C)** Hereditary angioedema is an autosomal dominant condition. The lesions are tense, rounded, nonpitting, and several centimeters in diameter. The edema, unlike urticaria, involves deeper tissue and is not pruritic. Edema of the glottis is the usual cause of death. *(Kasper, pp. 1951–1953)*

6. **(B)** Acquired immune deficiency syndrome (AIDS) is characterized by lymphopenia, with a selective diminution of helper T cells. Likely infectious complications and their appropriate prophylaxis can be predicted by the CD4 T-lymphocyte count. Lymphocyte dysfunction can occur even when severe lymphopenia is not yet present. *(Kasper, pp. 1104–1105)*

7. **(A)** Thymic tumors may be associated with myasthenia gravis, red cell aplasia, polymyositis, hemolytic anemia, pemphigus, and agranulocytosis. There is also an association with immunodeficiency and thymoma. These patients have B-lymphocyte deficiency and bacterial infections and diarrhea. Erythroid aplasia may develop as well. *(Kasper, pp. 2518–2522)*

8. **(C)** Autoantibodies can be demonstrated by immunofluorescence or electron microscopy on the basement membranes of glomeruli and alveoli in Goodpasture's syndrome. The disease is most common in young men but can strike at any age. The hemoptysis can be minimal or massive. The course of the hemoptysis is variable, but renal involvement is often progressive. Current therapy includes intensive plasma exchange, cytotoxic agents, and glucocorticoids. Other causes of lung-renal syndromes

such as various vasculitides, Wegener's granulomatosis, mixed essential cryoglobulinemia, Henoch-Schönlein purpura, and systemic lupus erythematosus (SLE) are not characterized by antibodies to basement membranes. *(Kasper, pp. 1560, 1676–1677)*

9. **(C)** Immune complexes are not detected in ATN, Wegener's, HUS, or Goodpasture's syndrome. Immune complexes with low complement levels can be seen in idiopathic and postinfectious glomerulonephritis, lupus, cryoglobulinemia, shunt nephritis, and bacterial endocarditis. Immune complexes with normal complement levels are found in IgA nephropathy and Henoch-Schönlein purpura. *(Kasper, pp. 1680–1681)*

10. **(E)** These systemic reactions are uncommon and easily managed in the office if detected, but if the patient leaves too soon, it could be dangerous. The exact mechanism of benefit for hyposensitization therapy is unclear. No single measurement of immune function correlates well with clinical efficacy, suggesting a complex of effects that likely includes a reduction in T-cell cytokine production. This type of therapy is reserved for clearly seasonal diseases that cannot be adequately managed with drugs. *(Kasper, pp. 1949–1950)*

11. **(C)** The symptoms of serum sickness are usually self-limited and may recur after apparent recovery. The natural course is 1–3 weeks. Recurrence can occur rapidly (12–36 hours) if repeat exposure to the offending antigen occurs. *(Kasper, pp. 319, 2013)*

12. **(E)** A positive skin test with *C. albicans* extract (erythema and induration of 10 mm or more at 48 hours) excludes virtually all primary T-cell defects. Lymphocyte enumeration and responses to mitogens are much costlier tests. Serum IgA levels are a good screening test for agammaglobulinemia, and the nitroblue tetrazolium assay is useful to detect killing defects of phagocyte cells. *(Kasper, pp. 1940–1941)*

13. **(E)** Although urticaria can involve any epidermal or mucosal surface, the palms and soles are usually spared. The associated itching indicates

stimulation of nociceptive nerves. The increased blood flow results in erythema that blanches on pressure. An ongoing, immediate hypersensitivity reaction in association with degranulation of mast cells is the most common cause. *(Kasper, pp. 1949–1950)*

14. **(D)** This represents a case of generalized heat urticaria or cholinergic urticaria rather than exercise-induced urticaria. The latter is characterized by larger lesions and possible anaphylactic reactions and is not triggered by hot showers. Although thought to be cholinergically mediated, atropine does not block symptoms in generalized heat urticaria. Because anaphylaxis does not occur and hydroxyzine is so effective, hot showers are not a great danger. *(Kasper, pp. 1951–1953)*

15. **(D)** Angioedema is often not itchy and, like urticaria, is transient; manifestation peaks in minutes to hours and disappears over hours to days. The fluid extravasates from deeper areas such as dermal and subdermal sites. Unlike other causes of edema, angioedema is not dependent and can involve all epidermal and submucosal surfaces, although the lips, tongue, eyelids, genitalia, hands, and feet are the most commonly involved. *(Kasper, p. 1951)*

16. **(E)** Anaphylaxis is characterized by an initial exposure followed by the formation of specific IgE antibody. Repeat exposure results in antigen combining with IgE bound to basophils and mast cells and subsequent degranulation. Anaphylactoid reactions, such as those to radiographic contrast media, are generally not immunemediated and do not require prior exposure. Insulin and folic acid rarely cause anaphylaxis. Similarly, erythromycin is not a common antibiotic to cause anaphylaxis. Nuts, eggs, seafood, and chocolate are among the many foods implicated in anaphylaxis. *(Kasper, pp. 1949–1950)*

17. **(D)** Even in advanced AIDS, only a minority of CD4$^+$ lymphocytes are actually infected. Numerous other factors, including "innocent bystander destruction" and autoimmune phenomena, might be implicated. Impaired soluble

antigen recognition by T lymphocytes can occur when absolute counts are still normal. Polyclonal activation of B cells, which occurs early in the disease, is unlikely to be triggered by direct HIV infection of B cells. Macrophages are felt to be particularly important in carrying the virus across the blood-brain barrier. Circulating immune complexes might help explain arthralgias, myalgias, renal disease, and vasculitis that occur in infected individuals. *(Kasper, pp. 1086–1087)*

18. **(B)** The three most common causes of focal brain lesion in HIV disease are toxoplasmosis, primary central nervous system (CNS) lymphoma, and progressive multifocal leukoencephalopathy (PML). Toxoplasmosis lesions are typically multiple, spherical, and ring-enhancing on CT scan. They are most likely located in the basal ganglia and the cortex. The symptoms develop characteristically over days and global brain dysfunction is common. Lymphoma presents with one or relatively few irregular weakly enhancing lesions more commonly in the periventricular area. PML presents with multiple nonenhancing lesions in the white matter. CMV, herpes, and *Cryptococcus* generally cause diffuse brain disease. Glioblastoma multiforme is not characteristic of HIV disease. *(Kasper, pp. 1115–1119)*

19. **(C)** There is a constant state of hyperreactivity of the bronchi, during which exposure to an irritant precipitates an asthmatic attack. A following subacute phase has been described that can lead to late complications. The presence of inflammation in the airways has resulted in increased usage of inhaled corticosteroids for maintenance therapy. Many cases of asthma have no discernible allergic component. *(Kasper, pp. 1508–1509)*

20. **(C)** Sulfites, used to keep salad greens fresh, can cause severe asthmatic reactions. Other sulfite-containing foods include fresh fruits, potatoes, shellfish, and wine. Aspirin, tartrazine (a coloring agent), and beta-adrenergic agonists also commonly provoke asthmatic attacks. *(Kasper, p. 1510)*

21. **(A)** Penicillin can cause numerous allergic reactions, including anaphylaxis, interstitial nephritis, rashes (the most common manifestation), urticaria, fever, pneumonitis, dermatitis, and even asthma in workers exposed to airborne penicillin. Hemolytic anemia is often IgG-mediated. Skin tests are reliable in predicting low risk (similar to general population) for those claiming previous penicillin reactions, and desensitization is feasible. The frequency of reactions to cephalosporins in penicillin-allergic patients is not definitely known. *(Kasper, pp. 1947–1951)*

22. **(B)** ACE inhibitors can cause angioedema of the face and oropharyngeal structures. This is felt to be a pseudoallergic reaction, possibly due to the drug's effect on the kinin system. It is thought that reactions may be more common in women, Blacks, and those with idiopathic angioedema. If this occurs, therapy with alternate ACE inhibitors should not be attempted. *(Kasper, pp. 1951–1953)*

23. **(C)** Aspirin frequently can precipitate asthma in susceptible individuals. At highest risk are asthmatics with chronic rhinosinusitis and nasal polyps. This is probably a pseudoallergic reaction related to inhibition of cyclooxygenase with a resultant enhancement of leukotriene synthesis or effect. Densensitization regimens have been developed. *(Kasper, p. 1510)*

24. **(A)** Ankylosing spondylitis and HLA B27 *(Kasper, pp. 1994–1995)*

25. **(F)** SLE is a multigenic disorder. *(Kasper, pp. 1960–1961)*

26. **(B)** Juvenile rheumatoid arthritis (RA) and HLA DR4 *(Kasper, p. 1968)*

27. **(C)** Type I diabetes mellitus and HLA DR3 *(Kasper, p. 2156)*

28. **(A)** Reiter syndrome and HLA B27 *(Kasper, pp. 1996–1997)*

29. **(B)** RA and HLA DR4 *(Kasper, p. 1968)*

30. **(A)** Reactive arthritis (e.g., *Shigella* or *Yersinia*) and HLA B27 *(Kasper, pp. 1996–1997)*

The relationship between HLA antigens and diseases is not absolute, but rather one of increased relative risk. The presence of HLA B27 increases the relative risk of ankylosing spondylitis by a factor of about 80, of Reiter syndrome by a factor of 40, and also increases the likelihood of reactive arthritis. The presence of HLA DR4 increases the likelihood of juvenile RA by a factor of 7 and RA by a factor of 6. The presence of HLA DR3 increases the likelihood of both SLE and insulin-dependent diabetes mellitus by a factor of approximately 3.

31. **(A)** Multiple myeloma and B-cell deficiency/dysfunction *(Kasper, pp. 656–657)*

32. **(C)** Hodgkin's disease and T-cell deficiency/dysfunction *(Kasper, pp. 654–655)*

33. **(A)** Chronic lymphocytic leukemia and B-cell deficiency/dysfunction *(Kasper, pp. 648–649)*

34. **(F)** SLE and complement deficiency *(Kasper, pp. 1960–1961)*

35. **(D)** Therapy for hematologic malignancy and neutropenia *(Kasper, p. 635)*

36. **(B)** Ataxia-telangiectasia and both T- and B-cell dysfunction *(Kasper, p. 2423)*

Multiple myeloma and chronic lymphocytic leukemia are two of the more common causes of B-cell deficiency/dysfunction. Hodgkin's disease, AIDS, sarcoidosis, and thymic aplasia or hypoplasia result in T-lymphocyte depletion/dysfunction. SLE has been associated with C3 deficiency, but most severe complement deficiencies result from inherited disorders. Ataxiatelangiectasia, common variable hypogammaglobulinemia, severe combined immunodeficiency, and Wiskott-Aldrich syndrome have mixed T- and B-cell deficiency.

CHAPTER 12

Diseases of the Respiratory System
Questions

DIRECTIONS (Questions 1 through 52): Each of the numbered items in this section is followed by answers. Select the ONE lettered answer that is BEST in each case.

1. A 33-year-old farmer complains of recurrent episodes of wheezing after working in a barn where hay is stored. On auscultation, there are bibasilar crackles and heart sounds are normal. His laboratory work is normal with no increase in eosinophils and the chest x-ray (CXR) reveals patchy lower lobe infiltrates. Which of the following is the most likely diagnosis?

   (A) asthma
   (B) chronic obstructive lung disease
   (C) hypersensitivity pneumonitis
   (D) bronchiectasis
   (E) sarcoidosis

2. A 57-year-old man with a 40-pack-per-year history of smoking experiences symptoms of shortness of breath on exertion. He has bilateral wheezes on expiration and increased resonance to percussion of the chest. Pulmonary function tests confirm the diagnosis of chronic obstructive lung disease (COPD). Which of the following is the best definition of this condition?

   (A) it is caused by bronchial asthma
   (B) it is preceded by chronic bronchitis
   (C) it is airflow limitation that is not fully reversible
   (D) it is due to destruction and dilatation of lung alveoli
   (E) is due to small airways disease only

3. An agitated and nervous 24-year-old woman has had severe wheezing and shortness of breath for 2 days. After receiving oxygen, steroids, and salbutamol (Ventolin) in the emergency room, her breathing improves. She is still wheezing and now feels tremulous and anxious with a pulse of 110/min and respirations 30/min. Arterial blood gases on oxygen reveal a pH of 7.40, P_{O_2} 340 mm Hg, P_{CO_2} 40 mm Hg, and bicarbonate of 24 mEq/L. She is hospitalized for further treatment. Which of the following treatments or medications should be avoided in her?

   (A) theophylline
   (B) sedatives
   (C) corticosteroids
   (D) sympathomimetic amines
   (E) intravenous (IV) fluids

4. A 29-year-old woman has a long history of mild asthma. She now has a flare and experiences recurrent episodes of bronchial obstruction, fever, malaise, and expectoration of brownish mucous plugs. On examination, there is bilateral wheezing. Infection is suspected and a CXR reveals upper lobe pulmonary infiltrates. The eosinophil count is 2000/mL, and serum precipitating antibodies to *Aspergillus* are positive. Which of the following is the most appropriate next step in management?

   (A) antihelminthic therapy
   (B) a short course of systemic glucocorticoid therapy
   (C) desensitization treatment
   (D) high-dose glucocorticoids by puffer
   (E) long-term systemic glucocorticoid therapy

5. A 31-year-old African American man presents with dyspnea on exertion. He also has fever and red tender rash on his shins. Physical examination reveals fine inspiratory crackles in both lower lung lobes and tender erythematous nodules on his legs. CXR shows bilateral hilar adenopathy and reticulonodular changes in both lungs. Transbronchial biopsy reveals noncaseating granulomas. Which of the following is the most appropriate next step in management?

(A) aspirin

(B) isoniazid (INH) and streptomycin

(C) steroids

(D) nitrogen mustard

(E) no therapy

6. A 53-year-old man with a long respiratory history is admitted to the hospital because of increasing shortness of breath and sputum production. He is started on antibiotics and inhaled bronchodilators and anticholinergic agents. The next day he is found in his room confused and sleepy. A P_{CO_2} determination reveals severe hypercarbia (P_{CO_2} 70 mmHg). Which of the following explanations regarding his elevated P_{CO_2} is correct?

(A) occurs only with CO_2 inhalation

(B) does not occur in obstructive lung disease

(C) does not occur in restrictive lung disease

(D) may worsen with oxygen administration

(E) occurs with chronic hypocapnia

7. A 63-year-old woman is seen in the emergency room with acute shortness of breath. There is no history of heart or lung problems in the past. She was recently diagnosed with breast cancer and is undergoing active treatment. On examination, her blood pressure is 120/80 mm Hg, pulse 100/min, and heart and lungs are normal. There are no clinical signs of deep venous thrombosis (DVT). Which of the following investigations is most likely to rule out a pulmonary embolism (PE)?

(A) normal CXR

(B) normal electrocardiogram (ECG)

(C) normal ventilation-perfusion lung scan

(D) normal ventilation scan

(E) normal magnetic resonance image (MRI)

8. A 40-year-old woman has been complaining of a 3-year history of increasing dyspnea and fatigue. She has no other medical illness. Physical examination reveals increased jugular venous pressure (JVP) with prominent *c-v* wave, and a reduced carotid pulse. Precordial examination reveals a left parasternal lift, loud P_2, and right-sided S_3 and S_4. There are no audible murmurs. CXR reveals clear lung fields and an ECG shows evidence of right ventricular hypertrophy. Pulmonary function tests show a slight restrictive pattern. Primary pulmonary hypertension is suspected. Which of the following is the most appropriate test to confirm the diagnosis?

(A) open lung biopsy

(B) pulmonary angiography

(C) cardiac catheterization

(D) noninvasive exercise testing

(E) electrophysiologic testing

9. A 63-year-old man is having symptoms of shortness of breath. As part of his workup, an arterial blood gas is done and the P_{CO_2} is 60 mm Hg. Which of the following is the most likely cause for the elevated P_{CO_2}?

(A) ventilation-perfusion ratio inequality

(B) right-to-left shunt

(C) impaired diffusion

(D) hypoventilation

(E) carbon monoxide poisoning

10. A 56-year-old man is evaluated for chronic cough. It is present most of the time and is progressively getting worse over the past 3 years. With the cough he usually has white to yellow sputum that he has to expectorate. There is no history of wheezing, asthma, congestive heart failure (CHF), or acid reflux disease. He currently smokes one pack a day for the past 25 years. On examination, his chest is clear. CXR is normal and his forced expiratory volume in

1 second (FEV1) and forced vital capacity (FVC) on spirometry are normal. Which of the following is the most likely diagnosis?

(A) chronic obstructive pulmonary disease (COPD)
(B) early cor pulmonale
(C) chronic bronchitis
(D) asthma
(E) emphysema

11. A 58-year-old man is recently diagnosed with bowel cancer. He now complains of vague chest discomfort and shortness of breath. On examination, he is unwell, blood pressure 90/50 mm Hg, pulse 110/min, respirations 26/min, and oxygen saturation 88%. His lungs are normal on auscultation, the JVP is 8 cm, and P_2 is loud. There is no edema or leg tenderness on palpation. A quantitative (ELISA) D-dimer assay is positive, ECG reveals sinus tachycardia, and cardiac enzymes are negative. The lung scan is read as high probability for PE. Which of the following tests is most likely to help in guiding emergent therapy?

(A) echocardiogram
(B) CT scan
(C) venous ultrasound of the legs
(D) contrast phlebography
(E) pulmonary function tests

12. A 40-year-old man has a routine CXR, which reveals a posterior mediastinal mass. Which of the following is the most likely diagnosis?

(A) lipoma
(B) neurogenic tumor
(C) esophageal cyst
(D) fibroma
(E) bronchogenic cyst

13. A 35-year-old man is evaluated for symptoms of shortness of breath. He reports no other lung or heart disease. He smokes half pack a day for the past 10 years. On examination, his JVP is 2 cm, heart sounds normal, and lungs are clear. A CXR shows hyperinflation and increased lucency of the lung fields. A chest CT reveals bullae and emphysematous changes, while

pulmonary function tests show an FEV1/FVC ratio of <70%. Evaluation of his family reveals other affected individuals. Which of the following is the most likely diagnosis?

(A) alpha1-antitrypsin deficiency
(B) beta-glycosidase deficiency
(C) glucose-6-phosphatase deficiency
(D) glucocerebrosides deficiency
(E) growth hormone deficiency

14. A 23-year-old man notices a gradual but progressive increase in breathing difficulty. He has a long history of back pain with prolonged morning stiffness. He has also had an episode of iritis in the past. On examination, there is reduced range of motion in the lumbar spine with forward flexion and pain on palpation of the sacroiliac joint and surrounding soft tissue. X-rays of the pelvis show erosions and sclerosis of the sacroiliac joint. Which of the following is the most likely pulmonary complication of this condition?

(A) fibrocavitary disease
(B) airflow obstruction
(C) bilateral lower lobe involvement
(D) pleural effusions
(E) hilar adenopathy

15. A 44-year-old woman has been complaining of a 4-year history of increasing dyspnea and fatigue. Physical examination reveals increased JVP and a reduced carotid pulse. Precordial examination reveals a left parasternal lift, loud P_2, and right-sided S_3 and S_4. There are no audible murmurs. CXR reveals clear lung fields and an ECG shows evidence of right ventricular hypertrophy. Pulmonary function tests show a slight restrictive pattern. A diagnosis of primary pulmonary hypertension is made. Which of the following is the most likely cause of death in this condition?

(A) intractable left ventricular failure
(B) intractable respiratory failure
(C) massive PE
(D) intractable right ventricular failure or sudden death
(E) myocardial infarction

16. A patient with hypoxemia, hypercapnia, and polycythemia is able to restore his blood gases to normal by voluntary hyperventilation. Which of the following is the most likely location for the abnormalities seen on his blood gases?

    (A) cerebral cortex
    (B) bone marrow
    (C) ventricular septum
    (D) respiratory center
    (E) cerebellum

17. A 63-year-old woman presents with dyspnea and coughing up foul smelling purulent sputum. She has had many similar episodes in the past. There are no other constitutional symptoms and she denies excessive alcohol intake. On physical examination, she appears chronically ill with clubbing of the fingers. Heart sounds are normal, JVP is measured at 4 cm, and there are inspiratory crackles heard at the lung bases posteriorly. There is no hepatosplenomegaly or any palpable lymph nodes. CXR shows scaring in the left lower lobe, which on chest CT scan is identified as cystic changes with airway dilatation and bronchial wall thickening. Which of the following is the most appropriate initial next step in management?

    (A) antibiotics and postural drainage
    (B) steroids
    (C) radiotherapy
    (D) aerosols
    (E) INH

18. A 32-year-old man develops symptoms of wheezing, cough, and shortness of breath. He has bilateral expiratory wheezes, and the rest of the examination is normal. Further evaluation with pulmonary function tests reveals a reduced FEV1/FVC ratio that corrects with bronchodilators. Which of the following statements about a diagnosis of idiosyncratic asthma (also called nonatopic) is correct?

    (A) known antigenic stimulus
    (B) adult onset
    (C) history of atopy

    (D) positive skin tests
    (E) high immunoglobulin E (IgE) levels

19. A 20-year-old African American woman presents with mild dyspnea on exertion and joint discomfort in her knees, wrists, and ankles. She also has a fever and red tender rash on her shins. Physical examination reveals hepatosplenomegaly, generalized lymphadenopathy, corneal opacities, and tender erythematous nodules on her legs. CXR shows bilateral symmetric hilar adenopathy. Transbronchial biopsy reveals noncaseating granulomas. Which of the following is the most likely cause for the eye lesion?

    (A) uveitis
    (B) diabetic complications
    (C) steroids
    (D) congenital origin
    (E) infectious infiltration

20. A 74-year-old man with a history of smoking notices blood in his chronic daily sputum production. He has no fever or chills, but has lost 10 lb in the past 6 months. On examination, he has bilateral expiratory wheezes, and his fingers are clubbed. There are no lymph nodes and the remaining examination is normal. CXR reveals a left hilar mass. Which of the following suggests that the tumor is a small cell lung cancer?

    (A) syndrome of inappropriate antidiuretic hormone (SIADH) secretion
    (B) acanthosis nigricans
    (C) Cushing's syndrome
    (D) leukemoid reaction
    (E) Stevens-Johnson syndrome

21. A 66-year-old man with chronic alcoholism has had a low grade fever and cough for several weeks. His heart sounds are normal and there are crackles in the left lower base. A CXR reveals a left lower lobe lung abscess. Which of the following is the most appropriate therapy?

    (A) penicillin
    (B) clindamycin
    (C) ceftriaxone

(D) metronidazole

(E) metronidazole plus respiratory fluoroquinolone (levofloxacin)

22. A 44-year-old woman presents with increased shortness of breath, cough, and sputum production. She has had asthma since childhood and uses her medications as directed. Recently, she noticed that her peak flow readings were decreasing after the symptoms started. On examination, she is in moderate respiratory distress, respirations 25/min, there are bilateral wheezes and oxygen saturation is 90% on room air. On her blood gas, the P_{CO_2} is 50 mm Hg. Which of the following is the most likely mechanism for her carbon dioxide retention?

(A) impaired diffusion syndromes

(B) right-to-left shunt

(C) hyperventilation

(D) ventilation-perfusion ratio inequality

(E) mechanical ventilation at fixed volume

23. A previously well 53-year-old man develops progressive shortness of breath. Pulmonary function tests reveal a restrictive defect and a high-resolution CT suggests pulmonary fibrosis. Which of the following is the most likely role of transbronchial biopsy in this condition?

(A) assess disease severity

(B) assess possible bronchiolar narrowing

(C) diagnose specific causes of interstitial lung disease

(D) determine degree of inflammation

(E) diagnose possible cancer

24. A 28-year-old man presents with coughing up blood and sputum. He gives a history of recurrent pneumonias and a chronic cough productive of foul-smelling purulent sputum. He has no other past medical history and is a lifetime nonsmoker. On physical examination, there are no oral lesions, heart sounds are normal, and wet inspiratory crackles are heard at the lung bases posteriorly. He also has clubbing of his fingers, but there is no hepatosplenomegaly or any palpable lymph nodes. CXR show fibrosis and pulmonary infiltrates in the right lower lung. Which of the following is the most appropriate initial diagnostic test?

(A) chest CT scan

(B) bronchoscopy

(C) bronchography

(D) open thoracotomy

(E) bronchoalveolar lavage

25. A 38-year-old woman has been complaining of a 2-year history of increasing dyspnea and fatigue. Physical examination reveals increased JVP and a reduced carotid pulse. Precordial examination reveals a left parasternal lift, loud P_2, and right-sided S_3 and S_4. There are no audible murmurs. CXR reveals clear lung fields and an ECG shows evidence of right ventricular hypertrophy. Pulmonary function tests show a slight restrictive pattern. Primary pulmonary hypertension is diagnosed. Which of the following treatments is helpful in this condition?

(A) corticosteroids

(B) nitrates

(C) alpha-adrenergic blockers

(D) calcium channel blockers

(E) angiotensin-converting enzyme (ACE) inhibitors

26. A 64-year-old woman is admitted to the hospital with right lobar pneumonia and sepsis syndrome. She becomes progressively more short of breath and hypoxemic requiring intubation and mechanical ventilation. Her repeat CXR in the intensive care unit now shows diffuse pulmonary infiltrates and a diagnosis of acute respiratory distress syndrome (ARDS) is made. Which of the following mechanisms is the most likely cause for the early "exudative" phase of ARDS?

(A) increased lung compliance

(B) increased interstitial fibrosis

(C) increased vascular permeability to fluid and proteins

(D) decreased pulmonary perfusion

(E) decreased ventilatory dead space

27. A 23-year-old man is experiencing a flare of his asthma. He is using his salbutamol inhaler more frequently than usual and despite increasing his inhaled steroids he is still short of breath. Previously his asthma was considered mild with no severe exacerbations requiring oral steroids or hospitalization. With his flare, he has recurrent episodes of bronchial obstruction, fever, malaise, and expectoration of brownish mucous plugs. On examination, there is bilateral wheezing. The heart, abdomen, neurologic, and skin exams are normal. CXR reveals upper lobe pulmonary infiltrates; the eosinophil count is 3000/mL, and serum precipitating antibodies to *Aspergillus* are positive. Which of the following is the most likely diagnosis?

   (A) ascaris infestation
   (B) allergic bronchopulmonary aspergillosis
   (C) Churg-Strauss allergic granulomatosis
   (D) Löeffler's syndrome
   (E) hypereosinophilic syndrome

28. A 34-year-old African American man presents with mild dyspnea on exertion and joint discomfort in his knees, wrists, and ankles. He also has a fever and red tender rash on his shins. Physical examination reveals hepatosplenomegaly, generalized lymphadenopathy, and tender erythematous nodules on his legs. CXR shows bilateral symmetric hilar adenopathy. Which of the following laboratory findings is not characteristic of this condition?

   (A) hyperglobulinemia
   (B) elevated ACE level
   (C) elevated sedimentation rate (ESR)
   (D) elevated serum calcium
   (E) normal gallium scan

29. A 66-year-old man has progressive shortness of breath due to COPD. He is currently able to do his activities of daily living, but has trouble walking more than one block. His physical examination reveals hyperinflation, increased resonance to percussion, and bilateral expiratory wheezes. He is on appropriate medical therapy for his stage of COPD. Which of the

following is also indicated in the management of this condition?

   (A) meningococcal vaccination
   (B) yearly influenza vaccination
   (C) weight reduction if obese
   (D) *Haemophilus influenzae B* vaccination
   (E) pneumococcal vaccination

30. A 45-year-old woman has severe symptoms of epigastric and abdominal pain after eating. A trial of acid suppression therapy with proton pump inhibitors (PPI) only partially improved her symptoms. She undergoes elective outpatient upper endoscopy, which is positive for a small duodenal ulcer. Two hours later, she is short of breath and complaining of severe anterior chest pain, which is made worse with deep inspiration. On examination, she looks unwell, blood pressure is 150/90 mm Hg, pulse 110/min, and lungs are clear. Heart sounds are normal but an extra "crunching" type sound is intermittently heard. CXR demonstrates air surrounding the heart. Which of the following is the most likely diagnosis?

   (A) acute pericarditis
   (B) acute cardiac ischemia
   (C) acute mediastinitis
   (D) aortic dissection
   (E) pneumothorax

31. Which of the following is most likely associated with cystic fibrosis in an adult patient?

   (A) spontaneous remission
   (B) good pancreatic exocrine function
   (C) hemoptysis
   (D) rectal polyps
   (E) normal sweat chloride

32. A 55-year-old woman is in the intensive care unit on a ventilator for hypoxemia following "flash" pulmonary edema. Her Po_2 on the blood gas prior to intubation was 44 mm Hg, and now while breathing 100% oxygen on the ventilator her repeat blood gas reveals a Po_2 of 80 mm Hg. Hypoxemia while receiving

100% oxygen indicates which of the following problems?

(A) ventilation-perfusion ratio inequality

(B) right-to-left shunt

(C) hypoventilation

(D) impaired diffusion

(E) interstitial lung disease

33. A 31-year-old man with severe kyphoscoliosis due to cerebral palsy is experiencing worsening shortness of breath with exertion. On examination, he has a severe scoliosis to the left and decreased air entry to that side. His right lung is clear, JVP is 3 cm, and heart sounds are normal. Pulmonary function tests are performed. Which of the following is the most likely abnormality to be seen on the pulmonary function tests?

(A) increased total lung capacity (TLC)

(B) increased functional residual capacity (FRC)

(C) decreased TLC

(D) increased compliance

(E) increased vital capacity (VC)

34. A 67-year-old woman has pulmonary function tests performed to evaluate symptoms of dyspnea. The most prominent finding is a reduction of the ratio of FEV1/FVC. Which of the following is the most likely diagnosis?

(A) COPD

(B) ankylosing spondylitis

(C) pickwickian syndrome

(D) scleroderma of the chest wall

(E) lobar pneumonia

35. Which of the following statements concerning asbestosis is correct?

(A) the type of asbestos fiber is crucial in determining whether asbestos-related lung disease occurs

(B) moderate rather than severe obstruction to airflow is characteristic of asbestosis

(C) mesothelioma is the common malignancy associated with asbestosis

(D) pleural effusions are invariably associated with malignancy in asbestosis

(E) short-term (i.e., 1–2 years) exposure can result in serious sequelae decades later

36. A 52-year-old man develops sudden-onset shortness of breath on postoperative day 4 after a hemicolectomy for colon cancer. His surgery went well with no operative complications. He reports no cough, sputum, or pleuritic chest pain. His blood pressure is 155/90 mm Hg, pulse 100/min, temperature 37.8°C, lungs are clear, and heart sounds normal. He has bilateral pedal edema, but no discomfort in his legs. His CXR and ECG are normal. A chest CT with contrast reveals a thrombus in his right upper lobe artery. Which of the following statements concerning the management of this condition is most likely correct?

(A) continuous IV heparin or subcutaneous low-molecular-weight heparin (LMWH) therapy is indicated

(B) urgent thrombolytic therapy is indicated

(C) urgent inferior vena cava (IVC)

(D) filter insertion is indicated

(E) confirmation of the diagnosis with bilateral ultrasound leg Dopplers

37. A 55-year-old woman presents with coughing up blood and sputum. She gives a history of recurrent pneumonias and a chronic cough productive of foul-smelling purulent sputum. The sputum production is worse on lying down and in the morning. On physical examination, she appears chronically ill with clubbing of the fingers. Wet inspiratory crackles are heard at the lung bases posteriorly. There are no hepatosplenomegaly or any palpable lymph nodes. CXR shows scaring in the right lower lobe, which on chest CT scan is identified as airway dilatation, bronchial wall thickening, and grapelike cysts. Which of the following is a recognized precursor to this patient's condition?

(A) bronchial asthma

(B) cigarette smoking

(C) lung infection and impairment of drainage

(D) lung cancer

(E) silicosis

38. A 50-year-old man presents with excessive day-time sleepiness and a history of snoring. One week ago, he fell asleep while driving his car and got into a minor accident. On examination, he is obese (body mass index [BMI] >30) and his blood pressure is 160/90 mm Hg. His lungs are clear and heart sounds are distant. Which of the following is the most likely explanation for the symptoms associated with this condition?

    (A) related to cardiac dysfunction
    (B) neuropsychiatric and behavioral
    (C) pulmonary
    (D) gastrointestinal (GI)
    (E) musculoskeletal

39. Which of the following statements concerning hypoxemia in COPD is correct?

    (A) erythrocytosis is an appropriate compensation for hypoxemia, and phlebotomy will worsen symptoms
    (B) nocturnal oxygen therapy is effective in producing symptomatic and hemodynamic improvement in severe hypoxia
    (C) a P_{O_2} of 58 mm Hg is an indication for continuous oxygen therapy
    (D) a P_{O_2} of 65 mm Hg or below is an indication for supplemental oxygen during air travel
    (E) continuous supplemental oxygen improves functional ability but does not alter the natural history of obstructive airways disease with severe hypoxemia

40. A 58-year-old steam pipe worker presents with a vague ache in the left chest and mild dyspnea of several months' duration. There is dullness on percussion of the left chest associated with diminished breath sounds. His CXR is shown in Fig. 12–1. Which of the following is the most likely diagnosis?

    (A) pleural metastases
    (B) Paget's disease
    (C) mesothelioma and asbestosis
    (D) pleural effusion
    (E) multiple myeloma

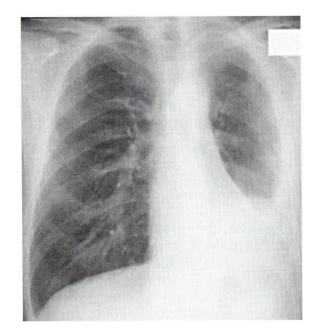

Figure 12–1.

41. A 23-year-old man presents with coughing up blood and sputum. He gives a history of recurrent pneumonias and a chronic cough productive of foul-smelling purulent sputum. The sputum production is worse when lying down and in the morning. On physical examination, he appears chronically ill with clubbing of the fingers. Wet inspiratory crackles are heard at the lung bases posteriorly. There are no hepatosplenomegaly or any palpable lymph nodes. CXR shows scaring in the right lower lobe, which on chest CT scan is identified as airway dilatation, bronchial wall thickening, and grapelike cysts. Which of the following is sometimes seen in this condition?

    (A) lung cancer
    (B) dextrocardia
    (C) fungal infection
    (D) carcinoid syndrome
    (E) Hodgkin's disease

42. A 27-year-old man presents with chest pain and feeling unwell. He describes cough with blood-tinged sputum, chills, and fever of 2 days' duration. Physical findings reveal dullness and moist rales in the left lower chest. His CXR is shown in Fig. 12–2. Which of the following is the most likely diagnosis?

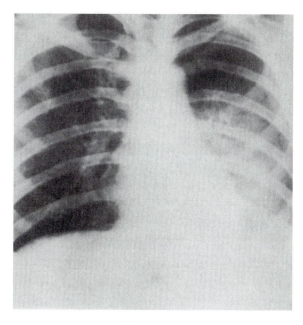

Figure 12–2.

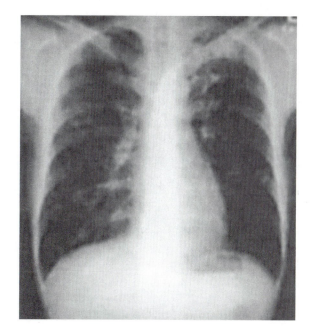

Figure 12–3.

(A) pneumonia, left lower lobe
(B) atelectasis, left lower lobe
(C) PE
(D) tuberculosis
(E) sarcoidosis

43. A 40-year-old man is seen for an insurance assessment. He has no past medical history and feels well. His compete physical examination is normal. His biochemistry, complete blood count (CBC), ECG, and urinalysis are also normal. His CXR is abnormal and presented in Fig. 12–3. Which of the following is the most likely diagnosis?

(A) hamartoma of the lung
(B) tuberculous granuloma of the left apex
(C) osteochondroma of the left 4th rib
(D) bronchogenic carcinoma
(E) pulmonary metastases

44. A 21-year-old man has a nonproductive cough, shortness of breath, and chest pain, which changes with breathing. He also has pain in the left arm. On examination, there is tenderness over the left shoulder, heart sounds are normal, and the lungs are clear. CXR reveals a lytic lesion in the left humerus and reticulonodular opacities in the upper and middles lobes

(Fig. 12–4). The eosinophil count is normal. Which of the following is the most appropriate initial diagnostic test?

(A) lung biopsy
(B) humerus bone biopsy
(C) CT scan of chest
(D) bronchoscopy
(E) pulmonary function tests

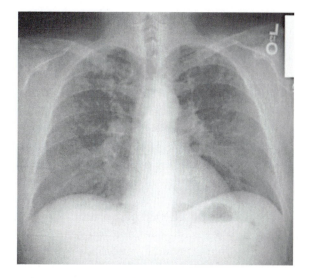

Figure 12–4.

45. The pulmonary function studies shown in Table 12–1 are of a 65-year-old man with severe dyspnea and cough. Which of the following is the most likely diagnosis?

    (A) emphysema
    (B) lobar pneumonia
    (C) chronic bronchitis
    (D) acute bronchitis
    (E) CHF

TABLE 12–1.   PULMONARY FUNCTION STUDIES

FEV1:	60% predicted
FVC:	110% predicted
FEV1/FVC:	60%
TLC:	120% predicted
RV:	130% predicted
DCO:	60% predicted

Abbreviations: FEV1—forced expiratory volume in 1 second; FVC—forced vital capacity; TLC—total lung capacity; RV—residual volume; DCO—diffusing capacity for carbon monoxide.

46. A 33-year-old woman, otherwise perfectly well, presents with recurrent episodes of hemoptysis. She has no fever, weight loss, cough, or sputum production. Her physical examination is entirely normal. Her CXR, biochemisty, CBC, and coagulation profile are also normal. Which of the following is the most appropriate initial diagnostic test?

    (A) echocardiogram
    (B) gallium scan
    (C) CT scan of chest
    (D) bronchoscopy
    (E) pulmonary function tests

47. A 34-year-old woman is complaining of progressive and worsening shortness of breath. Her symptoms first started 3 years ago, and she now gets dyspneic and fatigued while doing her activities of daily living. Her past medical history is not significant and she not taking any medications. Physical examination reveals increased JVP and a reduced carotid pulse. Precordial examination reveals a left parasternal lift, loud P_2, and right-sided S_3 and S_4. There are no audible murmurs. CXR reveals clear lung fields and an ECG shows evidence of right ventricular hypertrophy. Pulmonary function tests are normal. Which of the following is the most likely diagnosis?

    (A) asthma (without wheezing)
    (B) primary pulmonary hypertension
    (C) pulmonary veno-occlusive disease
    (D) pulmonary leiomyomatosis
    (E) "silent" tricuspid valve disease

48. An 83-year-old man with Parkinson's disease presents with low-grade fever and cough for several weeks. Lately, he has been experiencing more rigidity and difficulty with his walking. He is on a levodopa/carbidopa combination for treatment for the past 5 years. On examination, his gait is shuffling and slow. He has a tremor in his left hand at rest, and there is cogwheel rigidity of the forearm. There are crackles in the left lower lung field. CXR reveals a lung abscess in the left lower lobe. Which of the following is the most likely bacteriologic diagnosis for the lung abscess?

    (A) oropharyngeal flora
    (B) tuberculosis
    (C) *Staphylococcus aureus*
    (D) *Pseudomonas aeruginosa*
    (E) *Candida albicans*

49. A 28-year-old African American woman presents with mild dyspnea on exertion. She reports no coughing, sputum production, or wheezing symptoms, but has noticed a red tender rash on her shins. Physical examination reveals hepatosplenomegaly, generalized lymphadenopathy, and tender erythematous nodules on her legs. CXR shows bilateral symmetric hilar adenopathy. Her pulmonary function tests reveal a mild restrictive pattern. Which of the following tests will most likely make a definitive diagnosis?

    (A) tuberculin skin test
    (B) bronchoscopy with transbronchial biopsy
    (C) elevated ACE level
    (D) serum hypercalcemia
    (E) increased uptake on gallium scan

50. A 69-year-old woman has recently returned on an overnight flight from Europe. She now complains of vague chest discomfort and shortness of breath. On examination, she is comfortable, blood pressure 130/80 mm Hg, pulse 90/min, respirations 18/min, and oxygen saturation 97%. Her heart and lungs are normal on auscultation, and there is no edema or leg tenderness on palpation. A quantitative (ELISA) D-dimer assay is positive. Which of the following statements regarding the D-dimer assay is correct?

   (A) it is sensitive but not specific
   (B) it is specific but not sensitive
   (C) it is neither specific nor sensitive
   (D) a negative result suggests myocardial ischemia
   (E) it is both sensitive and specific

51. A 24-year-old African American woman presents with mild dyspnea on exertion, fever, and a rash on her legs. Her symptoms have come on gradually and she reports no pleuritic chest pain, hemoptysis or sputum production. She has no significant past medical history, smokes 10 cigarettes/day and is not taking any medications. Physical examination reveals generalized lymphadenopathy and tender erythematous nodules on her legs. CXR shows bilateral symmetric hilar adenopathy and reticulonodular changes in both lungs. She has a restrictive lung disease pattern on pulmonary function testing. Which of the following is the most likely diagnosis? (See Fig. 12–5)

   (A) Hodgkin's disease
   (B) tuberculosis
   (C) rheumatic fever
   (D) sarcoidosis
   (E) rheumatoid arthritis (RA)

52. A 30-year-old man presents with coughing up blood and sputum. There is no associated dyspnea, fever, or pleuritic chest pain. His past

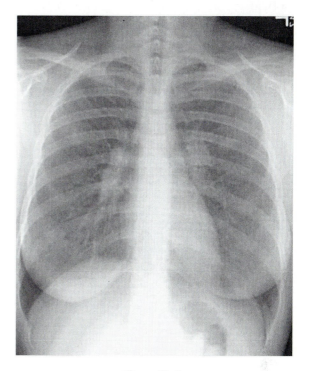

Figure 12–5.

medical history is significant for recurrent pneumonias and a chronic cough productive of foul-smelling purulent sputum. The sputum production is usually worse when lying down and in the morning. He quit smoking 5 years ago and started when he was 18 years old. On physical examination, he appears chronically ill with clubbing of the fingers. Wet inspiratory crackles are heard at the lung bases posteriorly. CXR shows scaring in the right lower lobe, which on chest CT scan is identified as airway dilatation, bronchial wall thickening, and grapelike cysts. Which of the following is the most likely diagnosis? (See Fig. 12–6.)

   (A) bronchiectasis
   (B) chronic bronchitis
   (C) disseminated pulmonary tuberculosis
   (D) pulmonary neoplasm
   (E) chronic obstructive emphysema

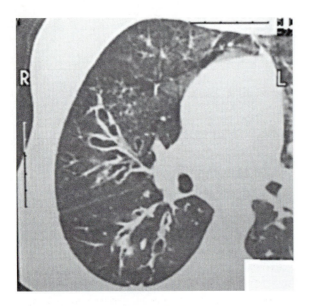

Figure 12–6.

DIRECTIONS (Questions 53 through 62): Each set of matching questions in this section consists of a list of lettered options followed by several numbered items. For each numbered item, select the appropriate lettered option(s). Each lettered option may be selected once, more than once, or not at all. **EACH ITEM WILL STATE THE NUMBER OF OPTIONS TO SELECT. CHOOSE EXACTLY THIS NUMBER.**

Questions 53 through 57

   (A) acute asthmatic attack

   (B) complete pneumothorax

   (C) large pleural effusion

   (D) atelectasis

   (E) lobar pneumonia

For each patient with abnormal pulmonary physical findings, select the most likely diagnosis.

53. A 64-year-old woman is admitted to the hospital after the acute onset of left-sided weakness. She has had a large right cerebral stroke and is confined to bed. On the fifth hospital day, her oxygen saturation is noted to be reduced to 90% on room air. She feels fine, the neurologic weakness is unchanged, blood pressure is 130/90 mm Hg, and pulse 80/min. Examination of the chest reveals decreased fremitus, dullness to percussion, and absent breath sounds in the left lower lung. There is also a tracheal shift towards the left side. (SELECT ONE)

54. A 72-year-old man with COPD develops acute shortness of breath and presents to the hospital. He appears uncomfortable: blood pressure is 120/90 mm Hg, pulse 100/min, oxygen saturation 85% on room air. On examination of the chest, there is absent fremitus, absent breath sounds, and hyperresonant percussion of the right lung. The trachea is shifted to the left. (SELECT ONE)

55. A 45-year-old woman comes to the emergency department because of increased shortness of breath. Examination of the chest reveals decreased fremitus, low diaphragms, and prolonged expiration phase. (SELECT ONE)

56. A 24-year old woman notices increasing shortness of breath after recent treatment for right lower lobe pneumonia. She has no fever, cough, or sputum production. On examination, the pertinent findings are decreased fremitus, dullness on percussion, and absent breath sounds of the right lower lung. In addition, the trachea has shifted to the left. (SELECT ONE)

57. A 61-year-old man is not feeling well because of shortness of breath and left-sided chest pains that increase with breathing. His examination reveals increased fremitus, dull to percussion, and bronchophony on the left side. His heart sounds are normal. (SELECT ONE)

Questions 58 through 62

   (A) squamous cell carcinoma

   (B) adenocarcinoma

   (C) large cell carcinoma

   (D) small cell carcinoma

   (E) bronchioloalveolar carcinoma

For each patient with lung cancer, select the most likely cell type based on clinical description.

58. A 66-year-old man with a 40-pack-per-year history of smoking is investigated for hemoptysis. CXR reveals a central 3-cm mass near the left bronchus. His serum biochemistry is abnormal for elevated calcium, but there is no boney metastasis on the bone scan. Biopsy of the mass is positive for a type of lung cancer associated with paraneoplastic hypercalcemia. (SELECT ONE)

59. A 55-year-old woman presents with symptoms of fever, chills, and colored sputum production. She is a former 40-pack-per-year smoker. Her CXR is abnormal for a 2-cm right hilar mass and right lower lobe infiltrate. She is started on antibiotics and a biopsy of the hilar mass is positive for a type of lung cancer responsive to cytotoxic chemotherapy. (SELECT ONE)

60. A 71-year-old man is having an elective left total knee replacement, when a routine preoperative CXR finds a solitary lung mass. He has no other symptoms related to the lung mass. His surgery is cancelled and a biopsy of the lung mass is positive for a type of cancer that can potentially be cured by surgery. (SELECT FOUR)

61. A 58-year-old woman has a witnessed generalized seizure. She has no prior history of seizures, and her only new symptoms are weight loss and anorexia. She looks unwell and cachectic, and the remaining examination is normal. Her serum sodium is 112 mEq/L, osmolality 260 mOsm/kg, and urine osmolality 420 mOsm/kg. Her CXR is abnormal for a large left hilar mass. She has a 30-pack-per-year history of smoking. Biopsy of the mass is positive for a lung cancer most commonly associated with ectopic endocrine syndromes. (SELECT ONE)

62. A 58-year-old man comes to the emergency department because of left shoulder pain radiating down his left arm. His only risk factor for cardiac disease is hypertension and a 30-pack-per-year smoking history. On examination, his blood pressure is 150/90 mm Hg in both arms, pulse 100/min, and heart sounds are normal. He also has ptosis of his left eyelid and a left pupil that is smaller than the right. ECG is normal, and a CXR shows a large left apical mass with 1st and 2nd rib destruction. A biopsy of the mass is consistent with lung cancer most commonly associated with Pancoast's syndrome. (SELECT ONE)

Answers and Explanations

1. **(C)** Hypersensitivity pneumonitis is an inflammatory disorder of the lungs involving alveolar walls and terminal airways that is caused by repeated exposure to organic agents. In this example of "farmer's lung," the inhalation of antigens present in moldy hay such as thermophilic actinomyces or *Aspergillus* species are the causative agents. When exposure to moldy hay is stopped, symptoms and signs of farmer's lung all tend to abate and complete recovery usually follows. In acute syndromes, the presentation is 4–8 hours after exposure. Symptoms include fever, chills, malaise, cough, and dyspnea without wheezing. The rate of disease depends on rainfall (which promotes fungal growth) and agricultural practices related to turning and stacking hay. In acute and subacute presentations, removing exposure to the antigen will result in complete recovery. *(Kasper, p. 1516)*

2. **(C)** COPD is defined as a disease state that is characterized by airflow limitation that is not fully reversible. Emphysema and chronic bronchitis are closely related, and the term COPD is often used to encompass both. Chronic bronchitis is a clinical syndrome defined as excessive tracheobronchial mucous production severe enough to cause productive cough for at least 3 months of the year for at least two consecutive years. Emphysema is defined as the distention of air spaces distal to the terminale bronchiole, with destruction of alveolar septa. It is primarily a histologic diagnosis. Smoking is the usual antecedent for COPD. *(Kasper, p. 1547)*

3. **(B)** Tranquilizers and sedatives should be avoided in prolonged asthma attacks. Bronchodilators, fluids, aminophylline, and steroids may be used. In acute situations, IV glucocorticoids are frequently used. Results of therapy should be monitored in an objective manner, with peak expiratory flow rates or FEV1. In acute asthmatic attacks, hypocarbia is usual on blood gas analysis. Normal or elevated $Paco_2$ is a bad sign and requires intensive monitoring and aggressive treatment. *(Kasper, pp. 1570–1571)*

4. **(E)** Allergic bronchopulmonary aspergillus usually requires long-term treatment with glucocorticoids. The major diagnostic criteria are bronchial asthma, pulmonary infiltrates, eosinophilia greater than 1000, immediate wheal and flare response to *Aspergillus fumigans*, serum precipitins to *A. fumigans*, elevated serum IgE, and central bronchiectasis. *(Kasper, p. 1520)*

5. **(C)** Relatively asymptomatic patients often require no treatment. Steroids are used with ocular (as in this case), CNS, or other serious complications. Although 50% of patients are left with permanent organ impairment, these are usually not symptomatic or significant. Only in 15–20% of cases does the disease remain active or recur. Glucocorticoids are the treatment of choice, but numerous other agents have been used. *(Kasper, p. 2023)*

6. **(D)** The administration of oxygen may worsen the syndrome of carbon dioxide narcosis because the chief stimulus to ventilation is often hypoxia, and when this is suddenly

relieved, the ventilation may drop quickly. Causes of the chronic hypoventilation syndrome include impaired respiratory drive (e.g., prolonged hypoxia, central nervous system [CNS] disease), neuromuscular disorders (e.g., motor neuron disease, myasthenia gravis), or impaired ventilatory apparatus (e.g., kyphoscoliosis, COPD). *(Kasper, p. 1570)*

7. **(C)** The perfusion lung scan is most valuable in ruling out a PE. If properly performed early in the course of symptoms, a normal scan rules out the diagnosis. High-probability scans are usually considered enough evidence of PE to warrant definitive treatment. Intermediate- or low-probability scans may require further investigation (e.g., with pulmonary angiography), depending on the prior probability of disease. More recent data suggest that a normal high-resolution chest CT with contrast rules out clinically significant PE and is replacing perfusion scanning since the lung images may provide an alternate diagnosis for the patient's symptoms. *(Kasper, p. 1562)*

8. **(C)** Open lung biopsy is not required. Pulmonary angiography is usually performed only if a lung scan suggests thromboembolic disease. Cardiac catheterization is useful to exclude an underlying cardiac shunt as the cause of the pulmonary hypertension. The pulmonary capillary wedge pressure is normal but can be difficult to obtain. *(Kasper, p. 1404)*

9. **(D)** Hypoventilation always causes both hypoxemia and hypercapnia. If the hypoventilation syndrome is caused exclusively by impaired respiratory drive (e.g., drug overdose), then the alveolar-arterial PaO_2 gradient remains normal. Often, hypoventilation results from more than one disorder in the respiratory system (e.g., COPD plus metabolic alkalosis secondary to diuretics and glucocorticoids). *(Kasper, p. 1569)*

10. **(C)** Chronic bronchitis is a clinical diagnosis defined by the presence of chronic productive cough for 3 months in each of 2 successive years in a patient in whom other causes of chronic cough have been excluded. Emphysema is a pathologic term describing the abnormal permanent enlargement of airspaces distal to the terminal bronchioles, accompanied by destruction of their walls without obvious fibrosis. Emphysema may be noted in patients with COPD. *(Kasper, p. 1549)*

11. **(A)** In most circumstances, treatment is anticoagulation to prevent further pulmonary emboli. However, hemodynamic instability may warrant primary therapy for the embolus (e.g., thrombolysis). Evidence of right ventricular hypokinesis on echocardiogram can be an indication for such primary therapy. *(Kasper, p. 1562)*

12. **(B)** Neurogenic tumors are the most common posterior mediastinal masses. Other posterior mediastinal masses include meningoceles, meningomyeloceles, gastroenteric cysts, and esophageal diverticula. Common anterior mediastinal masses include thymomas, lymphomas, teratomas, and thyroid masses. Middle mediastinal masses include vascular lesions, lymph nodes, and pleuropericardial and bronchogenic cysts. *(Kasper, p. 1568)*

13. **(A)** Most people have two MM genes and a resultant alpha1-antitrypsin level in excess of 2.5 g/L. Homozygotes with ZZ or SS genotypes have severe alpha1-antitrypsin deficiency and develop severe panacinar emphysema in the third or fourth decade of life. Smoking is an important cofactor in the development of disease. Heterozygotes (MZ or MS) have intermediate levels of alpha1-antitrypsin (i.e., genetic expression is that of an autosomal codominant allele). This heterozygous state is common (5–14% of general population), but it is unclear whether it is associated with lung function abnormalities. *(Kasper, p. 1551)*

14. **(A)** Ankylosing spondylitis is characterized by bilateral upper lobe fibrosis, which may be complicated by fibrocavitary disease. The pulmonary involvement is rare and is usually very slowly progressive. The cavities can be colonized by *Aspergillus*. *(Kasper, p. 1558)*

15. **(D)** The natural history of the disease is unclear because the disease is asymptomatic for a long period. Survival from diagnosis is dependent on the functional class of the patient. Functional class IV dyspnea suggests a mean survival of only 6 months. Death is usually the result of either intractable right heart failure or sudden death. *(Kasper, p. 1405)*

16. **(D)** The primary pathology is likely to be located in the respiratory center. Cyanosis, especially when asleep, is caused by a combination of polycythemia and hypoxia. The symptoms of alveolar hypoventilation are caused by both hypercarbia and hypoxemia. *(Kasper, p. 1570)*

17. **(A)** Antibiotics and postural drainage might be included in therapy. The choice of antimicrobial agents is guided by the sputum culture, but ampicillin and tetracycline are used if normal flora is found. The general principles of therapy include eliminating underlying problems, improved clearance of secretions, control of infections, and reversal of airflow obstruction. *(Kasper, p. 1543)*

18. **(B)** A significant portion of asthmatics have no known personal or family history of atopy and have normal IgE levels. Idiosyncratic asthma is more likely to have its onset in adult life. Upper respiratory infections can serve as triggers for idiosyncratic asthma. *(Kasper, p. 1508)*

19. **(A)** Acute granulomatous uveitis may be the initial manifestation of sarcoidosis. It can cause blindness. About 25% of patients with sarcoid have eye involvement—three-quarters have anterior uveitis and one-quarter have posterior uveitis. Involvement of lacrimal glands can lead to dry, sore eyes. *(Kasper, p. 2020)*

20. **(A)** Paraneoplastic syndromes are classified as metabolic, neuromuscular, connective tissue, dermatologic, and vascular. Stevens-Johnson syndrome usually follows drug allergy. Acanthosis nigricans and other cutaneous manifestations (e.g., dermatomyositis) are rare (<1%). Clubbing is common and occurs in up to 30% of non-small cell lung cancers. The various

endocrine syndromes occur in 12% of cases. At times, paraneoplastic syndromes may be the presenting finding in lung cancer or be the first sign of recurrence. Most occur with non-small cell lung cancer, but SIADH is more characteristic of small cell lung cancer. *(Kasper, p. 506)*

21. **(E)** Traditionally, penicillin was the treatment of choice for anaerobic lung disease. However, metronidazole plus either third-generation cephalosporin (ceftriaxone) or fluoroquinolone (levofloxacin) has a better spectrum of activity against oral anaerobes, Gram negatives, and *Streptococcus pneumoniae*. *(Kasper, p. 1535)*

22. **(D)** Carbon dioxide retention is seen in right-to-left shunt only with exercise and is uncommon in impaired diffusion syndromes. Disorders of the chest wall, lower airways, and lungs can cause an increased $PaCO_2$ because of severe ventilation-perfusion mismatching despite normal or increased minute volume of ventilation. *(Kasper, p. 1570)*

23. **(C)** Transbronchial biopsy helps differentiate idiopathic pulmonary fibrosis (IPF) from similar syndromes with specific treatments. These include chronic hypersensitivity pneumonitis, cryptogenic organizing pneumonia, and sarcoidosis. *(Kasper, pp. 1556–1557)*

24. **(A)** Bronchography has been superseded by a CT scan in defining the extent of bronchiectasis. Occasionally, advanced cases of saccular bronchiectasis can be diagnosed by routine CXR. The use of high-resolution CT scanning, in which the images are 1.5 mm thick, has resulted in excellent diagnostic accuracy. *(Kasper, p. 1542)*

25. **(D)** Patients frequently are subjected to test doses of short-acting vasodilators such as IV prostacyclin or adenosine, or inhaled nitric oxide. About half of these responders will then respond to high oral doses of nifedipine or diltiazem. Prostacyclin is also available as a treatment, but its applicability is limited by the necessity to administer it as a continuous IV infusion. *(Kasper, p. 1405)*

26. **(C)** The increased vascular permeability is the hallmark of the disease. Diagnostic criteria include acute onset, PaO_2/FiO_2 = 200 mm Hg (regardless of positive end-expiratory pressure [PEEP] level), bilateral infiltrate on frontal CXR, and pulmonary artery occlusion pressure = 18 mm Hg (or if not measured, no evidence of left atrial hypertension). *(Kasper, p. 1592)*

27. **(B)** Allergic bronchopulmonary aspergillosis (in asthmatics), parasitic reactions, and drugs are known causes of pulmonary eosinophilia. Idiopathic causes include Löeffler's syndrome (benign, acute eosinophilic pneumonia), chronic eosinophilic pneumonia, hypereosinophilic syndrome, and Churg-Strauss allergic granulomatosis. *(Kasper, p. 1520)*

28. **(E)** There is no diagnostic blood test, but two-thirds of patients with sarcoidosis will have an elevated level of ACE. Also there is an elevated ESR, hyperglobulinemia, and occasionally hypercalcemia, which are all nonspecific findings. A false-positive rheumatoid factor (RF) and antinuclear antibodies (ANA) antibodies can also be seen. The gallium scan is positive in patients with sarcoidosis. *(Kasper, p. 2022)*

29. **(B)** Yearly influenza vaccination is indicated for patients with COPD. Evidence for pneumococcal vaccination is not definitive but some advocate giving it as well. There is no role for vaccination with *H. influenzae B* or meningococcus in patients with COPD. Dietary support to prevent malnutrition and improve muscle strength can be helpful. Exercise programs seem to provide subjective improvement as well. Obviously, stopping smoking is crucial. *(Kasper, p. 1552)*

30. **(C)** Acute mediastinitis is a rare complication of upper endoscopy. It can also result from trauma to the trachea or esophagus, or dissection of the retroperitoneum. Clinical presentation may include substernal chest pain, subcutaneous emphysema, and Hamman's signs, a crunching or clicking noise synchronous with the heartbeat. *(Kasper, p. 1568)*

31. **(C)** Hemoptysis suggests infection in a patient with advanced lung disease. Pancreatic exocrine function is poor. Nasal polyps are common, but not rectal polyps. About 7% of cases of cystic fibrosis are diagnosed after age 18. Because of improved therapy, cystic fibrosis is no longer just a pediatric disease. Median survival is now 32 years for men and 29 years for women. *(Kasper, p. 1543)*

32. **(B)** Hypoxemia while receiving 100% oxygen indicates right-to-left shunt. Shunts permit circulation of blood that never passes through the ventilated lung. Shunting can occur within the lung (atelectasis, vascular abnormalities) or outside the lung (congenital cardiac malformations). The hypoxemia of ventilation-perfusion mismatch is more easily correctable by 100% oxygen. *(Kasper, pp. 1503–1504)*

33. **(C)** Bony deformities of the chest can lead to respiratory failure with raised PCO_2, as well as recurrent pulmonary infection. Most patients develop a restrictive lung disease pattern with decreased compliance, reduced TLC and VC. In addition, because of the reduced compliance, the resting position of the lung changes such that FRC is reduced. Finally, the net effect is an increase in the work of breathing. The pattern on pulmonary function testing is usually that of a restrictive pattern. *(Kasper, p. 1569)*

34. **(A)** The VC is reduced in emphysema, but the FEV1 is grossly reduced because of high airway resistance. In predominant emphysema, diffusing capacity is more profoundly decreased than in predominant bronchitis. *(Kasper, p. 1549)*

35. **(E)** All forms of asbestos fiber have been associated with lung disease. Restrictive, not obstructive, disease is characteristic. Lung cancer, either squamous cell or adenocarcinoma, is the most common malignancy and the risk is greatly increased by smoking. Benign pleural effusions can occur in both symptomatic and asymptomatic individuals. Reports

of mesothelioma 30–35 years after brief exposure to asbestos emphasize the importance of a complete occupational/environmental history. *(Kasper, p. 1522)*

36. **(A)** PE is an important postoperative complication, which requires urgent treatment. This man is hemodynamically stable and treatment consists of anticoagulation to prevent another PE or propagation of the clot. Thrombolytics are not indicated unless there is severe hemodynamic compromise, and especially in him since he has had recent surgery. The efficacy of IV heparin and LMWH is the same, and can be used with caution in the postoperative setting if there is no ongoing bleeding from the operative site. IVC filter would only be indicated if the patient could not be anticoagulated for some absolute contraindication. The thrust of management is therefore prevention. *(Kasper, p. 1561)*

37. **(C)** In the preantibiotic era, bacterial bronchopneumonia was the most common cause of bronchiectasis. Now it is felt that influenza and adenoviruses are the most common causes. Of the bacterial causes, *S. aureus*, *Klebsiella*, and anaerobes are the most common. Besides infection impaired drainage of the involved segment by bronchial obstruction (foreign body) or poorly functioning cilia is required. Other causes in some individual include poor host humeral immunity such as hypogammaglobulinemia. *(Kasper, p. 1542)*

38. **(B)** The description of a middle-aged man with daytime sleepiness, obesity, hypertension, and snoring suggests obstructive sleep apnea. Although nasal continuous positive airway pressure is effective treatment, simple oxygen therapy is not. Stopping sedative medications and avoiding alcohol improves symptoms. Restless sleep and sudden death have been described as part of the syndrome and surgery (uvulopalatopharyngoplasty or tracheostomy) has been used in severe cases. A wide variety of symptoms can occur, but neuropsychiatric and behavioral manifestations secondary to sleep disturbance are the most common. *(Kasper, p. 1573)*

39. **(B)** Nocturnal oxygen supplementation improves symptoms but is not as effective as continuous supplementation in prolonging life and decreasing hospitalization. Some symptoms of erythrocytosis, headaches, and fullness can be relieved by phlebotomy. In prolonged air travel, even those with P_{O_2} in the mid 70s should be considered for oxygen therapy. A P_{O_2} below 55 mm Hg is an indication for oxygen therapy, but between 55 and 60 mm Hg, associated evidence of right heart dysfunction should also be present before therapy is commenced. *(Kasper, p. 1552)*

40. **(C)** In asbestosis, there is moderate pleural thickening, with scalloped margins from apex to base. There is a similar finding in the mediastinal and diaphragmatic pleura. Furthermore, there is a plaque of pleural calcification in the base. The association of asbestosis with mesothelioma has long been known. As the neoplasm progresses, it may envelop the thorax. *(Kasper, p. 1552)*

41. **(B)** Kartagener's syndrome consists of situs inversus (with dextrocardia), bronchiectasis, and nasal polyps. The bronchiectasis results from impaired ciliary function. *(Kasper, p. 1542)*

42. **(A)** The diagnosis is pneumonia. There is consolidation of the left lower lobe. The increased density, presence of air bronchogram, and the silhouetting of the left diaphragm point to a parenchymal lesion. Pneumococcal infection, as in this patient, is still the most common etiology, although other bacterial infections such as *Klebsiella*, *Streptococcus*, or, *Staphylococcus* is often encountered. Viral and arthropod-borne diseases are also seen. *(Kasper, p. 1532)*

43. **(B)** There is a calcified nodule in the left apex. Obviously, a calcified tuberculous granuloma is the most common lesion. This may be from reinfection tuberculosis, where its preference for the apicoposterior segment is well-known. It is also possible that it may be a calcified Ghon's lesion. *(Kasper, p. 956)*

44. **(C)** Primary pulmonary Langerhans cell histiocytosis (PLCH), also called eosinophilic

granuloma of the lung, pulmonary Langerhans cell granulomatosis, and pulmonary histiocytosis X, is an uncommon interstitial lung disease that primarily affects young adults. There is a coarse, reticular pattern in the whole lung, somewhat more prominent in the upper lobes, suggesting a honeycomb appearance. It is the density here that is abnormal and not the lucency. The next most appropriate test would be a better definition of the lung findings with a high-resolution CT scan. The other more invasive investigations may be more appropriate after the CT. *(Kasper, p. 1520)*

45. **(A)** Because of the maintained increase in minute volume and the maintenance of arterial PaO_2, patients with emphysema are referred to as *pink puffers*. The relatively high PaO_2 and relatively low hemoglobin, as compared to chronic bronchitis, make cyanosis unusual in emphysema. *(Kasper, p. 1551)*

46. **(C)** This history suggests a benign bronchial adenoma. These are usually centrally located on CXR. The most appropriate next test would be a lung CT to demonstrate a lesion. The other tests are invasive and/or not appropriate for identifying the source of bleeding. *(Kasper, p. 207)*

47. **(B)** This presentation is characteristic of primary pulmonary hypertension. Pulmonary veno-occlusive disease is much less common. The predominant pathology, plexogenic arteriopathy, is characterized by medial hypertrophy associated with laminar intimal fibrosis and plexiform lesions. The thrombotic arteriopathy is characterized by eccentric intimal fibrosis with medial hypertrophy, fibroelastic intimal pads in the arteries and arterioles, and evidence of old recanalized thrombi. There is a female predominance, and the third or fourth decade is the most common age at presentation. By the time of diagnosis, the pulmonary hypertension is usually severe. *(Kasper, p. 1405)*

48. **(A)** Most lung abscesses and all anaerobic abscesses involve the normal flora of the oropharynx. Septic embolic usually contain *S. aureus*. Factors that predispose to Gram-negative colonization of the oropharynx

include hospitalization, debility, severe underlying diseases, alcoholism, diabetes, and advanced age. Impaired consciousness, neurologic disease, swallowing disorders, and nasogastric or endotracheal tubes all increase the likelihood of aspiration. *(Kasper, p. 1538)*

49. **(B)** Transbronchial biopsy, looking for noncaseating granulomas, is required to confirm the diagnosis of sarcoidosis in someone with the right clinical context. The other investigations are supportive of a diagnosis of sarcoidosis but not diagnostic of it, since many other conditions can cause an elevated ACE level or positive gallium scan. *(Kasper, p. 2023)*

50. **(A)** A negative D-dimer level rules out thromboembolic disease in patients with intermediate or low pretest probability for DVT/PE. When done by the enzyme-linked immunosorbent assay (ELISA) technique, it is relatively sensitive (i.e., a negative result helps rule out DVT or PE). When done by the latex agglutination method (qualitative assay), it is neither specific nor sensitive enough to guide therapy. *(Kasper, p. 1562)*

51. **(D)** Sarcoidosis is the most likely diagnosis. Granulomatous inflammatory changes of sarcoidosis may occur in almost any organ. About 90% of patients with sarcoid will have an abnormal CXR at some point. *(Kasper, p. 2022)*

52. **(A)** Bronchiectasis is defined as a permanent abnormal dilatation of large bronchi due to destruction of the wall. It is a consequence of inflammation, usually an infection. Other causes include toxins or immune response. Persistent cough and purulent sputum production are the hallmark symptoms. *(Kasper, p. 1542)*

53. **(D)**

54. **(B)**

55. **(A)**

56. **(C)**

57. **(E)**

Careful physical examination can be very useful in diagnosing many common pulmonary disorders. Atelectasis and large pleural effusions both can present with decreased fremitus, dullness or flatness to percussion, and absent breath sounds. In atelectasis, tracheal shift, if present, is toward the affected side, and the opposite for a large pleural effusion. Asthma's most typical manifestations are prolonged expiration and diffuse wheezing. However, impaired expansion, decreased fremitus, hyperresonance, and low diaphragms can also be found. A complete pneumothorax results in absent fremitus, hyperresonance or tympany, and absent breath sounds. Lobar pneumonia is characterized by consolidation with increased fremitus, dullness, and auscultatory findings of bronchial breathing, bronchophony, pectoriloquy, and crackles. *(Kasper, p. 1496)*

58.　**(A)** Hypercalcemia may be due to metastatic destruction of bone, ectopic formation of parathyroid hormone, or formation of other osteolytic substances. *(Kasper, pp. 506–507)*

59.　**(D)** Combination chemotherapy has produced promising results in lung cancer, particularly of the small cell anaplastic type. Alkylating agents and anthracyclines are active among other agents. *(Kasper, pp. 506–507)*

60.　**(A, B, C, E)** Early stage non-small cell lung cancer can be cured by surgery. However, 70% present with disseminated disease. *(Kasper, pp. 506–507)*

61.　**(D)** The most commonly encountered syndromes are SIADH, Cushing's syndrome, and gynecomastia. *(Kasper, pp. 506–507)*

62.　**(A)** Pancoast's syndrome (or superior sulcus syndrome) is found in apical lung tumors, usually epidermoid. Shoulder pain secondary to involvement of the eighth cervical and first and second thoracic nerves is characteristic. Horner syndrome frequently coexists. *(Kasper, pp. 506–507)*

CHAPTER 13

Clinical Pharmacology
Questions

DIRECTIONS (Questions 1 through 43): Each of the numbered items in this section is followed by answers. Select the ONE lettered answer that is BEST in each case.

1. A 72-year-old man is prescribed hydrochlorothiazide for hypertension. Which of the following is the most likely symptomatic side effect?

   (A) increased serum potassium
   (B) metabolic acidosis
   (C) sexual impotence
   (D) respiratory alkalosis
   (E) hypernatremia

2. A 73-year-old man with gastroesophageal reflux is prescribed ranitidine. Which of the following is the most likely effect of this medication?

   (A) stimulates acid secretion
   (B) acts on H1 receptors
   (C) acts on the columnar epithelium of the esophagus
   (D) increases bicarbonate production
   (E) decreases basal acid secretion

3. A 58-year-old man with a lung lesion develops hyponatremia (Na 127 mEq/L). He appears euvolemic clinically and urine electrolytes reveal a high Na (>20 mmol/L) and high osmolality. Which of the following is the most likely mechanism for the low serum sodium?

   (A) increased permeability of the proximal renal tubule to water
   (B) increased permeability of the distal renal tubule to water

   (C) decreased glomerular filtration rate
   (D) increased sodium excretion
   (E) active reabsorption of water from the loop of Henle

4. A 38-year-old woman develops palpitations, weight loss, and heat intolerance. On examination, she has a mild tremor, an enlarged thyroid, and resting tachycardia. Biochemical tests confirm the diagnosis and she is started on methimazole. Which of the following is the most likely mechanism of this drug?

   (A) inhibition of iodine uptake
   (B) inhibition of thyroidal organic binding and coupling reactions
   (C) lowering serum calcium
   (D) adrenal suppression
   (E) the same mechanism as perchlorate

5. A 69-year-old man with poorly controlled hypertension is on hydrochlorothiazide and metoprolol. Compliance with medications and salt restriction is reviewed with the patient and he is also prescribed nifedipine for optimal control of his blood pressure. Which of the following is the mechanism of action for this medication?

   (A) beta-adrenergic stimulation
   (B) interfering with calcium flux
   (C) inhibition of angiotensin 1
   (D) alpha-adrenergic blockade
   (E) direct smooth muscle relaxation

6. A 48-year-old man presents with fever, cough, and purulent sputum production. His chest x-ray (CXR) reveals a right middle lobe infiltrate and he is started on intravenous (IV) antibiotics after sputum and blood cultures are obtained. The following day his sputum cultures grow *Streptococcus pneumoniae*, which is sensitive to penicillin. He is better now so you step him down to oral treatment with amoxicillin rather than penicillin. Which of the following is the most likely reason why oral amoxicillin is preferred over penicillin?

(A) penicillin is not effective orally

(B) amoxicillin is not inactivated by penicillinase

(C) amoxicillin is acid stable

(D) amoxicillin is not effective against coliform organisms and therefore has a narrower spectrum

(E) amoxicillin is not allergenic

7. A 69-year-old man develops renal failure. Which of the following drugs requires a major adjustment in dosage?

(A) levofloxacin

(B) ceftriaxone

(C) amphotericin B

(D) clindamycin

(E) ampicillin

8. Which of the following are mechanisms of action for thiocyanate and perchlorate?

(A) inhibit thyroglobulin release

(B) increase basal metabolic rate (BMR)

(C) inhibit iodide transport

(D) inhibit thyroid organic binding

(E) increase thyroxin synthesis

9. A 63-year-old woman with hypertension is started on a beta-blocker. Which of the following conditions require caution in prescribing this medication?

(A) migraine headaches

(B) hypertrophic subaortic stenosis

(C) Marfan syndrome

(D) atrioventricular (AV) node dysfunction

(E) intermittent claudication

10. A 69-year-old woman, with poor dietary habits and alcoholism, is found to have a macrocytic anemia with hypersegmented neutrophils. Which of the following is the most appropriate diagnostic test?

(A) red blood cell vitamin levels

(B) plasma vitamin levels

(C) bone marrow

(D) Schilling test

(E) therapeutic trial

11. A 69-year-old man is given a multivitamin containing B_{12}. Which of the following is most characteristic of vitamin B_{12} absorption?

(A) totally dependent on the intrinsic factor

(B) best in the duodenum

(C) improved in folic acid deficiency

(D) best in the distal ileum

(E) prevented by antiparietal cell antibodies

12. A 19-year-old man takes an overdose of lysergic acid diethylamide (LSD). Which of the following clinical findings are mostly to be seen in this individual?

(A) pupillary dilatation

(B) pupillary constriction

(C) bradycardia

(D) blindness

(E) deafness

13. A 15-year-old boy is prescribed tetracycline for facial acne. Which of the following is the most common side effect of tetracycline?

(A) neutropenia

(B) allergic reactions

(C) hepatitis

(D) gastrointestinal (GI) symptoms

(E) polyuria

14. A 79-year-old man on quinidine for paroxysmal atrial fibrillation develops thrombocytopenia.

Which of the following is the most likely mechanism for this syndrome?

(A) it is due to bone marrow suppression

(B) it is due to sequestration in the spleen

(C) it is due to intravascular destruction of platelets

(D) it is immunologically mediated

(E) there is cross-reactivity with penicillin

15. A 28-year-old woman with bipolar disorder has a lithium level of 2.3 mEq/L (normal range 0.6–1.25 mEq/L). Which of the following side effects is most likely to occur?

(A) mania

(B) depression

(C) tremor

(D) hyponatremia

(E) leukopenia

16. A 69-year-old man with stable angina is given nitroglycerin. Which of the following is the most likely effect of this medication?

(A) dilating coronary arteries

(B) increasing cardiac venous return

(C) increasing cardiac output

(D) constricting peripheral veins and capillaries

(E) decreasing cardiac work

17. A 74-year-old man with a previous episode of gout is given allopurinol. Which of the following is the most likely mechanism of action for this medication?

(A) increasing uric acid production

(B) blocking excretion of uric acid by renal tubular mechanism

(C) inhibiting xanthine oxidase

(D) diminishing inflammation of acute gouty arthritis

(E) stabilizing lysozymes

18. A 29-year-old woman develops deep vein thrombosis (DVT) in the third trimester. Which of the following statements regarding heparin therapy is correct?

(A) is active by mouth

(B) affects hepatic synthesis of factors

(C) is monitored by prothrombin time (PT)

(D) is contraindicated in pregnancy

(E) may be neutralized by protamine

19. A 19-year-old college student smokes cannabis on a regular basis. Which of the following clinical findings is most likely to be seen an hour after inhalation?

(A) a decrease in heart rate

(B) an increase in intraocular pressure

(C) prolonged reaction time

(D) peripheral vasoconstriction

(E) an increase in intelligence quotient (IQ)

20. An 83-year-old woman has chronic congestive heart failure (CHF) due to grade IV left ventricular function (ejection fraction <20%). She requires 80 mg/day of furosemide as part of her treatment. Which of the following metabolic abnormalities is most likely to be seen while she is taking this medication?

(A) metabolic acidosis

(B) respiratory alkalosis

(C) metabolic alkalosis

(D) hyperkalemia

(E) hypernatremia

21. Three teenaged high school students develop meningitis. A classmate is concerned and comes to see you. Which of the following is the most appropriate next step in management?

(A) penicillin

(B) sulfonamides

(C) only reassurance and observation

(D) rifampin

(E) doxycycline

22. A 69-year-old man's dyspepsia is improved with ranitidine therapy. Which of the following is the best explanation for improvement in his symptoms?

    (A) almost totally abolishes acid secretion
    (B) blocks histamine-H1 receptors
    (C) is well-absorbed in the stomach
    (D) must be taken four times per day
    (E) has no neurologic side effects

23. A 68-year-old man presents with symptoms and signs of CHF. Which of the following is a contraindication to use furosemide?

    (A) has hypoalbuminemia
    (B) is oliguric
    (C) has acidosis
    (D) had a rash with trimethoprim-sulfamethoxazole
    (E) is on anticoagulants

24. A 43-year-old woman with breast cancer is being treated with doxorubicin. Which of the following is a limitation to therapy with doxorubicin?

    (A) neurologic toxicity
    (B) severe nausea
    (C) cystitis
    (D) neutropenia
    (E) heart failure

25. A 23-year-old homeless man is found to have consumed alcohol adulterated with methanol. He is started on treatment effective for minimizing the toxicity to methanol. Which of the following is the most likely explanation for the benefit of this treatment?

    (A) enhances renal excretion of methanol
    (B) prevents biotransformation of methanol
    (C) combines to form a nontoxic polymer
    (D) changes the toxin's volume of distribution
    (E) sedates the patient, thus preventing neurologic damage from methanol

26. A 69-year-old man with heart failure and paroxysmal atrial fibrillation is prescribed amiodarone for maintenance of sinus rhythm.

Which of the following is a known characteristic of amiodarone?

    (A) excellent oral absorption
    (B) a short half-life
    (C) an active metabolite
    (D) few drug interactions
    (E) a small volume of distribution

27. Which of the following features of barbiturate-induced coma is most likely correct?

    (A) requires at least 20–30 times the full sedative dose
    (B) is increasing in frequency
    (C) is characterized by an initial period of hyperventilation
    (D) causes death by depression of the cardiovascular system
    (E) causes death by pulmonary complications

28. Which of the following is a stimulus for insulin secretion?

    (A) hypoxia
    (B) hypothermia
    (C) severe burns
    (D) beta2-adrenergic receptor antagonists
    (E) ketones

29. Which of the following is the most deleterious effect of epinephrine infusion on cardiac function?

    (A) increased heart rate
    (B) increased stroke volume
    (C) increased cardiac output
    (D) arrhythmias
    (E) increased coronary blood flow

30. Which of the following is the most striking difference in the cardiac actions of epinephrine and norepinephrine?

    (A) heart rate
    (B) stroke volume
    (C) cardiac output
    (D) arrhythmias
    (E) coronary blood flow

31. Which of the following statements concerning the relative effects of epinephrine and norepinephrine infusion on peripheral circulation is correct?

    (A) both drugs increase total peripheral resistance
    (B) neither drug increases total peripheral resistance
    (C) neither drug increases renal blood flow
    (D) both drugs increase cutaneous blood flow
    (E) both drugs increase muscle blood flow

32. Which of the following statements concerning the use of isoproterenol and dobutamine for shock is correct?

    (A) isoproterenol is preferred because of its short half-life
    (B) neither drug will potentiate cardiac ischemia
    (C) dobutamine has a more prominent inotropic effect than chronotropic effect compared with isoproterenol
    (D) neither drug affects smooth muscle
    (E) isoproterenol raises blood pressure more than dobutamine

33. Which of the following is the most likely reason why beta2-selective adrenergic agonists are preferred to nonselective beta-adrenergic agonists in the treatment of asthma?

    (A) relax bronchial smooth muscle and thus decrease airway resistance
    (B) improve mucociliary function
    (C) suppress the release of leukotrienes and histamine from mast cells in lung
    (D) decrease microvascular permeability
    (E) have fewer side effects

34. Which of the following statements concerning innate tolerance to alcohol is correct?

    (A) it develops over many years of even moderate drinking
    (B) high levels of innate tolerance protect against the development of alcoholism
    (C) this is likely a result of polygenic inheritance

    (D) pharmacokinetic factors are not involved
    (E) it is not a factor in the development of alcoholism

35. Which of the following is the most likely reason for pharmacokinetic tolerance?

    (A) changes in absorption
    (B) changes in distribution
    (C) changes specific to that drug
    (D) changes in metabolism
    (E) renal adaptation

36. Which of the following is an example of learned tolerance?

    (A) avoiding alcohol when feeling unsteady
    (B) drinking alcohol only with food
    (C) walking a straight line when intoxicated
    (D) not driving when drunk
    (E) using vitamins to prevent alcohol damage

37. Which of the following best describes sensitization to a drug?

    (A) an allergic response
    (B) a purely behavioral effect
    (C) a shift to the right of a dose response curve
    (D) reverse tolerance
    (E) a response to an acute binge

38. The administration of which of the following drugs is most likely to result in sensitization?

    (A) heroin
    (B) cocaine
    (C) tobacco
    (D) alcohol
    (E) diazepam

39. Which of the following drugs is most likely to result in addiction among those who have ever used it?

    (A) alcohol
    (B) tobacco
    (C) cocaine
    (D) heroin
    (E) cannabis

40. Which of the following is a symptom of withdrawal from prolonged moderate dose benzodiazepine usage?

    (A) delirium
    (B) somnolence
    (C) seizures
    (D) decreased hearing
    (E) anxiety and agitation

41. Which of the following features concerning heroin withdrawal is correct?

    (A) it is frequently life-threatening
    (B) it starts about 24 hours after the last dose
    (C) pupillary constriction is present
    (D) irritability and restlessness
    (E) blood pressure is lowered

42. Which of the following opioid analgesics is most likely to cause central nervous system (CNS) disturbance?

    (A) heroin
    (B) morphine
    (C) meperidine
    (D) fentanyl
    (E) codeine

43. Which of the following is the most likely reason why fentanyl does not disturb cardiovascular stability as much as morphine?

    (A) is water soluble
    (B) is lipid soluble
    (C) does not stimulate histamine release
    (D) is long acting
    (E) is not as potent as morphine

DIRECTIONS (Questions 44 through 66): Each set of matching questions in this section consists of a list of lettered options followed by several numbered items. For each numbered item, select the appropriate lettered option(s). Each lettered option may be selected once, more than once, or not at all. EACH ITEM WILL STATE THE NUMBER OF OPTIONS TO SELECT. CHOOSE EXACTLY THIS NUMBER.

Questions 44 through 48

    (A) neutralizes gastric acid
    (B) works by binding to cysteine
    (C) inhibits gastrin release
    (D) irreversible H1-receptor blockade
    (E) synthetic analogue of prostaglandin E1
    (F) reversibly competes with histamine for binding to the H2 receptor on parietal cells
    (G) prevents hydrolysis of mucosal proteins by pepsin
    (H) can enhance gastric secretion
    (I) inhibition of the gastric H/K, adenosine triphosphatase (ATPase) pump

For each patient with an acid-peptic disorder, select the mechanism of action of the prescribed medication.

44. A 27-year-old woman occasionally uses calcium carbonate (Tums) for "heartburn" symptoms after a large meal. (SELECT ONE)

45. A 56-year-old man has intermittent symptoms of burning-type epigastric discomfort. The symptoms are not related to exertion and a recent cardiac evaluation is normal. He is felt to have gastroesophageal reflux disease (GERD) and is prescribed ranitidine for symptom relief. (SELECT ONE)

46. A 76-year-old woman with urosepsis becomes hypotensive and needs admission to the intensive care unit (ICU) for inotropic medications, mechanical ventilation, and monitoring. She is prescribed sucralfate for the prophylaxis of gastric stress ulcers. (SELECT ONE)

47. A 46-year-old man with rheumatoid arthritis (RA) takes naproxen (nonsteroidal anti-inflammatory drug [NSAID]) for the treatment of his joints inflammation and discomfort. He is prescribed misoprostol for NSAID-induced gastric ulcer prophylaxis. (SELECT ONE)

48. A 43-year-old man presents with presyncope and a history of very dark black stools starting 2 days ago. He also reports having nonspecific

abdominal discomfort for the past month. Upper endoscopy reveals a duodenal ulcer, and biopsies are positive for *Helicobacter pylori*. He is prescribed omeprazole as part of "triple therapy" for the eradication of *H. pylori*. (SELECT ONE)

Questions 49 through 53

(A) combines with cytochromes and catalase to block hydrogen and electron transport, thus producing tissue asphyxia

(B) methemoglobinemia

(C) vertigo, hyperventilation, tinnitus, and deafness

(D) bone marrow depression

(E) acute hepatic insufficiency

(F) severe renal injury

For each patient with a toxic ingestion or exposure, select the most likely clinical effect.

49. A 43-year-old man works in a factory where industrial solvents are frequently used to clean the equipment. (SELECT ONE)

50. A 75-year-old woman with rheumatoid arthritis (RA) takes aspirin for symptom control. She usually adjusts the dose of her own medications depending on how she is feeling. (SELECT ONE)

51. A young child ingests silver polish by accident. The local poison control center states that cyanide is a common ingredient of silver polish. (SELECT ONE)

52. A troubled youth has a long history of gasoline sniffing. (SELECT ONE)

53. A 45-year-old man with chronic alcoholism ingests antifreeze. (SELECT ONE)

Questions 54 through 57

(A) digitalis

(B) verapamil

(C) diltiazem

(D) beta-blockers

(E) adenosine

(F) quinidine

(G) flecainide

(H) propafenone

(I) nonsynchronized electric defibrillation

(J) sotalol

(K) procainamide

(L) disopyramide

(M) amiodarone

For each patient with an arrhythmia, select the most appropriate treatment.

54. A 37-year-old woman presents with palpitations and light-headedness. She has a history of palpitations and previously was told that she has "Wolff-Parkinson-White" (WPW) syndrome. Her blood pressure is 110/80 mm Hg and pulse 150 beats/min. Her lungs are clear and heart sounds are normal. The electrocardiogram (ECG) reveals a regular wide complex tachycardia at 150 beats/min and no P waves are visible. (SELECT ONE)

55. A 67-year-old man is brought to the hospital because of a witnessed syncopal event. His past medical history is significant for depression and he is taking amitriptyline. The past few days he has felt unwell from the "flu" and has been vomiting. His potassium is 2.4 mEq/L. While in the emergency room, he has another syncopal event and the monitor records polymorphic VT with increased QT interval (torsades de pointes). (SELECT ONE)

56. A 64-year-old man presents with increased shortness of breath. He has a past history of chronic obstructive pulmonary disease (COPD) and recently developed increased cough and sputum production but no fever or chills. He appears in mild respiratory distress, respirations are 26/min, pulse 120 beats/min, blood pressure 145/84 mm Hg, and oxygen saturation 90%. He has bilateral expiratory wheezes. His ECG reveals multifocal atrial tachycardia (MAT) (discrete P waves with at least three different morphologies). (SELECT ONE)

57. A 23-year-old woman presents with palpitations to the emergency room. The symptoms have been going on for 1 hour. There is no prior history of cardiac disease or family history of arrhythmias or sudden cardiac death. Her pulse is 170 beats/min, blood pressure 115/80 mm Hg, and respirations 16/min. The lungs are clear and heart sounds are normal. The ECG reveals a narrow complex regular tachycardia at 170/min, and no P waves are visible. (SELECT ONE)

Questions 58 through 61

 (A) Hodgkin's disease
 (B) acute lymphocytic leukemia
 (C) multiple myeloma
 (D) chronic lymphocytic leukemia
 (E) chronic granulocytic leukemia
 (F) malignant melanoma
 (G) breast cancer
 (H) colon cancer
 (I) hairy cell leukemia
 (J) choriocarcinoma
 (K) prostate cancer
 (L) ovarian cancer
 (M) Kaposi sarcoma

Match the chemotherapeutic agent with the diseases it is used in.

58. Melphalan (SELECT THREE)

59. Methotrexate (SELECT THREE)

60. Bleomycin (SELECT ONE)

61. Flutamide (SELECT ONE)

Questions 62 and 63

 (A) sensory loss
 (B) prolonged QT interval
 (C) Parkinson-like symptoms
 (D) action tremor
 (E) insomnia
 (F) increased refractory period
 (G) dystonic movements

For each patient on a specific medication, select the most likely side effects to occur.

62. A 74-year-old woman with Alzheimer's disease is treated with haloperidol. (SELECT TWO)

63. A 69-year-old woman being treated for dysrhythmias with quinidine (SELECT TWO)

Questions 64 through 66

 (A) albuterol
 (B) ethanol
 (C) amitriptyline
 (D) ipratropium bromide
 (E) NSAIDs
 (F) caffeine
 (G) propranolol

For each patient with a clinical symptom, select the most appropriate medication.

64. A 29-year-old woman presents with increasing shortness of breath and coughing. She had asthma as a child but has not required any treatment for the past 10 years. On examination, she has expiratory wheezes. Which of the above may cause bronchodilation? (SELECT TWO)

65. A 69-year-old man suffers from heartburn. Lately he has been experiencing more severe symptoms than usual including waking up at night with epigastric discomfort. His clinical examination is normal. Which of the above may increase gastric secretion? (SELECT TWO)

66. A 79-year-old woman complains of dry mouth. She reports no other symptoms and cannot recall the medications she is currently taking. Which of the above may be a factor? (SELECT ONE)

Answers and Explanations

1. **(C)** The most common symptomatic side effect in men is impotence, and it should be specifically looked for. The most serious complications relate to fluid and electrolyte imbalance and include hyponatremia, hypokalemia, and volume contraction. *(Brunton, p. 849)*

2. **(E)** Ranitidine is an H2-blocker that reversibly competes with histamine for binding to H2 receptors on gastric parietal cells. Its effect is profound on basal acid secretion, but it also has a significant effect on stimulated (e.g., food, hypoglycemia, vagal stimulation) acid production. *(Brunton, p. 971)*

3. **(B)** The mediator of hyponatremia is likely antidiuretic hormone (ADH). Although controlling water permeability is the main function under ADH control, there is some evidence that ADH influences sodium transport in the cortical collecting duct. ADH can also act as a neurotransmitter. Autonomic effects of ADH in the CNS include bradycardia, increase in respiratory rate, suppression of fever, and alteration of sleep patterns. *(Brunton, pp. 778–779)*

4. **(B)** Methimazole is an effective treatment for hyperthyroidism. Methimazole interferes with thyroid function mainly by inhibition of thyroidal organic binding and coupling reactions. In contrast to other agents such as perchlorate, the action of thioamides is not prevented by large doses of iodide. *(Brunton, pp. 1527–1528)*

5. **(B)** Nifedipine is a synthetic agent that is a potent, long-acting systemic vasodilator for the treatment of coronary vasospasm. It is also effective for hypertension. At doses used clinically, nifedipine does not block transmission through the AV node. The vasodilatation can result in a reflex increase in heart rate. *(Brunton, pp. 832–834)*

6. **(C)** Polar side chains added to penicillin molecules made these compounds acid stable and, therefore, improved absorption. Intake of food prior to ingestion of ampicillin will decrease absorption. In cases of severe renal impairment, the dose should be adjusted downward. *(Brunton, p. 1139)*

7. **(A)** Most of the fluoroquinolones are renally excreted and therefore require dose adjustment in renal failure. Exceptions are moxifloxacin and pefloxacin, which are metabolized by the liver. The other antibiotics do not require any adjustment for renal failure. Ampicillin needs to be adjusted only with severe renal failure. *(Brunton, p. 1121)*

8. **(C)** Because of their toxicity, neither drug is widely used in treatment, but both are effective in inhibiting iodide transport. They work by preventing the thyroid gland from concentrating iodide. Thiocyanate is produced following enzymatic hydrolysis of certain plant glycosides (e.g., cabbage), and may be a contributing factor to endemic goiter in certain parts of the world where iodide intake is low. *(Brunton, pp. 1530–1531)*

9. **(D)** Beta-blockers are frequently used in the treatment of hypertrophic cardiomyopathy and for migraine prophylaxis and might prevent aortic dilatation in Marfan syndrome. It rarely causes clinical problems in patients with claudication, but if AV conduction defects are present (either by disease or use of other drugs), life-threatening bradyarrhythmias can occur. *(Brunton, pp. 287–288)*

10. **(A)** Folate deficiency can be secondary to small bowel disease, alcoholism, inadequate intake, disease states with high cell turnover (hemolytic anemia), drugs (methotrexate), and pregnancy. The concentration of folate in plasma changes rapidly with changes in food intake, so the diagnosis of anemia secondary to folate deficiency is made more reliable by measuring red blood cell folate. *(Brunton, p. 1460)*

11. **(D)** Vitamin B_{12} absorption is best in the distal ileum. Receptors for the intrinsic factor are present in the distal ileum, but mass action absorption also occurs with large doses. However, the oral route is still felt to be unreliable if hematologic or neurologic effects are present. The Schilling test, with and without intrinsic factor, can help diagnose the exact cause of B_{12} deficiency. *(Brunton, pp. 1454–1455)*

12. **(A)** Sympathomimetic effects such as pupillary dilatation, piloerection, hyperthermia, and tachycardia are common in an overdosage of LSD. Other symptoms include dizziness, weakness, drowsiness, nausea, and paresthesias. The hallucinogenic effects can last for hours and are mainly visual. *(Brunton, pp. 624–625)*

13. **(D)** GI symptoms are the major side effects of tetracycline. Stomatitis, glossitis, and diarrhea are seen and may be related to superinfections. Hepatic toxicity has been reported but is rare except in massive doses or during pregnancy. Tetracyclines can cause discoloration of teeth in children and in fetuses of mothers given the drug during pregnancy. *(Brunton, p. 1178)*

14. **(D)** Thrombocytopenia usually occurs after weeks or months of therapy. It is due to formation of drug-platelet complexes that evoke a circulating antibody. Thrombocytopenia and bleeding can be severe but resolve rapidly on discontinuing the drug. The antibody is long-lasting, and reintroduction of quinidine, even in a small dose, can rapidly cause thrombocytopenia. Other hypersensitivity reactions to quinidine include hepatitis, bone marrow suppression, and a lupus syndrome. The most common side effects of quinidine are gastrointestinal and include nausea, vomiting, and diarrhea. *(Brunton, pp. 928–929)*

15. **(C)** Lithium is used primarily for bipolar affective disorder, either to treat mania or prevent recurrences of the bipolar disorder. It has also been used in severe unipolar depression. Acute intoxication can result in vomiting, diarrhea, tremor, ataxia, coma, and convulsions. Leukocytosis is also a side effect of lithium therapy. Polyuria and polydipsia secondary to acquired nephrogenic diabetes insipidus is a common side effect. Both acute and chronic intoxication can be lethal. The toxic and therapeutic levels of lithium are very close, and patients on lithium require close medical observation, including measurement of serum lithium levels. *(Brunton, pp. 487–488)*

16. **(E)** The benefit of nitroglycerin is probably due to diminution in cardiac output and work of the heart. Nitroglycerin generally dilates most veins and arteries, and this result in both a decreased preload and a decreased afterload for the heart. This leads to decreased myocardial oxygen requirements. Although coronary artery dilation also occurs, it is probably not as important in relieving anginal pain. *(Brunton, pp. 827–828)*

17. **(C)** Allopurinol effectively blocks uric acid production by inhibiting xanthine oxidase. Allopurinol is indicated in patients with a history of uric acid calculi of the urinary tract. In addition, it is often used in patients with malignancy (e.g., leukemia, lymphoma), particularly when chemotherapy or radiation therapy is being used. *(Brunton, pp. 708–709)*

18. **(E)** Heparin must be given parenterally (usually intravenously or subcutaneously) to be active, and its activity is monitored by the partial thromboplastin time (PTT), not the PT. It is safer than oral anticoagulants in pregnancy and does not deplete clotting factors as its mode of action. Rather, it potentiates the effect of antithrombin III on the clotting cascade. It can be neutralized by administration of protamine. Because protamine can cause a bleeding tendency by its own actions, it is used only when bleeding is severe, and in the lowest possible dose. When low-molecular weight-heparin is used, it has a more predictable pharmacokinetic profile which allows for a weight-adjusted

dosage without laboratory follow-up. *(Brunton, pp. 1471–1474)*

19. **(C)** The most common therapeutic use of cannabis is as an antiemetic during cancer chemotherapy. It might have some analgesic and anticonvulsant properties. Its ability to lower intraocular pressure has not been therapeutically useful in glaucoma. However, all the possible therapeutic effects of cannabis are accompanied by psychoactive effects, which include impaired cognition and perception, prolonged reaction time, and impaired memory and learning. *(Brunton, pp. 622–623)*

20. **(C)** In addition to dehydration, hypokalemia, hypochloremia, and alkalosis also result from excessive use of furosemide. Loop diuretics such as furosemide act primarily to inhibit electrolyte reabsorption in the thick ascending limb of the loop of Henle. The degree of diuresis is greater than in other classes of diuretics. *(Brunton, pp. 752–753)*

21. **(D)** This is likely an outbreak of meningitis secondary to *Neisseria meningitidis*. The first line of drugs used for treatment of acute disease includes cefixime, levofloxacin, and ceftriaxone. For prophylaxis, rifampin is the preferred agent. *(Brunton, pp. 1208–1209)*

22. **(A)** Ranitidine blocks histamine-H2 to receptors and is well-absorbed in the small intestine. It decreases all gastric secretion, not just acid, and is helpful in short bowel syndromes, whereas omeprazole is not. *(Brunton, pp. 971–972)*

23. **(D)** Furosemide is effective despite gross electrolyte disturbances or hypoalbuminemia. Excretion of large volumes of bicarbonate-poor urine leads to alkalosis, so an acidosis is not a contradiction in severe fluid and electrolyte depletion; a trial in oliguric states is often appropriate. Furosemide is related to sulfonamide, and severe allergic reactions can occur. *(Brunton, pp. 752–753)*

24. **(E)** Anthracyclines include daunorubicin and doxorubicin. The major site of metabolism is the liver, and the mechanism of action includes inhibition of deoxyribonucleic acid (DNA)-dependent ribonucleic acid (RNA) metabolism. The cardiomyopathy is characteristic of these drugs and is characterized by arrhythmias and cumulative dose-related CHF. *(Brunton, pp. 1358–1359)*

25. **(B)** Ethanol is the standard antidote for methanol. It inhibits the conversion of methanol to its toxic metabolite, formic acid, by alcohol dehydrogenase. *(Brunton, pp. 592–593, 599–600)*

26. **(C)** With prolonged treatment, the active *N*-desethyl derivative of amiodarone accumulates in plasma, and its concentration may exceed that of the parent compound. Amiodarone is poorly (approximately 30%) absorbed and there is marked interindividual variability. The half-life is long, 25–60 days, presumably because it is extensively bound to tissues, resulting in a large volume of distribution and a reservoir of drug. *(Brunton, pp. 920–921)*

27. **(E)** Most deaths from barbiturate-induced coma are caused by pulmonary complications (atelectasis, edema, bronchopneumonia) or renal failure. Hypoventilation is characteristic, and only 10 times the full reactive dose can cause severe poisoning. This low toxic-therapeutic ratio is one reason why barbiturate use (hence barbiturate coma) is declining. *(Brunton, pp. 414–420)*

28. **(E)** Ketones, glucose amino acids, and fatty acids promote insulin secretion. Stimulation of alpha2-adrenergic receptors inhibits insulin secretion, whereas beta2-adrenergic receptor stimulation enhances release of insulin. As a result, beta2-adrenergic receptor antagonists decrease insulin levels. Activation of the autonomic nervous system (hypoxia, hypothermia, severe burns, surgery) will also suppress insulin secretion. *(Brunton, pp. 1615–1616)*

29. **(D)** All the changes listed are correct, but the increased automaticity of the heart with the development of ventricular premature beats (or more serious ventricular arrhythmias) is the most prominent change. *(Brunton, pp. 243–245)*

30. (C) Epinephrine results in a more rapid heart rate and more powerful systolic contraction resulting in increased cardiac output. Norepinephrine results in an unchanged or even decreased cardiac output. *(Brunton, pp. 244–248)*

31. (C) Both epinephrine and norepinephrine decrease renal blood flow. Epinephrine decreases total peripheral resistance whereas norepinephrine increases total peripheral resistance. Both drugs decrease cutaneous blood flow and only epinephrine increases muscle blood flow. *(Brunton, p. 244)*

32. (C) The preferential effect of dobutamine on contractility makes it useful in low cardiac output states. Both drugs are very short-acting, can potentiate cardiac ischemia, and affect smooth muscle. Unlike isoproterenol, dobutamine frequently increases blood pressure quite significantly thus requiring dosage adjustment. *(Brunton, pp. 250–251)*

33. (E) Most of the side effects from the use of beta-adrenergic agonists in asthma come from stimulation of the beta1-receptors in the heart. Thus, beta2-selective agonists, which act primarily in the lung, are safer to use. Both selective and nonselective beta-agonists will decrease airway resistance. This is their major therapeutic effect. The effects on mucociliary transit, mast cells, and microvascular permeability occur with both nonselective and selective agonists, but the clinical importance of these effects is unclear. *(Brunton, pp. 251–253)*

34. (C) It is felt that innate tolerance is a polygenic characteristic. Frequently, variation in pharmacokinetic variables (absorption, metabolism, excretion), which can be inherited, are the cause of different levels of innate tolerance. Those who have high levels of innate tolerance are more likely to become addicted to alcohol. There is a higher concordance rate for alcoholism among identical twins than fraternal twins, but it is not 100%. *(Brunton, pp. 601–602)*

35. (D) The most common cause of pharmacokinetic tolerance is an increase in the metabolism of the drug. Since these same enzymes can then metabolize other drugs, this kind of tolerance is not necessarily specific to the drug that induced it. *(Brunton, pp. 609–611)*

36. (C) Learned tolerance refers to the reduction of the effect of a drug due to compensatory mechanisms that are learned. An example is walking a straight line despite the motor impairment caused by alcohol. This likely represents both acquisition of motor skills and the learned awareness of one's deficit; thus the person walks more carefully. *(Brunton, p. 610)*

37. (D) Sensitization is the reverse of tolerance. It refers to an increase in effect of the drug with repetition of the same dose. It does not occur during an acute binge. The dose response curve would be shifted to the left. *(Brunton, p. 611)*

38. (B) Cocaine and amphetamines are the drugs most likely to cause sensitization. It is poorly studied in humans, but it is thought that stimulant psychosis results from sensitization after prolonged use. *(Brunton, p. 611)*

39. (B) Almost one-third of people who have tried tobacco become addicted. In comparison, about 15% become addicted to alcohol. Heroin is also highly addictive (23% of users become addicted), but since so few people even try heroin, the addiction rate in society as a whole is quite low (0.4%). *(Brunton, pp. 608–609)*

40. (E) Muscle cramps, anxiety, insomnia, and dizziness are among the common side effects of withdrawal from moderate dose usage. Withdrawal seizures and delirium occur usually in withdrawal from high dosage. Withdrawal should be done gradually, often over many months. *(Brunton, pp. 614–615)*

41. (D) Craving for opioids, restlessness, irritability, and anxiety are common symptoms of heroin withdrawal. Piloerection, pupillary dilatation, sweating, tachycardia, and blood pressure elevation are frequently seen signs of heroin withdrawal. It starts within 6–12 hours of the last dose and is quite unpleasant, but not life-threatening. *(Brunton, pp. 618–619)*

42. **(C)** Meperidine has a half-life of 3 hours, but it has an active metabolite, normeperidine, which has a half-life of 15–20 hours. Therefore, accumulation of normeperidine with toxicity is common. The drug should not be used for prolonged periods (over 48 hours), and probably should not be used at all in those susceptible to delirium (e.g., the elderly). *(Brunton, p. 570)*

43. **(C)** Morphine releases histamine and can cause cardiovascular instability. Fentanyl does not release histamine, and causes only mild decreases in heart rate and blood pressure. Fentanyl, a lipid-soluble drug, has an elimination half-life between 3 and 4 hours. It is 100 times more potent than morphine. *(Brunton, p. 571)*

44. **(A)** Although doctors seldom prescribe antacids because of the availability of superior medications, patients still use them extensively. As well as neutralizing acid, calcium carbonate enhances secretion in the stomach. The release of CO_2 from bicarbonate can result in belching, nausea, and abdominal distension. Belching can exacerbate gastroesophageal reflex. *(Brunton, pp. 974–975)*

45. **(F)** Ranitidine inhibits acid production by reversibly competing with histamine for binding to H2 receptors on parietal cells. Ranitidine's most prominent effect is on basal acid secretion, but it still significantly suppresses stimulated (feeding, gastrin, etc.) acid production. *(Brunton, pp. 971–972)*

46. **(G)** After the mucosa is damaged by acid, further damage is caused by pepsin-mediated hydrolysis of mucosal proteins. Sucralfate, in an acid environment, forms a sticky protective gel over epithelial tissues and ulcer craters to prevent further damage by pepsin. This viscous layer can inhibit absorption of many drugs, so patients should wait for at least 2 hours after taking other medications before taking sucralfate. *(Brunton, pp. 973–974)*

47. **(E)** Prostaglandins have two effects on gastric mucosa: they inhibit acid secretion by binding to the EP3 receptor on parietal cells, and they have a cytoprotective effect by stimulating mucin and bicarbonate secretion and local mucosal blood flow. Misoprostol is a synthetic prostaglandin analogue, and has both an acid suppression and cytoprotective effect. *(Brunton, p. 973)*

48. **(I)** Omeprazole is a potent suppressor of acid secretion by the parietal cell. It inhibits the H, K-ATPase pump (proton pump) and reduces daily basal and stimulated acid secretion by 80–95%. Proton pump blockers are part of the regimen for the eradication of *H. pylori*. *(Brunton, pp. 969–970)*

49. **(E)** In chronically poisoned patients, neurologic symptoms and evidence of liver damage may develop. Many industrial solvents are chlorinated hydrocarbons and have been implicated in several deaths. Carbon tetrachloride was once used widely for medical purposes and as a cleaning agent. It has been replaced by safer alternatives. Hepatotoxicity of these compounds is exacerbated by concurrent ethanol ingestion. In lethal cases, death is usually due to deep narcosis, aspiration of vomitus, or cardiac arrhythmias. *(Brunton, pp. 625–626)*

50. **(C)** Salicylates are associated with vertigo, hyperventilation, tinnitus, and deafness. Excretion of salicylates is renal, and in the presence of normal renal function, about 50% will be excreted in 24 hours. Severe toxicity can cause severe acid-base abnormalities. It can be difficult to diagnose when the toxicity is secondary to a therapeutic regimen. *(Brunton, pp. 691–692)*

51. **(A)** Cyanide is contained in silver polish, insecticides, rodenticides, and some plants. Inhalation of hydrogen cyanide may cause death within a minute; oral doses act more slowly, requiring several minutes to hours. Cyanide combines with cytochromes and catalase to produce tissue asphyxia. The treatment for cyanide poisoning includes the administration of IV sodium thiosulfate, which hastens the transformation of the cyanide to thiocyanate, which is excreted in the urine. *(Brunton, p. 885)*

52. **(D)** Benzene is associated with bone marrow depression. Benzene is present to some extent in most gasolines, and poisoning may result from ingestion or vapors. Acute benzene poisoning can cause severe CNS symptoms such as blurred vision, tremors, shallow and rapid respiration, ventricular irregularities, paralysis, and loss of consciousness. *(Brunton, pp. 625–626)*

53. **(F)** Ethylene glycol is widely used as antifreeze. It causes CNS depression and renal toxicity characterized by oxalate crystals in the tubules. As in methanol poisoning, ethanol is used as a competitive substance for alcohol dehydrogenase to decrease the rate of formation of toxic metabolites. *(Brunton, pp. 599–600)*

54. **(K)** Digitalis and verapamil decrease the refractoriness of the accessory pathways in Wolff-Parkinson-White syndrome (WPW) and the ventricular rate can exceed 300/min. This can be life-threatening and is treated with IV procainamide or cardioversion. *(Kasper, pp. 1350–1351)*

55. **(I)** Numerous cardiac and noncardiac medications can cause torsades de pointes. Although it has been described with amiodarone, this is quite rare. The arrhythmia can result in sudden death. Unstable forms of this arrhythmia are treated with cardioversion. *(Kasper, p. 1353)*

56. **(B)** MAT usually occurs in the setting of advanced lung disease. Treatment involves withdrawing theophylline and improving lung function. There may be some role for treatment with verapamil. *(Kasper, p. 1350)*

57. **(E)** Adenosine is the agent of first choice for the termination of AV nodal or AV reentrant tachycardias that are not terminated by vagal maneuvers such as carotid sinus massage. IV beta-blockers and calcium channel blockers are second choice. Digitalis IV acts too slowly and is not recommended for this type of arrhythmia. *(Kasper, pp. 1347–1349)*

58. **(C, G, L)** Melphalan is an alkylating agent of the nitrogen mustard type. Although not curative therapy, it is particularly useful in the management of multiple myeloma, breast cancer, and ovarian cancer. *(Brunton, p. 1328)*

59. **(B, G, J)** Methotrexate is classified as an antimetabolite, and is a folic acid analogue. Other tumors where methotrexate has an effect include osteogenic sarcoma, mycosis fungoides, and lung cancer. *(Brunton, pp. 1338–1339)*

60. **(A)** Bleomycin, a naturally occurring antibiotic, is useful in Hodgkin's disease, non-Hodgkin's lymphoma, and cancers of the testes, head and neck, skin, esophagus, lungs, and genitourinary tract. *(Brunton, pp. 1361–1362)*

61. **(K)** Flutamide is an antiandrogen that is useful in prostate cancer. Leuprolide, a gonadotropin-releasing hormone analogue, and various estrogen compounds are the other hormonal-type agents used in prostate cancer therapy. *(Brunton, p. 1388)*

62. **(C, G)** Sensory loss is not a side effect of phenothiazines. Parkinson-like symptoms disappear when phenothiazine is withdrawn. Dystonic movements involve the mouth, tongue, and shoulder girdle. As well as having useful antipsychotic effects, phenothiazines are useful as antiemetics and antinausea agents. They can also potentiate the effects of sedatives, analgesics, and general anesthetics. Some phenothiazines are intrinsically sedating, but none of them commonly interfere with sleep. *(Brunton, pp. 477–480)*

63. **(B, F)** The increased refractory period accounts for the effect on tachycardia. Similar effects are seen with procainamide. The slowed repolarization can result in a prolonged QT interval. Life-threatening polymorphic ventricular tachycardias (torsades de pointes) can be provoked by quinidine. It is rarely used in modern practice. *(Brunton, pp. 928–929)*

64. **(A, D)** In susceptible individuals, the beta2-adrenergic blocking effect of propranolol can cause life-threatening bronchoconstriction. Ephedrine, isoproterenol, and albuterol are beta-adrenergic agonists and cause bronchodilatation.

Ipratropium bromide results in bronchodilatation by its anticholinergic effect. The other medications listed have no effect on bronchial airways. *(Brunton, pp. 195, 719–720)*

65. **(B, F)** Caffeine and other methylxanthines also stimulate acid production. Vagal cholinergic stimulation is a major stimulus for gastric secretion. Alcohol may increase secretion by stimulating gastrin and histamine release. *(Brunton, pp. 727–728)*

66. **(C)** Xerostomia (dry mouth) can result from the anticholinergic side effects of taking amitriptyline. The other medications on the list are not usually known to cause a dry mouth. *(Brunton, pp. 446–447)*

CHAPTER 14

Comprehensive Review
Questions

DIRECTIONS (Questions 1 through 100): Each of the numbered items in this section is followed by answers. Select the ONE lettered answer that is BEST in each case.

1. A 28-year-old man has purulent urethritis. A swab reveals Gram-negative diplococci within neutrophils. Which of the following is the most appropriate treatment?

   (A) intramuscular ceftriaxone plus oral doxycycline
   (B) oral penicillin G
   (C) intramuscular penicillin V
   (D) intramuscular ampicillin and oral penicillin V
   (E) intravenous (IV) tobramycin

2. Which of the following is a better characteristic feature of geriatric patients compared to younger patients?

   (A) medical problems are less complex
   (B) they spend less money on housing
   (C) homeostenosis is impaired
   (D) hepatic enzyme deterioration is a result of aging
   (E) senile dementia is a result of aging

3. A 72-year-old man is brought to the clinic by his daughter because she is concerned about his memory. A careful history, mini mental status, and physical examination confirm your suspicions of the patient having Alzheimer's disease. Which of the following investigations is included in the initial work up for reversible causes of dementia?

   (A) electroencephalogram (EEG)
   (B) urine tests for heavy metals
   (C) thyroid function tests
   (D) red blood cell (RBC) folate
   (E) urinary and plasma amino acids

4. A 74-year-old woman develops atrial fibrillation. She has no prior history of heart disease. Her thyroid-stimulating hormone (TSH) level is very low. Which of the following cardiac findings might also be seen in this condition?

   (A) aortic regurgitation
   (B) hypotension
   (C) soft S_1
   (D) systolic murmurs
   (E) soft S_2

5. A 74-year-old woman has metastatic bone disease on x-ray. Which of the following mediators is least likely to be involved?

   (A) interleukin-6 (IL-6)
   (B) ectopic parathyroid hormone (PTH)
   (C) tumor necrosis factor (TNF)
   (D) interleukin-1 (IL-1)
   (E) prostaglandins

6. A 30-year-old woman develops acute onset of erythema nodosum, fever, malaise, and anorexia. The chest x-ray (CXR) reveals bilateral hilar lymphadenopathy and a left paratracheal lymph node. Which of the following is the most likely diagnosis?

(A) acquired immune deficiency syndrome (AIDS)
(B) rheumatic fever
(C) sarcoidosis
(D) tuberculosis
(E) bronchogenic carcinoma

7. Which of the following imaging techniques is best able to measure regional brain substrate uptake and metabolic kinetics?

(A) magnetic resonance imaging (MRI)
(B) computed tomography (CT)
(C) positron emission tomography (PET)
(D) serial thallium scintigrams
(E) Doppler ultrasound

8. A 47-year-old man suddenly develops high fever and hypotension. He has a generalized erythematous macular rash, and over the next day, develops gangrene of his left leg. Which of the following is the most likely organism?

(A) *Corynebacterium diphtheriae*
(B) *Streptococcus* group C
(C) *Neisseria gonorrhoeae*
(D) *Streptococcus* group A
(E) *Salmonella enteritidis*

9. A 56-year-old woman presents to the hospital because of symptoms of dyspnea, blurry vision, and headaches. On examination, her blood pressure is 210/130 mm Hg, heart rate 100 beats/min, and oxygen saturation 95%. Her fundi reveal retinal hemorrhages and papilledema. The heart sounds are normal expect for an S_4, and the lungs have lower lobe crackles. Which of the following is the most appropriate agent to reduce her blood pressure?

(A) IV hydralazine
(B) IV labetalol
(C) oral methyldopa
(D) IV diazoxide
(E) sublingual nifedipine

10. A 56-year-old man complains of increased thirst and increased urinary volume and frequency. He has also noticed new symptoms of constipation and generalized aches and pains. He has no significant past medical problems and his physical examination is normal. Initial investigations consist of a normal complete blood count (CBC) fasting blood glucose and urinalysis. His sodium, urea, and creatinine are normal, but calcium is 12.4 mg/dL (8.4–10.2 mg/dL). Further testing reveals an elevated PTH level. Which of the following is the most likely mechanism for the polyuria in this condition?

(A) direct effect of PTH on the kidney
(B) hypercalcemia-induced renal tubular acidosis (RTA)
(C) hypercalcemia-induced chronic renal failure
(D) hypercalcemia-induced defect in renal concentrating ability (nephrogenic diabetes insipidus)
(E) hypercalcemia-induced defect in renal glucose handling

11. A 13-year-old boy has periods when he seems to be unresponsive, associated with blinking of his eyes. These are momentary, and he seems normal thereafter. Which of the following is the most effective treatment?

(A) phenytoin
(B) carbamazepine
(C) phenobarbital
(D) gabapentin
(E) ethosuximide

12. Which of the following lymphoid malignancies is invariably of B-cell origin?

(A) chronic lymphocytic leukemia (CLL)
(B) hairy cell leukemia
(C) Burkitt's lymphoma
(D) mycosis fungoides
(E) angioimmunoblastic lymphadenopathy

13. A patient with human immunodeficiency virus (HIV) infection has progressed to developing AIDS (clinical category C). Which of the following conditions is considered an AIDS-defining illness?

    (A) antibodies to HIV
    (B) palpable lymphadenopathy
    (C) Kaposi sarcoma
    (D) oral candidiasis (thrush)
    (E) herpes zoster (shingles)

14. Which of the following is more characteristic of ulcerative colitis when compared to Crohn's disease (regional enteritis)?

    (A) segmental involvement
    (B) granulomas
    (C) lymph node involvement
    (D) rectal bleeding
    (E) palpable abdominal mass

15. A 28-year-old pregnant woman develops sudden onset of dyspnea and tachycardia with no other physical findings. Which of the following is the most likely diagnosis?

    (A) pulmonary emphysema
    (B) pulmonary embolism
    (C) myocardial infarction
    (D) ventricular tachycardia
    (E) lobar pneumonia

16. A 60-year-old man from a poor socioeconomic environment is admitted with an acute illness characterized by mental disturbances. On examination, he has bilateral sixth nerve palsy and an ataxic gait. Which of the following is the most appropriate treatment?

    (A) thiamine
    (B) lecithin
    (C) vitamin D
    (D) phenytoin
    (E) diazepam

17. Which of the following is most characteristic of calcitonin?

    (A) it increases bone resorption
    (B) it decreases renal calcium clearance
    (C) it is produced by hepatocytes
    (D) it raises blood phosphate
    (E) it binds to osteoclasts

18. Following a severe sore throat, a 15-year-old boy feels unwell. He has had pain and swelling in his elbows and knees, and cardiac examination reveals new mitral regurgitation and tachycardia. Which of the following might also be seen on further examination?

    (A) chronic arthritis
    (B) involvement of spinal joints
    (C) subcutaneous nodules
    (D) erythema nodosum
    (E) meningeal irritation

19. For which of the following patients is a home total parenteral nutrition (TPN) program most likely to be useful?

    (A) an untreatable disease
    (B) a 4-day requirement for nutrition
    (C) short bowel syndrome
    (D) neoplasms with bowel obstruction
    (E) anorexia nervosa

20. Which of the following is the most important factor in selecting a patient as a potential heart transplant recipient?

    (A) absence of long-standing pulmonary hypertension
    (B) survival on mechanical assistance devices
    (C) availability of a human lymphocyte antigen (HLA)-compatible donor
    (D) age under 20 years
    (E) ventricular ejection fraction <20%

21. Which of the following features best characterizes CLL?

    (A) usually a T-cell disorder
    (B) a disease of children
    (C) responsive to splenectomy
    (D) frequently asymptomatic
    (E) most common in Asians

22. A 69-year-old man with alcoholic cirrhosis develops confusion and sleep disturbance. Which of the following is the most likely cause?

    (A) digoxin
    (B) furosemide
    (C) penicillin
    (D) gastrointestinal (GI) bleeding
    (E) stroke

23. An asymptomatic patient has proteinuria and hematuria that is glomerular in origin on a routine urinalysis. Which of the following is the most likely diagnosis?

    (A) diabetes mellitus (DM)
    (B) amyloidosis
    (C) immunoglobulin A (IgA) nephropathy (Berger's disease)
    (D) focal glomerulosclerosis
    (E) thalassemia minor

24. A 63-year-old man with a 60-pack-per-year history of smoking has been previously diagnosed as having emphysema. Which of the following features is most characteristic of this diagnosis?

    (A) mild dyspnea
    (B) copious purulent sputum
    (C) hematocrit over 55%
    (D) severe pulmonary hypertension at rest
    (E) decreasing diffusing capacity

25. A 26-year-old man with a recent diagnosis of rheumatoid arthritis (RA) complains of muscle weakness in his hands. On examination, he has multiple active joints in his hands and wrists. Strength in the hand muscles and wrist flexors and extensors is reduced (graded 4 out of 5). Strength in his legs is normal. Which of the

following features is characteristic of muscle weakness in RA?

    (A) occurring after several months of pain and immobility
    (B) showing a neutrophilic infiltrate on muscle biopsy
    (C) secondary to vasculitis
    (D) showing heavy mononuclear cell infiltrate on muscle biopsy
    (E) showing type II fiber atrophy and muscle fiber necrosis on muscle biopsy

26. An 18-year-old woman with a microcytic anemia is diagnosed with alpha-thalassemia. Formation of which of the following hemoglobins is increased in alpha-thalassemia?

    (A) H
    (B) A
    (C) F
    (D) A2
    (E) C

27. Which of the following is most characteristic of diabetic neuropathy?

    (A) it is usually bilateral
    (B) pain is not a feature
    (C) it most commonly affects the brain
    (D) it spares the autonomic system
    (E) it responds to meticulous control of blood glucose

28. A 57-year-old man, previously asymptomatic and on no medications, develops a painful left big toe. It is so painful that even the weight of his sheets is excruciating. On examination, there is a swollen red toe. Which of the following medications is relatively contraindicated?

    (A) indomethacin
    (B) colchicine
    (C) ibuprofen
    (D) allopurinol
    (E) naproxen

29. A 73-year-old woman is admitted to hospital with right-sided hemiparesis and expressive aphasia. CT scan of the brain reveals a stroke in

the right middle cerebral artery territory. Which of the following is the most common cause of ischemic stroke?

(A) cerebral hemorrhage
(B) cerebral embolism
(C) arteritis
(D) dissecting aneurysm
(E) hemorrhage into atherosclerosis

30. Which of the following is the next most common cause of blood transfusion-related hepatitis after hepatitis B?

(A) hepatitis A
(B) Epstein-Barr hepatitis
(C) hepatitis C
(D) hepatitis D
(E) HIV hepatitis

31. A 20-year-old man develops abrupt onset of hematuria and proteinuria, accompanied by azotemia and salt and water retention. Which of the following is the most likely diagnosis?

(A) nephrotic syndrome
(B) multiple myeloma
(C) diabetic nephropathy
(D) nephrolithiasis
(E) acute glomerulonephritis

32. A 36-year-old man is diagnosed with a duodenal ulcer after undergoing upper endoscopy. Which of the following is the most common symptom of duodenal ulcer?

(A) epigastric pain
(B) nausea
(C) melena
(D) anorexia
(E) midback pain

33. An elderly patient receiving a blood transfusion for myelodysplastic syndrome develops tachypnea, lumbar pain, tachycardia, and nausea. Which of the following is the most likely explanation?

(A) anxiety
(B) fluid overload

(C) hemolysis
(D) pulmonary embolism
(E) acute leukemia

34. A 23-year-old pregnant woman in her first trimester develops hyperthyroidism. Which of the following treatments is contraindicated?

(A) thyroid surgery
(B) propylthiouracil (PTU)
(C) drugs that cross the placenta
(D) radioactive iodine
(E) glucocorticoids

35. A 78-year-old woman is treated for depression with nortriptyline. Which of the following is the most common side effect of nortriptyline?

(A) impaired cardiac contractility
(B) heart block
(C) weight loss
(D) anticholinergic side effects
(E) diarrhea

36. A 23-year-old woman is diagnosed with mitral valve prolapse as seen on echocardiography for evaluation of a systolic murmur. Which of the following is most characteristic of mitral valve prolapse?

(A) a pansystolic murmur
(B) usually a benign course
(C) sudden death
(D) infective endocarditis
(E) highest incidence in men over age 50

37. A 14-year-old boy develops nephrotic syndrome. A renal biopsy shows foot process fusion and no deposits on the membranes under electron microscopy. Which of the following is the most likely diagnosis?

(A) mesangial proliferative glomerulonephritis
(B) minimal change disease
(C) focal glomerulosclerosis
(D) membranous glomerulonephritis
(E) Goodpasture's syndrome

38. A 65-year-old man presents with hemoptysis. His sputum cytology is positive for malignant cells, but the CXR is normal. Which of the following is the next best step in management?

    (A) annual CXR
    (B) unilateral pneumonectomy
    (C) blind percutaneous needle biopsies
    (D) bronchoscopic brushings and biopsies
    (E) mediastinoscopy and biopsy

39. A 34-year-old man presents with dyspnea and increasing peripheral edema. He recently had a "flu like" illness with intermittent sharp left-sided chest pain. On examination, his jugular venous pressure (JVP) is elevated at 8 cm, heart sounds are soft and the blood pressure (BP) is 125/80 mm Hg with a 20 mm Hg decrease in systolic arterial pressure during slow inspiration. Which of the following is the most likely diagnosis?

    (A) cardiac tamponade
    (B) pulmonary hypertension
    (C) ventricular septal defect
    (D) coarctation of the aorta
    (E) malignant hypertension

40. A 45-year-old man develops end-stage renal disease due to diabetic nephropathy. He undergoes a renal transplant with a kidney donated from his sister. Which of the following immune suppression therapies are usually used to prevent rejection in renal transplant patients?

    (A) splenectomy and irradiation
    (B) plasmapheresis and steroids
    (C) cyclosporine and steroids
    (D) azathioprine and plasmapheresis
    (E) steroids and thymectomy

41. A 42-year-old woman has a prior history of left eye pain and visual loss that resolved spontaneously. She now has diplopia and weakness with spasticity in her right leg. Which of the following is the most likely diagnosis?

    (A) cerebral emboli
    (B) subclavian steal syndrome
    (C) Guillain-Barré syndrome
    (D) recurrent transient ischemic attacks (TIAs)
    (E) multiple sclerosis

42. A 16-year-old female presents with abdominal pain, joint discomfort, and purpuric spots on the skin. On examination, the abdomen is tender, but there is no rigidity or rebound tenderness. There are multiple palpable purpuric lesions on her skin, and there are no acute joints. Laboratory investigation reveals a normal CBC, but an abnormal urinalysis with hematuria and proteinuria. Which of the following is the most likely diagnosis?

    (A) hemolytic-uremic syndrome
    (B) thrombotic thrombocytopenic purpura
    (C) heavy metal poisoning
    (D) subacute bacterial endocarditis (SBE)
    (E) Henoch-Schönlein purpura (HSP)

43. Which of the following drugs causes an increase in the effective refractory period of the atrioventricular (AV) node?

    (A) bretylium
    (B) amiodarone
    (C) procainamide
    (D) quinidine
    (E) disopyramide

44. A 74-year-old postmenopausal woman is found to have hypercalcemia due to hyperparathyroidism. She has multiple medical comorbidities and decides against having surgery. Which of the following treatments might she benefit from?

    (A) estrogen therapy
    (B) androgen therapy
    (C) calcium therapy
    (D) radioiodine
    (E) IV phosphate

45. A 23-year-old man of African descent is treated for malaria contracted on a recent trip. He develops anemia due to hemolysis after treatment is started. Which of the following is the most likely diagnosis?

(A) fulminant malaria

(B) paroxysmal nocturnal hemoglobinuria

(C) hereditary spherocytosis

(D) glucose-6-phosphatase dehydrogenase (G6PD) deficiency

(E) microangiopathic hemolysis

46. A 20-year-old woman presents with cough and yellow sputum production. On her chest x-ray, there is a right lower lobe infiltrate. Which of the following is the most appropriate treatment of community-acquired pneumonia?

(A) carbenicillin

(B) tobramycin

(C) levofloxacin

(D) methicillin

(E) tetracycline

47. A 60-year-old man presents with symptoms of polyuria and nocturia. Investigations reveal a normal fasting glucose and calcium level. His urine electrolytes suggest a renal transport defect. Which of the following is the most likely cause for his symptoms?

(A) acute nephritis

(B) acute renal failure (ARF)

(C) renal tubular defects

(D) nephrolithiasis

(E) systolic hypertension

48. A 62-year-old man is found to have severe erosive esophagitis on endoscopy and is started on the most effective treatment for this condition. Which of the following is the mechanism of action of this therapy?

(A) binds to the ulcer bed

(B) antagonizes H2 receptors

(C) inhibits acetylcholine

(D) stimulates mucin secretion

(E) inhibits parietal cell proton pump

49. A 70-year-old woman, previously in good health, is found to have an asymptomatic monoclonal immunoglobulin peak on serum electrophoresis. Which of the following is the most likely diagnosis?

(A) monoclonal gammopathy of uncertain significance (MGUS)

(B) multiple myeloma

(C) Waldenström's macroglobulinemia

(D) amyloidosis

(E) non-Hodgkin's lymphoma

50. A 30-year-old woman complains of symptoms of dry mouth and eyes. She also has parotid gland enlargement on examination. Her serum is positive for Ro/SS-A autoantibodies. Which of the following is the most likely diagnosis?

(A) ankylosing spondylitis

(B) mixed connective tissue disease

(C) systemic sclerosis

(D) thrombotic thrombocytopenic purpura

(E) Sjögren's syndrome

51. In an extreme emergency, patients may be transfused with unmatched blood. Which of the following is considered suitable for unmatched blood transfusion?

(A) blood type AB

(B) polycythemic individual

(C) a sibling of the recipient

(D) blood type O

(E) Lewis A positive

52. A 37-year-old woman presents with shortness of breath on exertion. She has a past history of rheumatic fever as a child. On cardiac auscultation, there is a loud S_1 and a mid-to-late low-pitched diastolic murmur. You suspect she has mitral stenosis. Which of the following findings is most likely to be seen on the CXR in someone with mitral stenosis?

(A) general enlargement of the heart

(B) Kerley B lines

(C) attenuation of pulmonary arteries

(D) straightening of the left heart border

(E) diffuse modulation of the lower lung fields

53. A 25-year-old woman presents with symptoms of fatigue and weakness. On examination, there is diplopia, ptosis, weakness, and fatigability of muscles on repeated use. Which of the following is the most likely diagnosis?

    (A) myasthenia gravis
    (B) multiple sclerosis
    (C) TIAs
    (D) muscular dystrophy
    (E) cerebral palsy

54. Which of the following women have the highest risk of developing breast cancer?

    (A) cousins of breast cancer patients
    (B) those receiving CXRs as children
    (C) those with late-onset menarche
    (D) multiparous
    (E) those who have already had one breast cancer

55. A 16-year-old man is newly diagnosed with cystic fibrosis (CF). Which of the following is correct for patients with CF diagnosed as an adult?

    (A) the reproductive system is not involved
    (B) heatstroke occurs
    (C) pulmonary hypertension is avoided
    (D) GI disease is mild
    (E) hypersplenism is prominent

56. A 25-year-old nonsmoking man has a 2-cm solitary pulmonary nodule in the left lower lobe, with a "popcorn ball" calcification pattern. Which of following is the most appropriate next step in management?

    (A) left lower lobe resection
    (B) serial CXRs
    (C) needle aspiration biopsy
    (D) left pneumonectomy
    (E) mediastinoscopy

57. A 60-year-old man with unstable angina pectoris fails to respond to heparin, nitroglycerin, and beta-adrenergic blockers. He continues to have ongoing chest pain symptoms. Which of the following is the most appropriate next step in management?

    (A) IV streptokinase
    (B) coronary angiography
    (C) exercise testing
    (D) oral aspirin
    (E) antihypertensive therapy

58. Which of the following is the major effect of glucocorticoids in asthma?

    (A) anti-inflammatory
    (B) bronchodilatory
    (C) sedative
    (D) mucus dissolving
    (E) antibacterial

59. A 56-year-old man with nephrotic syndrome undergoes a renal biopsy for diagnosis. The renal lesion is consistent with a diagnosis of focal and segmental glomerulosclerosis (FSGS). Which of the following changes are most likely to be seen on immunofluorescence studies of the renal biopsy in FSGS?

    (A) nodular deposits of immunoglobulin M (IgM) and complement 3 (C3)
    (B) linear deposits of immunoglobulin G (IgG)
    (C) nothing
    (D) granular deposits of IgG and complement 4 (C4)
    (E) extensive fibrin strands

60. A 26-year-old woman complains of burning retrosternal chest pain, radiating to the sides of the chest that is aggravated by bending forward. Which of the following is this pain most likely to arise from?

    (A) heart
    (B) lumbar spine
    (C) intercostal nerves
    (D) pancreas
    (E) esophagus

61. A 34-year-old woman has Raynaud's phenomenon associated with systemic sclerosis

(scleroderma). Which of the following is the most appropriate management for this condition?

(A) amphetamines

(B) ergotamines

(C) beta-blocking drugs

(D) warm clothing

(E) surgical sympathectomy

62. Which of the following is the most common presentation of hemophilia A?

(A) hematuria

(B) melena

(C) hemarthrosis

(D) pressure neuropathy

(E) intracerebral hemorrhage

63. Three weeks after surgery to implant a mechanical aortic valve, a 70-year-old man develops chest pain, fever, and leukocytosis. On examination, the JVP is increased, there is a mechanical S_2 sound, and a pericardial friction rub. Which of the following is the most likely diagnosis?

(A) infection in the aortic valve

(B) postpericardiotomy syndrome

(C) cytomegalovirus (CMV) infection

(D) pulmonary embolism

(E) acute myocardial infarction

64. Which of the following typically causes a macrocytic anemia?

(A) blind loop syndrome

(B) iron deficiency

(C) thalassemia

(D) chronic inflammation

(E) sideroblastic anemia

65. An 18-year-old woman develops weakness, weight gain, amenorrhea, abdominal striae, and behavioral abnormalities. Physical examination reveals lateral visual field loss. Which of the following is the most likely diagnosis?

(A) a functional pituitary tumor

(B) adrenal hyperplasia

(C) anorexia nervosa with bulimia

(D) glioblastoma multiforme

(E) multiple sclerosis

66. A 64 year-old man with Type II diabetes has his fasting lipid profile measured. Which of the following is the most common pattern of dyslipidemia in Type II diabetes?

(A) increased triglycerides only

(B) increased low-density lipoprotein (LDL) only

(C) increased high-density lipoprotein (HDL) only

(D) decreased triglycerides and increased HDL

(E) increased triglycerides and decreased HDL

67. A previously asymptomatic 62-year-old woman presents with sudden onset of severe midback pain. X-rays reveal an anterior compression fracture of T10. Other vertebral bodies show decreased density and prominent vertical striations. Which of the following is the most likely diagnosis?

(A) multiple myeloma

(B) metastatic breast cancer

(C) vitamin D deficiency

(D) osteoporosis

(E) Paget's disease of bone

68. A 70-year-old man, with no evidence of heart disease, develops transient right arm and leg weakness, which resolves within 1 hour. CT scan of the brain is normal and carotid ultrasound Doppler reveals 60% stenosis of left carotid artery. Which of the following is the most appropriate treatment for this patient?

(A) carotid endarterectomy

(B) aspirin

(C) beta-blockers

(D) nonsteroidal anti-inflammatory drugs (NSAIDs)

(E) calcium channel antagonists

69. A 60-year-old woman being investigated for menorrhagia is found on history to have lethargy, constipation, cold intolerance, and muscle stiffness. Which of the following is the most likely diagnosis?

    (A) uterine carcinoma
    (B) systemic lupus
    (C) hypothyroidism
    (D) severe iron deficiency
    (E) hypercalcemia

70. A 20-year-old patient with asymptomatic lymphadenopathy in the right supraclavicular area is found to have nodular sclerosing Hodgkin's disease on biopsy. There is no other evidence of disease on his imaging tests. Which of the following is the most appropriate next step in management?

    (A) combination chemotherapy with MOPP (mechlorethamine, vincristine [Oncovin], procarbazine, prednisone)
    (B) wide surgical excision following radiotherapy
    (C) combination chemotherapy with ABVD (adriamycin [doxorubicin], bleomycin, vinblastine, dacarbazine)
    (D) radiotherapy alone
    (E) observation until symptoms occur

71. A 45-year-old man presents with weakness, fever, weight loss, and abdominal pain. On examination, he is hypertensive, the heart sounds are normal, and lungs are clear. While being investigated, he has a focal seizure. Laboratory studies show a high erythrocyte sedimentation rate (ESR), anemia, ARF, and a positive test for hepatitis B surface antigen. Which of the following is the most likely diagnosis?

    (A) polyarteritis nodosa (PAN)
    (B) acute hepatitis B
    (C) SBE
    (D) multiple staphylococcal abscesses
    (E) chronic active hepatitis

72. Patients with AIDS can develop chorioretinitis with blindness, enteritis with intractable diarrhea, interstitial pneumonitis, and adrenalitis.

Which of the following infections is the most likely cause of these illnesses?

    (A) cryptosporidium
    (B) herpes zoster
    (C) *Toxoplasma*
    (D) pneumocystis carinii pneumonia
    (E) CMV

73. A 45-year-old man is evaluated for new onset of jaundice. Investigations reveal an extrahepatic biliary obstruction. Which of the following is most likely correct concerning his jaundice?

    (A) negative urine bilirubin
    (B) marked increase in conjugated bilirubin
    (C) normal unconjugated bilirubin
    (D) painless jaundice
    (E) decrease in glucuronyl transferase

74. A 19-year-old man has a pigmented skin lesion. Which of the following characteristics suggests a dysplastic nevus (atypical mole) rather than a benign acquired nevus?

    (A) uniform tan color
    (B) located on buttock
    (C) 4 mm in diameter
    (D) 20 similar lesions on body
    (E) located on back

75. A 73-year-old man is brought to the emergency department because of decreased urine output for the past 2 days. Which of the following urine values distinguishes prerenal azotemia from ARF?

    (A) urine osmolality <400
    (B) brown granular casts
    (C) urine creatinine <20
    (D) a high fractional excretion of filtered sodium
    (E) urine sodium of <20

76. Which of the following blood gas results is most likely in a patient with hyperventilation caused by anxiety?

    (A) increased P_{CO_2}
    (B) decreased P_{O_2}

(C) decreased pH

(D) decreased P_{CO_2}

(E) increased P_{O_2}

77. A 57-year-old woman presents to the hospital with a 2-hour history of retrosternal chest pain and dyspnea. Her electrocardiogram (ECG) reveals an acute myocardial infarction pattern. Which of the following ECG patterns is consistent with that interpretation?

(A) tall P waves

(B) prominent U waves

(C) small QRS complex

(D) elevated ST segments

(E) widened QRS complex

78. A 34-year-old man is brought to the emergency room by his family because of extreme lethargy. After further questioning, he admits to taking a large number of phenobarbital tablets. Which of the following is the most appropriate next step in management?

(A) acidification of urine to pH 3.0

(B) repetitive administration of activated charcoal

(C) ipecac to induce vomiting

(D) hemoperfusion

(E) hemodialysis

79. A 45-year-old man was exposed to high levels of radiation after an accident at a nuclear reactor 5 years ago. Which of the following illnesses is he at greatest risk of developing?

(A) aplastic anemia

(B) radiation dermatitis

(C) lung cancer

(D) multiple myeloma

(E) leukemia

80. Which of the following statements concerning progressive supranuclear palsy is correct?

(A) tremor is the usual presenting symptom

(B) superior gaze impairment is the most common gaze abnormality

(C) dementia is a rare consequence

(D) men are more frequently affected

(E) response to L-dopa therapy is usually dramatic

81. Which of the following diuretics will continue to induce significant diuresis after return of blood volume to normal levels?

(A) hydrochlorothiazide

(B) spironolactone

(C) triamterene

(D) furosemide

(E) metolazone

82. A 34-year-old man with HIV is taking isoniazid (INH) and rifampin for the treatment of tuberculosis. He has finished 4 months of therapy without any complications but now complains of numbness in his feet. Clinical examination confirms a symmetric peripheral neuropathy. Which of the following statements is correct regarding the polyneuropathy that occurs in association with INH treatment?

(A) acute

(B) demyelinating

(C) pure sensory

(D) vitamin sensitive

(E) pure motor

83. A patient with recurrent arthritis of the knees recalls an acute illness with fever and severe dermatitis 1 year earlier. Which of the following is the most likely diagnosis?

(A) RA

(B) Lyme disease

(C) syphilis

(D) PAN

(E) systemic lupus erythematosus (SLE)

84. Which of the following is zidovudine (AZT) a treatment for?

(A) retroviral infection

(B) pneumocystis carinii pneumonia

(C) Kaposi sarcoma

(D) toxoplasmosis

(E) herpes simplex of the genitals

85. Which of the following statements concerning women's health issues is correct?

   (A) breast cancer is the leading cause of death in American women

   (B) men benefit more from thrombolytic therapy than women

   (C) the mortality from acute myocardial infarction is greater in women than men

   (D) estrogen therapy decreases mortality in postmenopausal women primarily by its ability to prevent osteoporosis-related fractures

   (E) immune-related disorders are less common in women

86. Which of the following statements concerning hypertension during pregnancy is correct?

   (A) preeclampsia becomes manifest during the end of the middle trimester

   (B) angiotensin-converting enzyme (ACE) inhibitors are useful antihypertensives in pregnant women

   (C) pregnancy increases the risk for future renal impairment in women with essential hypertension

   (D) alpha-methyldopa is a useful antihypertensive in pregnant women

   (E) gestational hypertension infrequently recurs in subsequent pregnancies

87. Which of the following statements concerning pregnancy and infection is correct?

   (A) CMV is the most common cause of congenital viral infection

   (B) postpartum infections are the most common cause of maternal mortality in the United States

   (C) N. gonorrhoeae infection is transmitted to the child only during delivery

   (D) asymptomatic bacteriuria is common but unimportant in pregnant women

   (E) HIV infection in newborns is invariably contracted during the first trimester

88. A 35-year-old man presents with severe left-sided periorbital headaches associated with nasal stuffiness and tearing of the eye. He experiences 3 short-lived attacks a day, usually occurring at the same time of the day for the past 3 weeks. He has had similar headaches a year ago. Which of the following characteristics about these headaches is correct?

   (A) are likely tension headaches

   (B) are typical of common migraine (without an aura)

   (C) may be relieved by the vasodilation of alcohol

   (D) usually recur in cycles lasting several months to years

   (E) can be relieved by administration of oxygen

89. A 75-year-old woman presents with sudden onset of a communication disorder. She speaks fluently but in a series of incomprehensible syllables. She cannot read or repeat sounds or words. Which of the following is characteristic of this syndrome?

   (A) unlikely to improve with time

   (B) usually associated with hemiparesis of the dominant side

   (C) usually associated with hemiparesis of the nondominant side

   (D) usually in the distribution of the posterior cerebral artery

   (E) frequently associated with parietal lobe sensory defects

90. A 38-year-old man acutely develops severe retrosternal chest pain radiating to the back. It is aggravated by breathing and movement. He has always been in perfect health but did have a mild upper respiratory tract infection 1 week ago. His cardiogram is pictured in Fig. 14–1. Which of the following is the most likely cause for his condition?

   (A) occlusion of left anterior descending artery

   (B) occlusion of circumflex artery

   (C) a viral infection

   (D) dissection of the aortic artery

   (E) pneumococcal infection

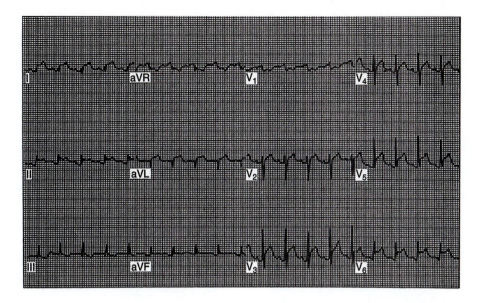

Figure 14–1.

91. A 27-year-old woman develops cough and fever with some sputum production. She is a nonsmoker and, although ill, is deemed to not require hospitalization. Her CXR is revealed in Fig. 14–2. Which of the following statements regarding her management is correct?

(A) a repeat CXR in 2 weeks

(B) a repeat CXR in 6 weeks

(C) antibiotic coverage for *Legionella* infection

(D) antibiotic coverage for *Mycoplasma* infection

(E) antibiotic coverage for Gram-negative infection

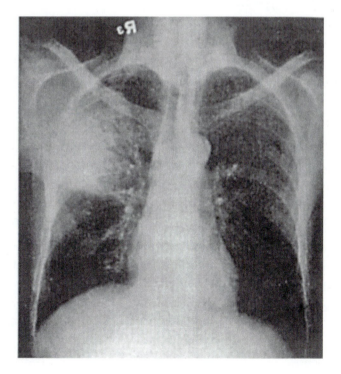

Figure 14–2.

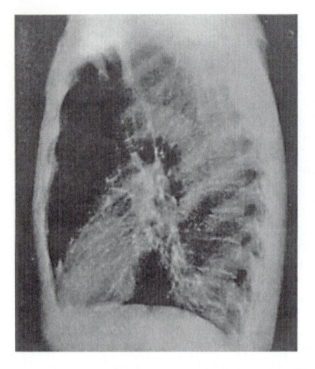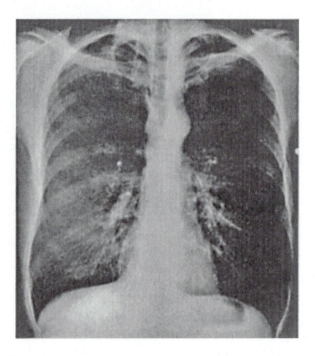

Figure 14–3.

92. A 63-year-old man has had significant short-ness of breath for 2 years. His CXR is revealed in Fig. 14–3. Which of the following is the most likely diagnosis?

(A) primary pulmonary hypertension
(B) right ventricular dysfunction
(C) left ventricular dysfunction
(D) emphysema
(E) mitral stenosis

93. A 42-year-old woman presents with fever, weight loss, and malaise. Physical examination reveals hypertension of 190/100 (normal 1 year earlier). Her ESR is 105 mm/h, and urinalysis reveals numerous RBCs. Her abdominal angiogram is revealed in Fig. 14–4. Which of the following the most likely diagnosis?

(A) Wegener's granulomatosis
(B) rapidly progressive glomerulonephritis
(C) renal artery stenosis
(D) hypernephroma
(E) PAN

94. A 29-year-old man complains of back pain for several months. It takes him over 2 hours to limber up in the morning. His x-ray is shown in Fig. 14–5. Which of the following is the most likely diagnosis?

(A) RA
(B) spondylolithiasis
(C) osteomalacia
(D) ankylosing spondylitis
(E) bone involvement with Hodgkin's disease

95. A 69-year-old man has had mild arthritis involving many joints for several years. Over 1 or 2 days, he develops severe pain and swelling of his knee. His x-ray reveals calcifications in his articular cartilage. Which of the following is the most likely diagnosis?

(A) acute gout
(B) RA
(C) pseudogout
(D) infectious arthritis
(E) torn ligament

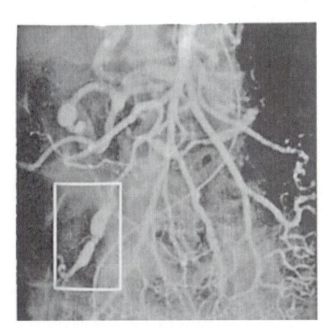

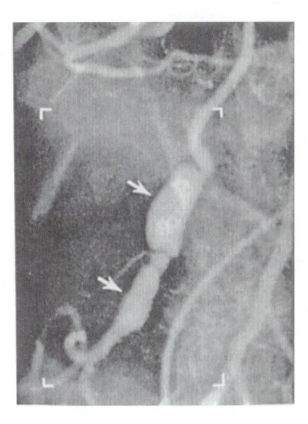

Figure 14–4.

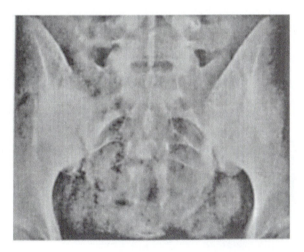

Figure 14–5.

96. A 75-year-old man complains of chronic dysphagia to fluids and solids. On occasion, he regurgitates food he has eaten 1 or 2 days before. Last year, he was hospitalized for pneumonia, but he is otherwise well. His barium swallow x-ray is shown in Fig. 14–6. Which of the following is the most appropriate next step in management?

(A) endoscopic dilatation

(B) myotomy

(C) balloon dilatation of lower esophageal sphincter

(D) surgical excision

(E) vigorous antireflux therapy with surgery if medical management fails

97. A 69-year-old woman is feeling fatigued. Blood work reveals hemoglobin of 9.0 g/dL (14 g/dL 1 year earlier). She has no other symptoms. Her blood film is shown in Fig. 14–7. Which of the following is the most appropriate next diagnostic test?

(A) serum B_{12} level

(B) hemoglobin electrophoresis

(C) colonoscopy

(D) bone marrow aspiration

(E) sickle cell preparation

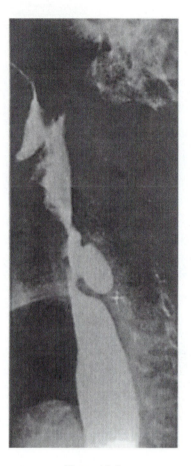

Figure 14–6.

98. A 94-year-old female nursing home resident is referred for evaluation of anemia of 8 g/dL. She has dementia, and adequate documentation of her past medical history is not available. She eats well and is cooperative. Examination reveals evidence of cognitive impairment, primitive reflexes, and a well-healed midline abdominal scar. Her blood film is shown in Fig. 14–8. You presume a relationship between the anemia and the previous surgery. Which of the following surgical procedures is most likely to cause her current anemia?

   (A) gastrectomy
   (B) vagotomy and pyloroplasty
   (C) cholecystectomy
   (D) right hemicolectomy
   (E) common bile duct exploration

99. A 42-year-old man suffers a myocardial infarction during coronary angiography. Which of the following is the approximate risk of this complication?

   (A) 1 in 10,000
   (B) 1 in 100
   (C) 1 in 100,000
   (D) 1 in 1000
   (E) unknown

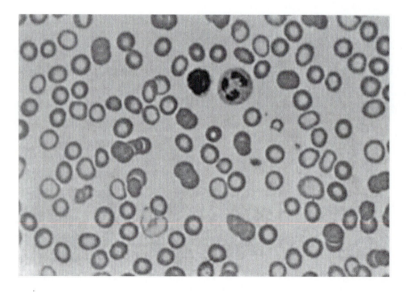

Figure 14–7.

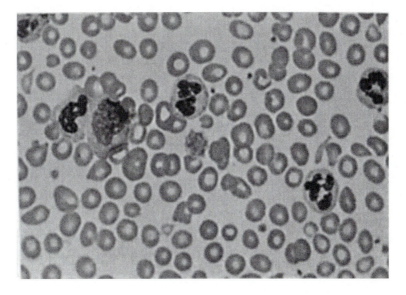

Figure 14–8.

100. An asymptomatic 59-year-old man is treated with oral anticoagulants for chronic atrial fibrillation. When reviewing the benefits of warfarin therapy, he asks about the risks of major bleeding while taking the medication. Which of the following is the best estimate of the major bleeding complication rate with warfarin anticoagulation?

(A) 5% per year
(B) 10% per year
(C) 1–3% per year
(D) unknown
(E) <1% per year

DIRECTIONS (Questions 101 through 113): Each set of matching questions in this section consists of a list of lettered options followed by several numbered items. For each numbered item, select the appropriate lettered option(s). Each lettered option may be selected once, more than once, or not at all. EACH ITEM WILL STATE THE NUMBER OF OPTIONS TO SELECT. CHOOSE EXACTLY THIS NUMBER.

Questions 101 through 105

(A) increased sensitivity with aging
(B) decreased sensitivity with aging
(C) altered excretion with aging
(D) altered metabolism with aging
(E) altered distribution with aging

Match the appropriate statement about pharmacology with each of the following medications.

101. Beta-blockers (SELECT ONE)

102. Nitrazepam (SELECT ONE)

103. Warfarin (SELECT ONE)

104. Lithium (SELECT ONE)

105. Fentanyl (SELECT ONE)

Questions 106 through 110

(A) selective serotonin reuptake inhibitors (SSRIs)
(B) mineral oil
(C) diuretics
(D) INH
(E) phenytoin and phenobarbital
(F) salicylates
(G) corticosteroids
(H) L-Dopa

For each of the following side effects, select the most likely medication to cause them.

106. Disinterest in food with protein/calorie malnutrition (SELECT ONE)

107. Zinc deficiency (SELECT ONE)

108. Vitamin B$_6$ deficiency (SELECT ONE)

109. Impaired calcium absorption (SELECT ONE)

110. Altered vitamin D metabolism (SELECT ONE)

Questions 111 through 113

    (A) sleep more than younger adults

    (B) increased arousals during the night

    (C) increased slow-wave sleep

    (D) sleep improved with alcohol

    (E) most common cause of excessive daytime sleepiness in the elderly

    (F) breakdown of normal temporal organization of sleep-wake cycling

For each of the following situations, select the most likely sleep disturbance.

111. A common change in sleep as people age (SELECT ONE)

112. Common in a 73-year-old woman with Alzheimer's disease (SELECT TWO)

113. Sleep apnea syndrome (SELECT ONE)

DIRECTIONS (Questions 114 through 118): Each of the numbered items in this section is followed by answers. Select the ONE lettered answer that is BEST in each case.

114. A 73-year-old man is brought into the hospital by his family. He is very confused, but collateral history reveals that this is new. Physical examination reveals crackles in his lungs, some abdominal distension, and bilateral asterixis. Which of the following is the most appropriate initial diagnostic test?

    (A) CT scan of head

    (B) CT scan of head with enhancement

    (C) CXR

    (D) MRI of head

    (E) spiral CT of chest

115. A 69-year-old woman is brought to the hospital under an order of medical evaluation after she was found confused in an unkempt apartment with five cats. Extensive investigation does not reveal a specific cause of confusion in this woman, and the medical service wonders whether the true diagnosis is dementia. Which of the following cognitive or behavioral impairments is more typical of delirium than dementia?

    (A) impaired long-term memory

    (B) paranoid behavior

    (C) language impairment

    (D) impaired attention

    (E) fluctuating performance

116. A 77-year-old man is brought to the hospital by his granddaughter for evaluation of confusion. He has no focal findings and his neuro-imaging studies are normal. Further investigations reveal a urinary tract infection, and the man improves somewhat after treatment, but still exhibits poor judgment and bizarre behavior. Pressing the family for information, the intern unearths a history of 8 years of progressive bizarre behavior. The man has undressed himself and made sexual advances to young female relatives, has urinated in hallways, and pushed food into his mouth with alarming speed. Which of the following is the most likely diagnosis?

    (A) Alzheimer's disease

    (B) frontotemporal dementia

    (C) dementia with diffuse Lewy bodies

    (D) vascular dementia

    (E) benign frontal tumor

117. A 68-year-old woman with frontotemporal dementia is being cared for at home by a supportive family. Which of the following is the most common reason for considering nursing home placement in this individual?

(A) inability to perform instrumental activities of daily living (IADLs)

(B) immobility

(C) forgetfulness

(D) intolerable behavior

(E) incontinence

118. A 69-year-old man has developed memory difficulty and is seen for further evaluation. Complete neurologic assessment is normal except for the Mini-Mental Status Examination (MMSE) where he sores 19/30. His laboratory and brain imaging investigations are normal, and there does not appear to be any reversible cause for the memory deficits. His clinical features are most compatible with a diagnosis of Alzheimer's disease. Which of the following pathologic changes are most likely to be seen in the brain of a patient with Alzheimer's disease?

(A) microangiopathic changes

(B) lacunar infarcts

(C) diffuse Lewy bodies

(D) pigmentary degeneration

(E) neurofibrillary tangles

Answers and Explanations

1. **(A)** This patient has gonorrhea, and since 1986, increasing penicillin resistance has meant that penicillin/ampicillin are no longer drugs of choice. Alternatives to ceftriaxone include ciprofloxacin, ofloxacin, or cefixime given orally, with 7 days of doxycycline, or a single 1 g dose of azithromycin in case of coinfection with *Chlamydia*. In Asia and the Pacific (as well as in California), quinolones are not considered first-line therapy because of the high rate of resistant organisms. In these locations, ceftriaxone is the drug of choice. In pregnant women, erythromycin replaces doxycycline. Disseminated gonococcal infection should be treated in a hospital with IV antibiotics. *(Kasper, pp. 860–862)*

2. **(C)** The impaired physiologic reserve of every organ system is characteristic of aging. The term *homeostenosis* has been used to describe this phenomenon. Decline in most systems starts in the third decade and is gradual and progressive. Decrements in each organ system seem independent of other systems and are influenced by diet, environment, personal habits (e.g., exercise), and genetic factors, as well as just chronologic age. At times, it can be difficult to differentiate between age-related physiologic change and age-related diseases. *(Kasper, pp. 44–45)*

3. **(C)** Other tests to rule out reversible disease might include serum electrolytes, B_{12} levels, CBC, Venereal Disease Research Laboratory (VDRL), and CT or MRI. Diagnosis of Alzheimer's disease remains a diagnosis of exclusion. However, the insidious and subtle onset, with few focal signs (except for higher mental functioning) and a slowly progressive course are characteristic. Careful attention to the pattern of cognitive defects also improves diagnostic accuracy. The intensity of investigation will depend on numerous factors, including age, presence of atypical findings, and the timing of presentation. There is as yet no definite consensus on the most appropriate plan of investigation. *(Kasper, pp. 2397–2398)*

4. **(D)** This patient has hyperthyroidism. Cardiac complications are more common in the elderly patient and may dominate the clinical presentation. There is often a wide pulse pressure, systolic murmurs, increased intensity of the first heart sound, and cardiomegaly. Sinus tachycardia and atrial fibrillation are the most common arrhythmias. A to-and-fro high-pitched sound in the pulmonic area (Means-Lerman scratch) can mimic a pericardial friction rub. *(Kasper, p. 1423)*

5. **(B)** A whole host of locally produced hormones and cytokines, as well as ectopically produced hormones, are implicated in local osteoclastic hypercalcemia. Parathormone-related protein is often elevated in malignant hypercalcemia (with or without bony metastases), but ectopic PTH production in malignancy is quite rare. *(Kasper, pp. 561–562)*

6. **(C)** Sarcoidosis presents as an asymptomatic CXR in at least 10–20% of cases in the United States, but more frequently in countries where pre-employment CXRs are mandatory. At least 40% of patients present with acute symptoms and hilar lymphadenopathy. Approximately 90% will have an abnormal CXR at some point

in their illness. Only a small proportion develops progressive disease. *(Kasper, pp. 2019–2022)*

7. **(C)** PET scans use glucose analogues to demonstrate metabolic activity. They are rarely available, however, and functional MRI scans are now being used extensively to assess areas of brain activity. *(Kasper, p. 2355)*

8. **(D)** *Streptococcus* group A can cause a toxic shock-like syndrome, and has been increasing in frequency in North America. Streptococcal toxic shock-like syndrome was so named because of its similarity to staphylococcal toxic shock syndrome. The illness includes fever, hypotension, renal impairment, and the respiratory distress syndrome. It is usually caused by strains that produce exotoxin. It may be associated with localized infection as well; the most common associated infection is a soft tissue infection such as necrotizing fasciitis. The mortality is high (up to 30%), usually secondary to shock and respiratory failure. The rapid progression of the disease and its high mortality demand early recognition and aggressive treatment. Management includes fluid resuscitation, pressor agents, mechanical ventilation, antibodies, and, if necrotizing fasciitis is present, surgical débridement. *(Kasper, pp. 827–828)*

9. **(D)** Diazoxide acts immediately in malignant hypertension and is the easiest to administer for no individual titration of dosage is required. Nitroprusside is more effective, but requires an IV infusion. Labetalol is also useful but has more contraindications. It is particularly useful in the setting of angina or myocardial infarction. Regardless of which drug is selected, early administration of medications for long-term control is mandatory. *(Kasper, p. 1480)*

10. **(D)** This man has primary hyperparathyroidism. Hypercalcemia induces a tubular concentrating defect by interfering with ADH-mediated water pore function (aquaporin-2 channel) on distal tubular cells. This results in the polyuria and polydipsia symptoms of diabetes insipidus. Chronic hypercalcemia can also cause renal stones, type 1 (distal) RTA and

chronic renal failure but these effects are not directly responsible for the polyuria. PTH has no direct effect on the concentrating ability of the distal tubule. *(Kasper, pp. 1694–1701)*

11. **(E)** Ethosuximide and valproic acid are common medications used to treat petit mal epilepsy. Side effects of ethosuximide include GI irritation, skin rash, and bone marrow suppression. *(Kasper, p. 2367)*

12. **(B)** Hairy cell leukemia is a B-cell malignancy. Burkitt's lymphoma is of T-cell origin 5% of the time. CLL can be of T- or B-cell origin. Mycosis fungoides and angioimmunoblastic lymphadenopathy are of T-cell origin. *(Kasper, p. 642)*

13. **(C)** The current case definition of AIDS in a patient with HIV infection is done by symptoms and CD4$^+$ T-lymphocyte cell count. Any category C symptoms (e.g., cervical cancer, mycobacterium avium infection, CMV, retinitis, Kaposi sarcoma, etc.) indicates frank AIDS as does a CD4$^+$ T-cell count <200/µL regardless of symptoms. Shingles and thrush are category B symptoms. *(Kasper, p. 1076)*

14. **(D)** Rectal bleeding is more characteristic of ulcerative colitis, as is malignancy with long-standing disease, but both can occur in regional enteritis. Transmural involvement, lymph node involvement, skip lesions, granulomas, and anorectal complications (abscesses, fistulas, fissures) are characteristic of Crohn's disease. *(Kasper, pp. 1778–1779)*

15. **(B)** Sudden onset of unexplained dyspnea is the most common and often the only symptom of pulmonary embolism. Findings on physical examination may be deceptively normal, but tachycardia is a consistent finding. Pleuritic chest pain and hemoptysis suggest a peripheral embolism adjacent to the pleura. *(Kasper, p. 1561)*

16. **(A)** The patient has Wernicke's encephalopathy and requires treatment with thiamine. A delay of a few hours may permit progression to psychosis. The eye findings in Wernicke's

encephalopathy include bilateral (but not necessarily symmetrical) abductor weakness or paralysis, horizontal diplopia, strabismus, and nystagmus. The nystagmus is most frequently horizontal or vertical gaze-evoked nystagmus. (*Kasper, p. 1636*)

17. **(E)** Calcitonin is secreted by cells in the thyroid. Calcitonin reduces bone resorption and increases renal calcium clearance. The inhibition of osteoclast-mediated bone resorption and the stimulation of renal calcium clearance are mediated by receptors on osteoclasts and renal tubular cells. Other receptors to calcitonin are present in the brain, GI tract, and immune system. (*Kasper, p. 2251*)

18. **(C)** Major manifestations of rheumatic fever include carditis, migratory polyarthritis, chorea, erythema marginatum, and subcutaneous nodules. Minor manifestations include arthralgia, fever, elevated acute phase reactants (ESR, C-reactive protein), and prolonged PR interval. The diagnosis is made with two major or one major and two minor criteria, and evidence of group A streptococcal infection (positive throat culture or rapid streptococcal antigen test, or rising antibody titers). (*Kasper, p. 1978*)

19. **(C)** Home parenteral nutrition is usually helpful in extreme short-bowel syndrome, chronic obstruction due to adhesions, and severe radiation enteritis. Placement of a central venous catheter, careful calculation of fluid and nutritional requirements, and meticulous monitoring are required in a long-term parenteral nutrition program. (*Kasper, p. 418*)

20. **(A)** In selecting a heart for transplantation, size, ABO match, negative lymphocyte cross-match, and other disease states are important factors. The presence of severe pulmonary hypertension can result in intraoperative death. In the United States, it is estimated that only 2000 potential donor hearts become available each year for 20,000 potential recipients. This means that careful recipient selection is very important. The optimal candidates will have a high likelihood of return to a high level of function,

to be mentally vigorous and medically compliant. (*Kasper, pp. 1378–1379*)

21. **(D)** CLL is frequently discovered on routine evaluation of elderly patients and may not require treatment for several years. Splenomegaly, when present, rarely leads to symptoms. It is usually a disorder of B cells and is very indolent in its course. Most therapeutic regimens are designed for symptom control, not cure. Common reasons for treatment include hemolytic anemia, cytopenias, disfiguring lymphadenopathy, symptomatic organomegaly, or systemic symptoms. Chlorambucil is easy to administer, but fludarabine is considerably more effective. It requires IV administration. Maintenance therapy is not helpful. (*Kasper, pp. 648–649*)

22. **(D)** GI bleeding is the most common precipitating factor for hepatic encephalopathy. Furosemide, by causing hypokalemia, is another common cause. Narcotics and sedatives are also frequently implicated. (*Kasper, pp. 1867–1868*)

23. **(C)** Other causes of asymptomatic hematuria, with or without proteinuria, include sickle cell disease, Alport's syndrome, resolving glomerulonephritis, and thin basement disease. Berger's disease is characterized by immunoglobulin A (IgA) deposits in the mesangium. It most commonly affects older children and young adults, and is more common in Blacks than Whites. Macroscopic hematuria may occur with intercurrent illness or vigorous exercise. The prognosis is variable but tends to progress slowly. Spontaneous remissions are more common in children than in adults. About 20–50% of patients develop end-stage renal disease within 20 years of diagnosis. (*Kasper, p. 1690*)

24. **(E)** Chronic obstructive pulmonary disease (COPD) due to emphysema usually demonstrates severe dyspnea, scanty mucoid sputum, normal hematocrit, and decreased diffusing capacity on pulmonary function testing. Chronic bronchitis is characterized by milder dyspnea, greater sputum production, more frequent hypercarbia and polycythemia, and

more evidence of cor pulmonale and pulmonary hypertension. *(Kasper, p. 1551)*

25. **(E)** Muscle weakness in RA is common and can occur within weeks of onset of RA. It is most apparent in muscles adjacent to involved joints. There is not usually a vasculitis present, although a mononuclear infiltrate may be present. The most common finding on biopsy is type II fiber atrophy and muscle fiber necrosis. *(Kasper, pp. 1970–1971)*

26. **(A)** Alpha-thalassemia involves a decrease in alpha-chain production and leads to the formation of beta-globin tetramers known as hemoglobin H. Individuals normally inherit four alpha-chain genes. The clinical syndrome depends on how many genes are deleted. Deletion of one gene results in a silent carrier state. Deletion of all four is the most severe and presents as hydrops fetalis. This condition is incompatible with life. *(Kasper, p. 599)*

27. **(A)** Diabetic neuropathy usually presents as peripheral polyneuropathy, usually bilateral, including symptoms of numbness, paresthesia, severe hyperesthesia, and pain. Impairment of proprioceptive fibers can lead to gait abnormalities and Charcot's joints. Mononeuropathy is less common and is often spontaneously reversible. Common syndromes include wrist or foot drop and third, fourth, or sixth cranial nerve palsies. Autonomic neuropathy may cause gastroesophageal dysfunction, bladder dysfunction, and orthostatic hypotension. *(Kasper, pp. 2165–2166)*

28. **(D)** Uricosuric drugs and allopurinol have no role in the treatment of acute gouty arthritis. Salicylates are also not used in the treatment of gout. The treatments of choice are colchicine, NSAIDs, and intra-articular steroid injection. Response is best when initiated early in the disease. Colchicine can be given intravenously to avoid GI distress. A short course of systemic corticosteroids is also quite effective therapy. Allopurinol is started only when all inflammation is gone and colchicine prophylaxis has been started. It is not always required. *(Kasper, pp. 2046–2047)*

29. **(B)** The two broad categories of ischemic stroke are embolic and thrombotic. Emboli can originate from an arterial atheroma (e.g., common carotid bifurcation) or from the heart. In the latter case, anticoagulants are often indicated. On occasion, emboli occur without obvious source (e.g., hypercoagulable states, malignancy, eclampsia). *(Kasper, pp. 2375–2376)*

30. **(C)** Screening for antibodies to hepatitis C has reduced the incidence of this infection, but numerous chronic cases remain. Treatment options include interferon and ribavirin. The hepatitis C virus is a linear, single-stranded ribonucleic acid (RNA) virus. There are at least six distinct genotypes. *(Kasper, pp. 666–667)*

31. **(E)** Causes of acute glomerulonephritis include infectious diseases, especially *Streptococcus*, vasculitides, and primary glomerular disease. The acute nephritic syndrome consists of the abrupt onset of hematuria and proteinuria, often accompanied by azotemia and renal salt and water retention. Oliguria may be present. *(Kasper, pp. 1679–1680)*

32. **(A)** The pain may be described as sharp, burning, or gnawing, usually 90 minutes to 3 hours after eating, relieved by food or antacids. The pain frequently awakens the patient at night. Symptoms are usually episodic and recurrent. Periods of remission are usually longer than periods with pain. The ulcer crater can recur or persist in the absence of pain. Only a minority of patients with dyspepsia are found to have an ulcer on endoscopy. *(Kasper, pp. 1751–1752)*

33. **(C)** Intravascular hemolysis from blood transfusion is usually due to ABO incompatibility, often from human error. Symptoms of intravascular hemolysis include flushing, pain at the infusion site, chest or back pain, restlessness, anxiety, nausea, and diarrhea. Signs include fever and chills, shock, and renal failure. In comatose patients, hemoglobulinuria or bleeding from disseminated intravascular coagulation can be the first sign. Management is supportive. Acute hemolysis can also result from antibodies directed against other RBC

antigens such as Rh, Kell, or Duffy. *(Kasper, pp. 665–666)*

34. **(D)** Radioactive iodine is contraindicated both in scanning and treatment as it damages the fetal thyroid. Propylthiouracil crosses the placenta, but is safe and effective in pregnancy. The lowest effective dose should be used. Hyperthyroidism is hardest to control in the first trimester and easiest in the third trimester. *(Kasper, pp. 35–36, 2116)*

35. **(D)** Antihistamine side effects (sedation) and anticholinergic side effects (dry mouth, constipation, urinary hesitancy, blurred vision) are the most common side effects. Orthostasis is probably the most common serious side effect and is difficult to manage. Severe cardiac toxicity is uncommon and diarrhea and weight loss are associated with SSRI antidepressants. *(Kasper, pp. 2554–2555)*

36. **(B)** The most common pathogenic mechanism is thought to be excessive or redundant mitral leaflet tissue, with the posterior leaflet more commonly involved. Myxomatous degeneration can also be seen on pathologic examination. Reassurance regarding the benign nature of the disease is the mainstay of management. When a murmur is present, antibiotic prophylaxis for endocarditis is warranted. *(Kasper, pp. 1395–1396)*

37. **(B)** Little or no changes are seen on light microscopy in this syndrome. The disease is most common in children. Spontaneous remission is common in children and is enhanced by steroid therapy. Over 95% of children achieve remission within 8 weeks of institution of prednisone therapy. Therefore, in children with nephrotic syndrome, empiric therapy is frequently employed, rather than initial renal biopsy. Only 50% of adults will remit, and thus biopsy is more frequently required. Relapse is common in both children and adults. *(Kasper, p. 1685)*

38. **(D)** Over 90% of lesions can be localized by fiberoptic bronchoscope in the sedated, but awake, patient and collection of a series of differential brushings and biopsies. When lesions are found, conservative resection is usually performed. Five-year cure rates in such lesions approach 60%, but second primaries are common (5% per patient per year). There is no evidence that screening programs based on sputum examination will decrease mortality. *(Kasper, p. 509)*

39. **(A)** The drop in systolic pressure with inspiration is an important clue to cardiac tamponade, called paradoxical pulse. When severe, the arterial pulse may weaken on palpation during inspiration. Pulsus paradoxus is uncommon in constrictive pericarditis and rare in restrictive cardiomyopathy. It is commonly found in severe asthma as well. *(Kasper, pp. 1415–1417)*

40. **(C)** Cyclosporine A blocks production of interleukin-2 (IL-2) by helper-inducer (CD4$^+$) T cells. It works alone but is more effective in combination with glucocorticoids. The use of cyclosporine has improved 1-year cadaveric survival rates to the 80–85% range. Side effects include hepatotoxicity, hirsutism, tremor, and gingival hyperplasia, but only the nephrotoxicity presents a serious management problem. *(Kasper, pp. 1670–1671)*

41. **(E)** Typically, multiple sclerosis presents with optic neuritis. There is usually a history of at least two episodes of neurologic deficit at more than one site. Other common presenting symptoms include weakness, sensory loss, and paresthesias. *(Kasper, pp. 2462–2463)*

42. **(E)** This patient has HSP; other symptoms include arthralgia and GI function abnormalities. Renal biopsy shows immunoglobulin deposits. There is an underlying vasculitis. The prognosis is generally good, although relapses can occur before the final remission. *(Kasper, pp. 2010–2011)*

43. **(B)** Amiodarone causes a decrease in the sinus rate and an increase in the effective refractory period in the atrium, the AV node, and the ventricle. The pharmacology of amiodarone is complex and incompletely understood. *(Kasper, pp. 1346–1348)*

44. **(A)** Estrogen therapy may retard demineralization of the skeleton and may also reduce blood and urinary calcium levels. However, there is insufficient evidence for a formal recommendation. There is no clear consensus on when asymptomatic hyperparathyroidism requires surgery. Many experts will elect to follow elderly patients with mild hyperparathyroidism who are asymptomatic and have normal renal function and bone mass. (*Kasper, pp. 2254–2255*)

45. **(D)** Other drugs, besides antimalarials, that precipitate hemolysis in G6PD deficiency include dapsone, phenacetin, doxorubicin, and nalidixic acid. The disease is sex-linked and thus most common in males. About 11% of people of African descent have an abnormal allele. Female heterozygotes have a dual population of red cells and, depending on the proportion, may develop symptoms. During hemolysis, older red cells with the lowest enzyme levels are destroyed, and diagnostic tests done at this time may be falsely normal. They should be repeated some time after the hemolysis has resolved. (*Kasper, pp. 610–611*)

46. **(C)** Levofloxacin would be effective for most strains of *Streptococcus pneumoniae*, *Legionella pneumophila*, and other likely pathogens. Other commonly used drugs for community-acquired pneumonia are amoxicillin, cefuroxime, trimethoprim-sulfamethoxazole, and doxycycline. Theoretically, empiric therapy should be guided by knowledge of local resistance patterns. (*Kasper, pp. 1534–1535*)

47. **(C)** Other clues to renal tubule defects include electrolyte disorders, renal osteodystrophy, large kidneys, and proteinuria. Categories of tubulointerstitial kidney disease include toxins (exogenous and metabolic), neoplasia, immune diseases, vascular disorders, infections, and hereditary renal diseases. Defects in urinary acidification and concentrating ability are frequently the most troublesome manifestations of tubulointerstitial kidney disease. (*Kasper, pp. 1694–1698*)

48. **(E)** Proton pump inhibitors (e.g., omeprazole and lansoprazole) are the most effective treatments for ulcerative esophagitis. Antacids, sucralfate, and H2-blockers are all useful in less severe reflux disease. (*Kasper, pp. 1742–1743*)

49. **(A)** MGUS is vastly more common than multiple myeloma, occurring in 1% of the population over age 50. Patients with MGUS have smaller M components (usually <20 g/L); no urinary Bence Jones protein; <5% marrow plasmacytosis; and no anemia, renal failure, lytic bone lesions, or hypercalcemia. About 25% of patients with MGUS will go on to develop multiple myeloma. (*Kasper, pp. 658–659*)

50. **(E)** Sjögren's syndrome is an immunologic disorder characterized by progressive destruction of the exocrine glands leading to mucosal dryness. Pathology reveals lymphocytic infiltration. About one-third develop systemic (nonglandular) symptoms. The most common systemic manifestation is arthritis or arthralgia. If vasculitis occurs, purpura, urticaria, skin ulcers, and mononeuropathy are its most common manifestations. (*Kasper, pp. 1991–1992*)

51. **(D)** The type O donor may contain sufficient anti-A or anti-B to destroy some of the patient's RBCs, but this is seldom clinically significant. Generally, however, crystalloid or colloid solutions are sufficient for volume replacement until properly matched blood is available. (*Kasper, pp. 662–663*)

52. **(D)** Other early changes in mitral stenosis include prominence of the main pulmonary arteries and backward displacement of the esophagus. CXR changes are caused by enlargement of the left atrium. Severe disease can cause pulmonary congestion (Kerley B lines) and enlargement of the right ventricle, right atrium, and superior vena cava. (*Kasper, pp. 1391–1392*)

53. **(A)** The distribution of muscle weakness is characteristic with early involvement of the cranial nerves, especially the lids and extraocular muscles. Women are more frequently affected than men (3:2 ratio), and the age for

peak incidence in women is in the third or fourth decade. *(Kasper, pp. 2518–2519)*

54. **(E)** History of one breast cancer is a risk factor for a second tumor. Risk of breast cancer is increased in women with a family history, early menarche, late menopause, nulliparity, and late age at first pregnancy. Obesity, alcohol, and dietary fat are other possible risk factors. *(Kasper, p. 517)*

55. **(D)** Patients with minimal or absent GI symptoms and atypical respiratory symptoms may be diagnosed as adults. This accounts for 7% of cases. Moreover, because of modern therapy, about 36% of CF patients in the United States are over 18 years of age, and 12% are over 30. *(Kasper, pp. 1544–1545)*

56. **(B)** Signs of benignity of a solitary pulmonary nodule are lack of growth over a prolonged period and certain patterns of calcification. "Popcorn" calcification does suggest a benign hamartoma. A search for previous CXRs can provide a definitive diagnosis. In nonsmokers under age 35, >1% of solitary pulmonary nodules are malignant. *(Kasper, pp. 512–513)*

57. **(B)** A period of 24–48 hours is usually allowed to attempt medical therapy. Cardiac catheterization and angiography may be followed by bypass surgery or angioplasty. For those who do settle down, some form of subsequent risk stratification (e.g., exercise ECG) is indicated. *(Kasper, pp. 1446–1448)*

58. **(A)** Glucocorticoids are not bronchodilators, and their major use is in reducing airway inflammation. It is difficult to provide precise recommendations for their use, and a wide range of systemic and inhaled doses are used. *(Kasper, pp. 1513–1514)*

59. **(C)** Immunofluorescence is usually negative. By electron microscopy, focal basement membrane collapse and denudation of epithelial surfaces are noted. The course is generally progressive in adults. It is believed that remission of proteinuria with steroid therapy will improve the prognosis. Cytotoxic drugs and cyclosporine have also been used in treatment. The degree of proteinuria correlates with the likelihood of developing renal failure. The disease recurs rapidly in transplanted kidneys, suggesting a humoral factor in pathogenesis. *(Kasper, pp. 1686–1687)*

60. **(E)** Heartburn is a characteristic symptom of reflux esophagitis and may be associated with regurgitation. Odynophagia and atypical chest pain also occur in esophageal disease. *(Kasper, p. 1739)*

61. **(D)** Surgical sympathectomy usually provides only temporary improvement and does not prevent progression of the vascular lesion. Nifedipine is now the drug of choice for treating symptoms not responding to local warming measures (gloves, mitts) and avoidance of smoking and cold. Reserpine, alpha-methyldopa, and prazosin may also be useful. *(Kasper, p. 1490)*

62. **(C)** The most common presentation is with pain in a weight-bearing joint such as the hip, knee, or ankle. Hematuria is also common. Bleeding can occur at almost any site without prior trauma. *(Kasper, pp. 680–681)*

63. **(B)** The principal symptom is the pain of acute pericarditis that usually develops 1–4 weeks following the cardiac surgery but could appear after months. It can also occur after myocardial infarction (Dressler's syndrome) or after trauma to the heart (stab wound, blunt trauma). The syndrome can remit and recur for up to 2 years. The acute symptoms usually subside in 1–2 weeks. *(Kasper, pp. 1417–1418)*

64. **(A)** Blind loop syndrome leads to megaloblastic anemia and macrocytosis because of B_{12} deficiency. The deficiency is caused by colonization with bacteria that takes up ingested cobalamin before it can be absorbed. The other conditions generally cause microcytic or normocytic anemias. *(Kasper, pp. 601–604)*

65. **(A)** The patient has Cushing's syndrome secondary to an adrenocorticotropic hormone (ACTH)-secreting pituitary tumor. Relatively

few of such patients have a large pituitary tumor that affects the visual pathways. Over 50% have a microadenoma, which is under 5 mm in diameter. *(Kasper, pp. 2135–2136)*

66. **(E)** Elevated triglycerides are the most common dyslipidemia in DM. However, the LDL particles in DM are more atherogenic than in non-diabetics, even though they are not elevated by DM alone. DM frequently results in lower HDL levels as well. *(Kasper, pp. 2167–2168)*

67. **(D)** The vertebral bodies in osteoporosis may become increasingly biconcave because of weakening of the subchondral plates. This results in "codfish" vertebra. When vertebral collapse occurs, the anterior height of the vertebra is usually decreased. Plain x-rays are insensitive diagnostic tools because up to 30% of bone mass can be lost without any apparent x-ray changes. Dual-energy x-ray absorptiometry (DEXA) and CT scan are more sensitive tests for bone loss, but their exact clinical role has not been clearly established. *(Kasper, pp. 2268–2269)*

68. **(B)** Aspirin is given in low doses such as 325 mg/day, although the initial studies were done with higher doses. Carotid endarterectomy is the best treatment for stenoses of 70% or more. *(Kasper, pp. 2367–2377)*

69. **(C)** Later symptoms of hypothyroidism include loss of intellectual and motor activity, declining appetite, dry hair and skin, and deepening voice. In the elderly, hypothyroidism can be misdiagnosed as due to aging or to other diseases such as Parkinson's disease, Alzheimer's disease, or depression. *(Kasper, pp. 2108–2111)*

70. **(D)** Radiation therapy in stage lA Hodgkin's disease has a very high cure rate. Patients must be followed for hypothyroidism. The long-term disease-free survival is 80%. Mantle irradiation can result acutely in transient dry mouth, pharyngitis, fatigue, and weight loss. The most common long-term effect is hypothyroidism (in 30% of cases), but radiation pneumonitis and fibrosis or pericardial disease can occur.

Although radiotherapy alone would be acceptable in this case, there is a trend to add chemotherapy as well. *(Kasper, pp. 654–655)*

71. **(A)** PAN may be associated with hepatitis B antigenemia in 30% of cases, suggesting immunologic phenomena in the pathogenesis of the disease. Aneurysmal dilatations along involved arteries are characteristic and their presence in small- and medium-sized arteries in renal, hepatic, and visceral vasculature is diagnostic. Biopsy of involved areas can also be diagnostic. *(Kasper, pp. 2007–2008)*

72. **(E)** CMV can also cause neurologic complications from CNS infection. Treatment is with ganciclovir, foscarnet, or cidofovir. Relapse rates are high with both drugs, and therefore maintenance therapy is mandatory. *(Kasper, pp. 1104–1123)*

73. **(B)** Most patients have fever, pain, chills, elevated alkaline phosphatase, as well as increased conjugated bilirubin. Mechanical obstruction is most commonly due to stones, tumors, or strictures. For reasons that are unclear, the serum bilirubin tends to plateau and rarely exceeds levels of 600 mmol/L (25 mg/dL). *(Kasper, pp. 238–240)*

74. **(B)** Dysplastic nevi and benign acquired nevi are both most common on sun-exposed areas such as the back. Atypical moles can occur on the scalp, breasts, and buttocks, rare areas for benign acquired nevi. Both lesions are usually associated with similar lesions (10–40 on average for benign nevi, often >100 in the case of dysplastic nevi). Dysplastic nevi are larger (>6 mm) and have irregular pigmentation and borders. *(Kasper, p. 501)*

75. **(E)** Prerenal azotemia usually has urine osmolality over 500, urine creatinine over 40, and fractional excretion of sodium <1. The urinary sediment in prerenal azotemia reveals hyaline casts. In intrinsic renal azotemia, muddy brown granular casts are seen. *(Kasper, pp. 247–248)*

76. **(D)** The behavioral respiratory control system of the brain drives the hyperventilation, which leads to decreased P_{CO_2} and increased pH. If alkalemia is present with the hypocarbia, symptoms can be quite significant. They include dizziness, visual impairment, syncope, and seizures secondary to cerebral vasoconstriction; paresthesias, carpopedal spasm, and tetany (secondary to decreased free serum calcium); muscle weakness (secondary to hypophosphatemia); and cardiac arrhythmias (secondary to alkalemia). *(Kasper, pp. 1572–1573)*

77. **(D)** Early ischemic changes are tall, peaked T waves that then develop into inverted T waves. Elevated ST segments and Q waves also occur early. *(Kasper, pp. 1448–1449)*

78. **(B)** Renal elimination of phenobarbital is enhanced by alkalinization of the urine to a pH of 8 with sodium bicarbonate and fluids. Hemodialysis and hemoperfusion are reserved for extreme cases with refracting hypotension. Short-acting barbiturates are metabolized in the liver, so fluid administration and alkalinization are not helpful. Activated charcoal absorbs barbiturates very effectively and is useful in decontamination of the GI tract. *(Kasper, p. 2589)*

79. **(E)** Exposure to ionizing radiation is more likely to cause cancer if it occurs at an early age. Radiation-induced malignancy tends to occur at the same age as the same malignancy in the general population. This suggests that radiation is not the only factor. *(Kasper, pp. 486–488)*

80. **(D)** Men are affected twice as frequently as women. The most apparent sign of the supranuclear ophthalmoplegia is failure of voluntary saccadic gaze in the downward direction. Tremor is unusual, but dementia is common. Medications may help somewhat, but their impact is limited and rarely sustained. *(Kasper, pp. 2413–2414)*

81. **(D)** The loop diuretics inhibit tubular reabsorption of sodium, potassium, and chloride in the loop of Henle and can continue to cause diuresis even during volume contraction. The likely site of action of furosemide is in the thick ascending limb of the loop of Henle. *(Kasper, pp. 1373–1374)*

82. **(D)** INH acts as a pyridoxine antagonist and causes polyneuropathy in slow acetylators. Both sensory and motor involvement occurs. Treatment with pyridoxine can improve symptoms. *(Kasper, pp. 947–948)*

83. **(B)** The first stage of Lyme disease is an acute infection with the spirochete *Borrelia burgdorferi*, usually transmitted by tick bite. It is most common in the summer in rural, wooded areas. About 60% of patients who have not received antibiotic therapy will develop arthritis months later. The typical pattern is intermittent attacks of oligoarthritis lasting weeks to months. The knees are the most common joints involved. *(Kasper, pp. 996–997)*

84. **(A)** AZT is beneficial to patients with HIV infection, but the best time at which to commence therapy is still controversial. Common side effects include fatigue, macrocytic anemia, neutropenia, and myopathy. Treatment regimens now include protease inhibitors as well. Monotherapy with AZT results in development of resistance. *(Kasper, pp. 1124–1125)*

85. **(C)** The mortality from acute myocardial infarction is greater in women, particularly African American women. It is unclear whether this correlation is independent of age and disease severity. Ischemic heart disease, not breast cancer, is the leading cause of death in American women. The relative benefit of thrombolytic therapy seems similar in men and women. Estrogen therapy's major effect in decreasing mortality is via its reduction (40–50%) in deaths due to ischemic heart disease. This has not yet been verified in prospective trials. Estrogen therapy has not been shown to be beneficial in secondary prevention of heart disease in women. Immune-related disorders (RA, lupus, multiple sclerosis, thyroid disease) are usually more common in women. *(Kasper, pp. 29–30)*

86. **(D)** Alpha-methyldopa has been used extensively throughout pregnancy, with no evidence of harm to the fetus. ACE inhibitors are associated with increased fetal loss. Preeclampsia and eclampsia are diseases of the end of pregnancy. There is no evidence that pregnancy affects the course of essential hypertension. Gestational hypertension has a high rate of recurrence in subsequent pregnancies. *(Kasper, pp. 32–33)*

87. **(A)** CMV is the most common congenital viral infection, affecting 1–2% of all American newborns. Only a small minority of these infants are abnormal. *N. gonorrhoeae* infection can be transmitted in utero, during delivery, or in the postpartum period. Asymptomatic bacteriuria occurs in up to 7% of all pregnancies. Treatment can prevent about 75% of all acute pyelonephritis in pregnancy; thus, screening is warranted. HIV infection is usually transmitted during the perinatal period. Although postpartum infections are a significant cause of maternal mortality, the most important are thromboembolic disease, hypertension, ectopic pregnancy, and hemorrhage. *(Kasper, pp. 36–38)*

88. **(E)** This story of daily attacks of periorbital pain with annual recurrence in a man between age 30–50 is typical of cluster headaches. The recurrent bouts last days to weeks. The headaches can be provoked by alcohol and relieved by oxygen administration. Prophylactic treatment, however, is preferred. *(Kasper, pp. 93–94)*

89. **(E)** Wernicke's aphasia involves disease (most commonly infarction) in the distribution of the lower division of the middle cerebral artery. It is frequently associated with parietal lobe sensory deficits and hemianopsia; motor disturbance is not part of the syndrome. The condition may improve with time. *(Kasper, pp. 146–147)*

90. **(C)** The ECG reveals diffuse ST elevation with characteristic concave upward shape and PR depression in the precordial leads. This is more typical of pericarditis than of myocardial infarction. The presentation, symptoms, and age of the patient are all typical for viral pericarditis. *(Kasper, pp. 1414–1415)*

91. **(B)** Community-acquired pneumonia in previously healthy young people is commonly caused by *S. pneumoniae*, *Mycoplasma*, viruses, or *Chlamydia*. The pattern of dense right upper lobe consolidation in this case strongly suggests a typical bacterial pneumonia, such as *S. pneumoniae*. A follow-up CXR in 6 weeks is appropriate to ensure that no underlying abnormality is the cause of the problem. *(Kasper, p. 1536)*

92. **(D)** The CXR is typical of COPD, with flattened diaphragms, hyperlucent lungs, and increased retrosternal air space. *(Kasper, p. 1551)*

93. **(E)** Renal, musculoskeletal, and peripheral nerve involvement are the most common manifestations of PAN. Generally, if no tissue is easily available for biopsy, an arteriogram is a better diagnostic test than a blind biopsy. This arteriogram reveals multiple aneurysmal dilatations, the classic finding in PAN. *(Kasper, pp. 2007–2008)*

94. **(D)** The x-ray reveals typical evidence of sacroiliitis, with widening of the joints, sclerosis, and evasions. Similar findings can be seen in psoriatic and enteropathic spondyloarthropathy. *(Kasper, pp. 1993–1995)*

95. **(C)** The articular calcification chondrocalcinosis is typical for pseudogout or calcium pyrophosphate disease (CPPD). The most common joint involved is the knee, but the wrist, shoulder, ankle, elbow, and hand are also frequently involved. Definitive diagnosis depends on finding typical rhomboid-shaped crystals with weak-positive birefringence in the synovial fluid, but chondrocalcinosis in the correct setting allows a presumptive diagnosis. Numerous diseases are associated with CPPD, but the most common predisposing factor is advancing age. *(Kasper, pp. 2047–2048)*

96. **(B)** The x-ray reveals a Zenker's diverticulum. Halitosis, aspiration (perhaps explaining his pneumonia), regurgitation of old meals, and dysphagia are typical symptoms. Surgical treatment involves a cricopharyngeal myotomy.

At times, a diverticulectomy is also required. *(Kasper, p. 1745)*

97. **(C)** The film shows hypochromic, microcytic red cells, suggesting iron deficiency. Although thalassemia can mimic iron deficiency, the normal hemoglobin 1 year earlier makes this unlikely. Anemia of chronic disease is unlikely because there are no signs of such a chronic disease. Thus, blood loss from the GI tract is the most likely cause. *(Kasper, pp. 589–590)*

98. **(A)** The macrocytic cells and hypersegmented neutrophil are characteristic of megaloblastic anemia. Vitamin B_{12} and folate deficiency are the most common cause. Lack of intrinsic factor because of gastrectomy will eventually result in B_{12} deficiency. *(Kasper, p. 604)*

99. **(D)** Coronary angiography is a relatively safe procedure in the right individual. There are complications associated with this procedure that must be reviewed with the patient while obtaining informed consent. The risk of stroke and myocardial infarction is 1 in 1000 with coronary angiography. Other complications are arrhythmias, allergic reaction to the dye, and renal dysfunction. *(Kasper, pp. 1327–1328)*

100. **(C)** The major bleeding complication rate with long-term warfarin anticoagulation is approximately 1–3% per year when the target international normalized ratio (INR) is 2–3. *(Kasper, pp. 689–690)*

101. **(B)** Beta-adrenergic receptors become less sensitive with advancing age. Higher rates of isoproterenol infusion are required in the elderly to achieve an increased resting heart rate. Clinically, higher doses of propranolol have been shown to be required in the elderly to achieve similar degrees of beta-blockade as in the young. *(Grimley Evans, pp. 132–133)*

102. **(A)** The response to benzodiazepines is more pronounced in the elderly, even when corrected for pharmacokinetics. Prior impairment is a factor in this response. *(Grimley Evans, pp. 132–133)*

103. **(A)** Despite similar pharmacokinetics, the dose of warfarin to provide effective anticoagulation is lower in the elderly. *(Grimley Evans, p. 132)*

104. **(E)** The elderly have more body fat and less body water. A water-soluble drug such as lithium will have a considerably smaller volume of distribution. Thus, dosages should be decreased in the elderly to prevent toxicity. *(Grimley Evans, p. 130)*

105. **(A)** Failure to correct for the elderly patient's increased sensitivity to narcotics can result in significant toxicity. *(Grimley Evans, p. 132)*

106. **(A)** Tricyclic antidepressants and SSRIs are both effective treatments for depression, but their side effect profiles are different. Tricyclics can promote weight gain while weight loss is more common with SSRIs. *(Grimley Evans, pp. 993–994)*

107. **(C)** Diuretics promote urinary losses of magnesium, zinc, and potassium. Zinc deficiency is also seen in liver cirrhosis, Type II diabetes, and lung cancer. *(Grimley Evans, p. 163)*

108. **(D)** INH can result in pyridoxine (vitamin B_6) deficiency, particularly in malnourished individuals. It is recommended that patients who are elderly, or have DM, poor nutrition, alcoholism, seizure diathesis, or uremia, take pyridoxine while on INH. *(Grimley Evans, p. 538)*

109. **(G)** Corticosteroids impair calcium absorption. They are useful in managing hypercalcemia, but bisphosphonates are the usual drug of choice. *(Grimley Evans, p. 183)*

110. **(E)** Both phenytoin and phenobarbital can cause altered vitamin D metabolism and can even result in osteomalacia. Calcium absorption from the gut is also blocked directly. *(Grimley Evans, p. 628)*

111. **(B)** Sleep becomes more shallow with the loss of deep stages of sleep, resulting in more frequent arousals. Specific sleep disturbances such as sleep apnea and periodic leg movements

increase with advancing age as well. *(Grimley Evans, p. 758)*

112. **(B, F)** Neurodegenerative disorders can cause a change in normal circadian rhythm by causing a breakdown in the temporal organizing of sleep-wake cycling. This alteration in time of sleeping can be very disruptive to family members. The sleep pattern can be polyphasic, with multiple irregularly distributed periods of sleep, rather than one long sleep period at night. This can result in the patient's awakening during the night, which is also very disruptive. *(Grimley Evans, pp. 756–758)*

113. **(E)** Sleep apnea syndrome is the most common cause of daytime sleepiness in the elderly. The prevalence (at least in sleep disorder centers) increases with advancing age. Narcolepsy (usually having started earlier in life) and periodic limb movement disorder (restless legs) are other common causes of excessive daytime sleepiness. *(Grimley Evans, p. 750)*

114. **(C)** The lack of focal neurologic findings suggests that the confusion is secondary to delirium. Bilateral asterixis is frequently seen in metabolic encephalopathy, particularly in cases of hepatic encephalopathy, hypercapnia, or drug ingestion. In this case, the most urgent investigations would be to rule out pneumonia with respiratory failure. *(Kasper, pp. 1627–1629)*

115. **(E)** Although impaired attention is the hallmark of delirium (along with impaired consciousness), it can also be impaired in dementia. In very mild cognitive impairment, deficits in attention might differentiate delirium from dementia, but in the usual hospitalized patient, fluctuation in performance (particularly with regard to attention and level of consciousness) is probably more helpful. *(Kasper, pp. 1624–1625)*

116. **(B)** The progressive nature of the disorder suggests a degenerative dementia, and the predominance of disinhibited behavior suggests the frontal lobes are involved. Frontal dementias can result from trauma, tumor, or ischemia, but this history suggests a degenerative disorder. Alzheimer's can involve the frontal lobes and mimic a frontal dementia. *(Kasper, pp. 2401–2402)*

117. **(D)** In frontal dementia, and others as well, behavioral disturbances are often the reason for institutionalization. *(Kasper, pp. 2405–2406)*

118. **(E)** Alzheimer's disease is the most common cause of dementia in Western countries. Microscopically, there are neuritic plaques containing A-beta-amyloid in the neuronal cytoplasm. These plaques stain silver and are referred to as neurofibrillary tangles (NFT). There is also accumulation of A-beta-amyloid in arterial walls of cerebral blood vessels. *(Kasper, pp. 2398–2400)*

References

Brunton LL, Lazo JS, Parker KL. *Goodman and Gilman's The Pharmacological Basis of Therapeutics.* 11th ed. New York, NY: McGraw-Hill; 2006.

Devita VT, Hellman S, Rosebenberg SH. *CANCER Principles and Practice of Oncology.* 6th ed. Philadelphia, PA: Lippincott Williams & Wilkins; 2001.

Felig P, Frohman LA. *Endocrinology & Metabolism.* 4th ed. New York, NY: McGraw-Hill; 2001.

Fuster V, Alexander RW, O'Rourke RA, et al. *Hurst's the Heart.* 11th ed. New York, NY: McGraw-Hill; 2004.

Grimley Evans J, Williams TF, Beattie BL, et al. *Oxford Textbook of Geriatric Medicine.* 2nd ed. Oxford: Oxford University Press; 2000.

Kasper DL, Braunwald E, Fauci AS, et al. *Harrison's Principles of Internal Medicine.* 16th ed. New York, NY: McGraw-Hill; 2005.

Lichtman MA, Beutler E, Kipps TJ, et al. *Hematology.* 7th ed. New York, NY: McGraw-Hill; 2006.

Ropper AH, Brown RH. *Adams and Victor's Principles of Neurology.* 8th ed. New York, NY: McGraw-Hill; 2005.

Wolff K, Johnson RA. *Fitzpatrick's Colour Atlas & Synopsis of Clinical Dermatology.* 5th ed. New York, NY: McGraw-Hill; 2005.

Index